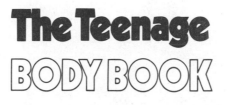

The Teenage
BODY BOOK

Charles Wibbelsman M.D.
and Kathy McCoy

The Teenage
BODY BOOK

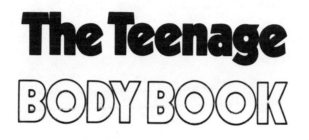

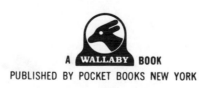

A WALLABY BOOK
PUBLISHED BY POCKET BOOKS NEW YORK

POCKET BOOKS, a Simon & Schuster division of
GULF & WESTERN CORPORATION
1230 Avenue of the Americas, New York, N.Y. 10020

ISBN: 0-671-79012-9

First Wallaby printing January, 1979

10 9 8 7 6 5 4 3 2

Trademarks registered in the United States and other countries.

Printed in the U.S.A.

ACKNOWLEDGMENTS

Our Special Thanks to

- Susan Ann Protter, our agent, for believing in us—and our book.
- Harriet Bell, our editor at Pocket Books, for her help and warm encouragement.
- Bob Stover, who not only provided the book's illustrations, but also volunteered for the tasks no one wanted (like proofreading the entire original manuscript—in triplicate—and double-checking all the phone numbers in the Appendix!).
- Diane Stafanson, R. N., Tony Greenberg, M.D., Michael McCoy, Mary Connolly, and Karen Rhodes for their invaluable comments and suggestions.
- Lynn Bowers, Rose Blake, and Sid Keith for their help in setting up interviews.
- Henk Newenhouse of Perennial Education, Inc., and Alice Snyder and Beth Blaisell of Northwestern University for their enthusiasm and generosity.
- All of the health professionals interviewed on these pages who gave generously of their time and special knowledge.
- The many teen-agers and young adults whose questions and personal stories comprise an important part of what you are about to read. To these very special young people, we want to say an extra note of thanks . . . thanks for taking the risk of asking . . . thanks for sharing your thoughts and feelings with us!

CONTENTS

The Teenage
BODY BOOK

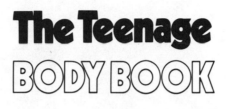

"Dear Young Adult . . ."

I'm a 20-year-old virgin who doesn't feel ready to have sex yet. Most of my friends do. Is there something wrong with me?

Concerned

I'm 16, male, and afraid I may be a homosexual. There's no one I can talk to about this. Will you help me to find out who I am? Please! I have no one to turn to!

Desperate

I'm 17 and have never had a date because I'm so overweight. I want to lead a normal life, but I can't stick to any diet. I hate myself! Help!

Hopeless

I'm a guy, 19, and I have ugly white pimples on my penis. Could this be a long-lasting form of VD?

Wondering

I'm a young diabetic and sometimes I just feel like I'm ready to give up.

Lonely

Dear Concerned
  Desperate
  Hopeless
  Wondering
  Lonely
Dear Young Adult Who Needs to Know . . .

It's a frustrating, frightening, and lonely feeling when you have questions and feelings you find difficult—if not impossible—to share with those close to you. There may be so many things you need to know BUT:

- You're afraid to ask your parents
- You're embarrassed to ask your doctor
- You hesitate to ask your friends.

Sometimes it's easier to ask a stranger. If you feel this way, so do thousands of teen-agers and young adults who deluged us with questions in letters, hotline calls, questionnaires, and anonymous question cards in school health and sex education classes. Perhaps many of their questions are *your* questions, too.

Your questions and feelings are of special concern to us.

As an adolescent medicine specialist, Dr. Wibbelsman has treated, counseled, and listened to thousands of young adults in clinics, hospitals, schools, and college health centers.

As a writer and a former editor of 'TEEN Magazine, Kathy McCoy has reached out to and shared feelings with thousands more young people who plead for correct information about all aspects of growing toward adulthood.

The purpose of this book is to give you that correct information and to explore with you all aspects of your health and sexuality in these vital transition years.

Before we begin our exploration together, we're going to make you some promises.

WE WILL NOT:

- Give you sermons
- Superimpose hangups
- Give you judgmental hassles
- Pass on myths and half-truths
- Give you absolute proclamations to replace the individual care that only your own doctor can provide for you.

WE WILL:

- Give you frank, straightforward answers to your questions
- Expose myths, false information, and old wives' tales
- Explore the special problems—and possibilities—you face
- Try to help you help yourself to grow toward self-acceptance, self-love, knowing and caring for your body, accepting and appreciating your sexuality, and, ultimately, developing the capacity to know yourself and to share who you are with another person in an intimate relationship.

Perhaps as you learn more about your health, your sexuality, and who you are, there will be promises you'll want to make to yourself.

Learning about and knowing your body is the first step toward accepting and loving who you are and determining who you will become. This self-discovery is, in a sense, a journey without end. We are delighted to be sharing this part of your journey with you.

Best wishes,
KATHY McCoy
CHARLES WIBBELSMAN, M.D.

CHAPTER ONE

"Dear Doctor: Am I Normal?"

Do you ever feel weird?

Out of it?

Always on the outside looking in?

Like a one-of-a-kind freak with problems you wouldn't dare discuss—even with your friends?

If so, believe it or not, you're far from alone!

Susan, 14, worries about some new desires she is feeling.

"My problem is my body," she wrote to us on a note card during a sex education class. "I have a large sex drive, but don't do anything about it because I'm afraid of getting pregnant. What can I do? My body has blossomed into a fully grown woman already. Is this *normal* for a girl my age?"

Thirteen-year-old Doug finds after-gym showers excruciating because "I don't seem to have grown as much in the penis or developed as much pubic hair as the other guys in my class. I really feel out of it. Am I normal?"

Susan, a 19-year-old college sophomore, told us about her problem in a letter.

"I'm scared of doctors—practically petrified!" she wrote. "Do other people feel this way, too? Am I strange? How do I get over this and become a normal person?"

A 16-year-old boy, who signed himself "Lost and Alone" wrote to us about his conflicting feelings.

"I wonder if it's normal to have mixed feelings about your parents?" he asked. "One minute I think they're the greatest and the next, I can't stand them. Is this a normal kind of thing for my feelings to change from one minute to the next?"

"Am I normal?" is, perhaps, the most frequent question teen-agers and young adults ask.

It's so easy—yet agonizing—to feel different, strange, lost, and alone at this time in your life.

You may feel different because of the changes in your body and increased sexual desires.

You may be suffering from an attack of the peer comparison blues.

Conflicting feelings, too, may make you seem alone and apart.

Your changing feelings about your parents may be especially confusing. You've always heard that people aren't supposed to feel hate or scorn for their parents. But sometimes you do hate them and feel embarrassed by them, even though you love them.

These feelings may be tough to talk about.

"I hate my parents sometimes!" may sound rather harsh and absolute. Yet, it may be just as difficult to say "I love you."

These conflicts may leave you wondering if you're normal.

You're normal.

It *is* normal, particularly at this time in your life, to feel different, lost, and alone at times.

It *is* normal, in the midst of all the changes you're experiencing, to feel scared sometimes.

Also, it may help to realize that *normal* is a very flexible word, especially now. Change is the natural order of things in adolescence and young adulthood. In fact, the Latin root of the word *adolescence* is "esso," which means "becoming."

This period of "becoming" is a long transition time between childhood and adulthood.

To be "becoming" may mean dramatic physical changes if you're in your early teens.

If you're in your late teens and early twenties, "becoming" may mean changes in life-styles and in social position as you assume more and more adult responsibilities.

To be in the process of "becoming" is synonymous with change. Yet, searching for some order in the middle of these changes, most young people seek some frame of reference for what is normal—besides the mere fact of change.

You may be among them.

"OK. It's normal for my body, my feelings, my social relationships, and my life in general to be in a state of change," you may be saying. "But surely there's some normal rate of change, some kind of normal progress I should be making."

It's a huge temptation to look at someone who is your age and say, "Now *that* person seems to be normal. But I'm not like him/her, so I'm *not* normal!"

You can be different *and* normal. Normal covers an incredibly wide spectrum.

Your body, too, has its own unique timetable for growth toward the destination of adulthood. This timetable is *not* a matter of having to be at certain stages at definite ages.

Time isn't the only variable as you journey toward adulthood. How, and in what sequence, your changes occur is a highly individual matter.

Some adolescents will go through emotional changes sooner than others. Other teens may experience physical changes before emotional maturity. There are probably striking examples of both in your class at school. You probably know people with the body of an adult and the emotional responses of a child as well as emotionally mature classmates who look much younger than they think or act. And then there are those in between.

Wherever you may find yourself at the moment, chances are you have felt, are feeling, or will feel some growing pains.

Growing pains, both physical and emotional, are *real*. They come in all varieties.

When a teen-ager complains of a backache or pains in the legs, for example, a physician, after a thorough examination, may attribute these sensations to growing pains.

Similarly, girls just beginning to ovulate and menstruate may have severe cramps and heavy menstrual flows.

A guy who is shorter than his male or female classmates and who is ridiculed because of this may feel a definite variety of pain.

An adolescent boy or girl who feels unpopular with peers and rejected by the opposite sex may experience a great deal of pain.

It may also hurt to feel different.

Yet, in the midst of changes, you can't *help* feeling different.

At this time in life, everyone feels different and very conscious of the progress or nonprogress others are making in the journey toward adulthood. Comparisons with peers are constant and inevitable.

In school shower rooms, boys may compare penis sizes, chest hair, and beards. Girls may compare the size and shape of breasts and menstrual experiences (or lack of them). Such comparisons—mingled with fear of being different—start early. We have had frantic letters from 11- and 12-year-old girls, for example, who are worried because their best friends have all started to menstruate—and they haven't.

Since essential changes never seem to happen at the same rate or in quite the same sequence, you can't help but worry about what is really normal.

Most people are normal.

Most people are different.

These are *not* contradictory terms. Your body—like your personality—isn't quite like anyone else's.

Somehow, though, we all seem more tolerant of personality differences. After all, we come from widely varied backgrounds, homes, and heritages.

Many of these same factors, however, also influence physical growth, development, and appearance.

Due to your heritage, you may be short instead of tall, have curly rather than straight hair, and have a rounded rather than angular figure.

Due to your genetic inheritance, you may also experience a slower—albeit normal—rate of physical development. Research has shown that if one or both of your parents happened to be "late bloomers," you may be, too.

If you're like most people, however, the physical aspects of your genetic legacy may be harder to live with. Here, the differences are so *obvious*.

Our 1975 study of the mostly female readers of *'TEEN Magazine*'s "Dear Doctor" column revealed that physical change problems—including delayed menstruation, delayed or small breast development, irregular menses, vaginal discharge, appearance of external genitalia, acne, overweight, sexual anxieties, and use of tampons ("Am I the *only* girl who can't seem to wear them?" was a recurring lament)—were, by far, the most frequently asked questions by readers who bombarded the column with hundreds of letters a month.

An earlier study of adolescent boys in the Los Angeles area junior high schools revealed similar concerns: penis size and appearance, delayed secondary sex characteristics, sexual anxieties, and self-proclaimed height and build deficiencies.

In both studies, the boys and girls generally concluded their questions with "Am I normal—or not?"

More recently, we did an informal poll of young adults in their twenties and early thirties. ALL reported that, when they were adolescents, they seriously questioned their normality in a number of ways. Worries about everything from penis size to perspiration, personality to popularity played a huge part in their lives as they were growing and changing.

Now, most of these adults can report their former fears frankly, saying that the self-acceptance that time and maturity can bring makes such anxieties less acute. Virtually all, however, report that once, not so long ago, they felt very different and very much alone.

"Why couldn't we talk about this when we were in high school?" one young adult asked a former high school classmate. "It would have helped me so much to talk!"

Talking about what you fear most or what hurts most may be difficult, however, especially when you're actually experiencing these growing pains. Talking about what's really going on with you can constitute an awesome risk as you look around at your classmates and friends. Sometimes, it may seem that everyone else has all—or most of—the answers. No one else seems to have quite the array of uncertainties that you do—or do they?

They do, but you may never know, unless you are able to take the risk of sharing. In sharing your feelings and experiences, you may learn some surprising facts, not only about your classmates, but also about their perceptions of you.

How do you come across to others?

Their answers may surprise you.

Fifteen-year-old Beverly, who felt extremely shy and out of it, was stunned to discover during an impromptu moment of truth with a classmate that the other kids saw her as sophisticated and as a bit of a snob.

And how you assume that others feel may not be how they feel at all!

Yes, it would be mortifying to reveal your feelings of being different and alone, your lack of self-confidence in certain situations, anxieties about your sexuality or conflicting feelings to a friend and to watch in agony as he/she recoils with shock and says loudly (for anyone within the radius of two miles to hear) "Oh, really? Well, *I've* never felt that way! You're sure weird!"

Such a reaction, however, is unlikely, especially if you share such confidences selectively, with people you genuinely care about and who care about you.

Being able to identify some of the pains and pressure points you're feeling, and sharing them with others may help a great deal.

You may see that things that used to seem abnormal are looking more normal all the time.

You may find, for example, that others feel a confusing mixture of love, hate, guilt, and tenderness for their parents as they struggle for independence.

You may find that many worry about being short or tall or embarrassingly out-of-balance with a romantic interest. Young teen-age girls, who tend to approach their maximum height at a younger age than their male classmates, and the young adolescent boys who lag temporarily behind may ALL feel a little uneasy as their lopsided growth patterns are displayed all too prominently at a junior high school dance. However, it is normal, at this stage, for many of the girls to be taller than the boys.

It is also normal for individuals of the same age and sex to experience widely different growth of sexual organs and development of secondary sexual characteristics (like underarm and pubic hair).

It is normal, too, at this time, to feel much more comfortable with (and maybe even physically attracted to) those of your own sex. Crushes on teachers, older schoolmates, relatives, and friends are common as you look for essential role models and for warmth and reassurance outside your immediate family circle.

Some young people may find early sexual experimentation much less threatening with those of their own sex. Some, especially in the early teens, may compare genitals out of mutual—and normal—curiosity. Experimentation may play a major role in your discovery of your own sexuality and sexual orientation.

To experiment, of course, means to try out. In adolescence, you may try on lots of ideas and different types of behavior to see what is for you—and what isn't. Your present social preferences, sexual development, and height, for example, are part of your life now. The rest of your life, as you grow and change, may be quite different.

That is the often comforting, yet confusing, thing about being in the process of "becoming." It is also the reason why it's so important not to put labels on yourself, especially during this time of change.

At this time of change and confusion, sharing your feelings and experiences with others can help a lot.

Of course, just because we say that sharing may be helpful doesn't necessarily make it any easier for you to do. Even if you're willing to try, it may be hard to know how to start.

So let's try an experiment.

Share with us first.

It's a no-risk situation.

Sit back in the privacy of your room or wherever you are and listen to others for a while. See what the other teen-agers and young adults, who contributed questions and comments to this book, are experiencing.

Such no-risk sharing may help you not only to accept many concerns as normal, but also to take the risk of sharing who you are and what you're experiencing with those close to you (once you learn that you're OK after all!). This experiment may also help you to grow in tolerance and appreciation not only of others, but also of yourself as a distinct individual.

Not only are you normal. You're also *special*.

When you can see yourself as, basically, a *normal* person who is experiencing normal changes, you may begin to recognize and appreciate some of your own unique qualities.

You may begin to appreciate who you are and who you may grow to become.

You may begin to give yourself permission *not* to be perfect!

You may even begin to see in a new light some of

your anxieties about your changing body and changing life. It's perfectly normal and OK to be concerned about what's happening. It's good to be aware of what you're experiencing now, to learn your health needs and how to care for your growing body.

As you read this book and explore with us the answers to many of these normal concerns that most young people have, you may be surprised. You may make a lot of discoveries about you, the normal person!

You may realize that, although you are a unique individual, you are, in many ways, just like anyone else you know.

You're *not* alone!

CHAPTER TWO

Woman's Body / Woman's Experience

When I started to menstruate . . .
"I felt proud!"
"I felt ashamed."
"I felt angry!"
"I felt, at last, like everyone else!"
"I felt nothing."

I feel that my breasts are . . .
"pretty!"
"too small."
"too large."
"inconvenient."
"just another normal part of me!"
"droopy and UGLY!"
"I never really thought about them."

When I think of touching or looking at my genitals . . .
"I feel OK. Genitals are just another part of my body, too!"
"Yuck! It's *dirty* down there!"
"GUILTY!!!"
"I'm curious, but afraid . . ."

As these statements from young women testify, living with and experiencing your own body is a highly subjective experience: What might be a proud moment for one might be humiliation for another; what might be a natural inclination for one woman might be unthinkable for the next.

Some young women feel at ease with their bodies. Others don't.

You may find yourself among the latter.

You may enjoy the fact that you're female (or simply accept it) and yet dislike what you see as the inconvenience of menstrual periods. You may wish for bigger breasts. If you have large breasts, you may cringe with embarrassment when people notice.

You may have new and urgent sexual feelings that can be pleasurable, yet mingled with the pleasure, there is pain.

You may feel the pain of guilt, of fear, of frustration.

You may feel at ease with your body and your sexual feelings, yet feel uncomfortable with the traditional roles that many women still fill.

You may feel ill at ease simply with the relative suddenness of your transition from girl to young woman (even though your body has been quietly preparing for puberty for years).

What were YOUR feelings when your body began to mature? Were you glad? Self-conscious? Angry? Mixed up?

If you felt a bit confused, if you don't know all you'd like to know, if your body is still something of a mystery to you, you have lots of company.

Some questions you may have may be hard for your parents or your friends to answer. And there may be some questions that you feel are impossible to ask.

Nothing can be more frustrating than needing to know so much and not being able to get some answers.

We hope to give you some answers that may help clear up some confusion and anxiety you may have about what it means to be a woman—biologically and psychologically.

We hope to share some ideas and information with you and to help alleviate some of the pain that confusion can bring.

Ignorance about your body and the way it works and grows *can* be painful.

Her letter is plaintive and stained with tears:

I'm 14 and I'm scared! Nobody ever told me anything about my body and how it is supposed to be, but I have a feeling that it isn't like anyone else's. I'm too embarrassed to ask my friends. My parents don't like to talk about these things. I feel different and scared and hate my body sometimes. What's supposed to be happening to me?

Worried Sick in Idaho

"Worried Sick" is far from alone with her fears about her body and its changes. Sadly, some young people have very little accurate information about the dramatic, natural, and wonderful changes of adolescence. With ignorance comes fear. And we've received some letters filled with genuine terror.

Help! Something is wrong. I think I have cancer cuz I bleed from my vagina about three days a month.

It's really yuk, but it goes away every time. I'm too scared to go to my doctor. Help!

Scared

Some teens worry about basic anatomy.

I'm 15 and have a very serious problem: My genitals are on the outside rather than the inside . . . I know lots of girls with this problem!

Judy

Judy seems unaware that only part of a woman's genital system is inside. All women also have external genitalia.

Perhaps "Worried Sick" and Judy are unusually unaware young people. You may be well-informed about the changes you have experienced. Yet you may have some questions or feel a bit unclear about some things.

In order to answer as many of your possible questions as we can, and to give you a really thorough understanding of the long process of changes your body is experiencing, we'll begin with basic anatomy and the process of puberty.

You're probably well into adolescence as you read this, but knowing the basics—and where you've been—may help you to understand better where you are right now.

GENITALIA

First, we'd like to help you get acquainted with the part of your body that you may be least likely to see: your genital area. You may know a lot more than Judy, but you may still have questions about the names—and functions—of various parts of your genital system, both external and internal. Let's do some exploring and clear up some of these mysteries about the female body now!

You can read this part of the chapter several ways.

You may not have the privacy nor the inclination to compare your own genitals with our illustrations. That's OK. Comparing the illustrations and our written descriptions may help you a great deal.

However, if you feel comfortable about exploring your own body as you read this, that's fine, too. A small mirror held between your legs, close to your

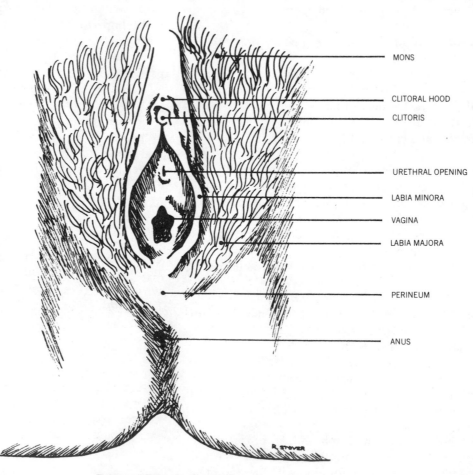

MONS

CLITORAL HOOD

CLITORIS

URETHRAL OPENING

LABIA MINORA

VAGINA

LABIA MAJORA

PERINEUM

ANUS

External Female Genitalia

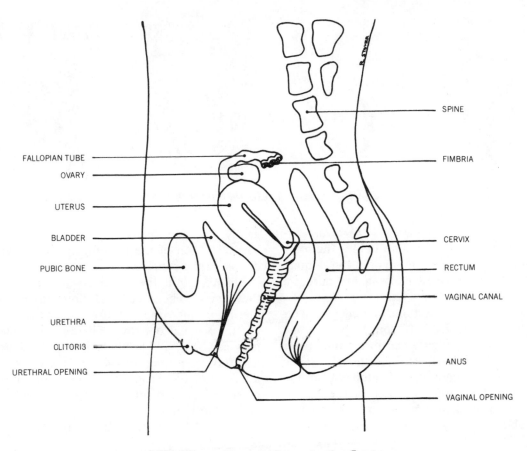

FALLOPIAN TUBE

OVARY

UTERUS

BLADDER

PUBIC BONE

URETHRA

CLITORIS

URETHRAL OPENING

SPINE

FIMBRIA

CERVIX

RECTUM

VAGINAL CANAL

ANUS

VAGINAL OPENING

Side View of Female Reproductive System

genital area, will help you to see and identify everything better.

Generally, the entire area between a woman's legs is called the *vulva*. This is another name for "external genitalia."

If you look closely, you will discover two sets of lips. The *labia majora*—or big lips—will be covered with hair if you have reached a certain stage of development. These outer lips serve as protection for the genital area within and may meet, covering that entire area. If this is the case, part them and you will notice the *labia minora,* or small lips. These lips are not always small. Sometimes, in fact, they will protrude from the outer lips. They vary a lot in color, too, from pink to brown. They may be wrinkled or smooth. There are many varieties of *normal* genitals.

The labia minora have no hair or fat padding, but do have oil and scent glands, tissue and blood vessels. At the juncture where the labia minora connect, they surround the *clitoris,* tiny but acutely sensitive and rich with nerve endings. The clitoris can play a vital role in sexual arousal.

How do you find your clitoris?

Trace the labia minora up to the area where they seem to meet. If you can see your clitoris, it is a small organ, the female counterpart of the penis. It may be

about the size of the tip of a pencil eraser. In many women, however, the clitoris may be hidden in the folds of the labia. If so, press down. If you begin to feel a rather pleasurable sensation, you've found it!

Although your clitoris has been sensitive since birth, you may be more aware of it now, as your genitals and sexual feelings grow.

Below the clitoris is the *urethra,* or urinary opening. It may feel—and look—like a small dimple.

Beneath the urethra is the *vaginal opening* (also called the *vaginal introitus*). This opening may be ringed or partially covered by the *hymen* (also called the maidenhead). The hymenal ring may be very evident or hardly visible. It may have one opening or several. (See illustration.)

The presence or absence of a hymen is not definitive proof of virginity. A virgin is a person who has not had sexual intercourse, period. Some women who are virgins may have been born without a noticeable hymen or may have stretched the hymen during vigorous sports activities or masturbation or petting. Other women who are having sexual intercourse may have intact, though stretched, hymens. The remnants of a hymen may even be found in a woman who has given birth to a baby.

Only in very rare instances is there *no* opening in

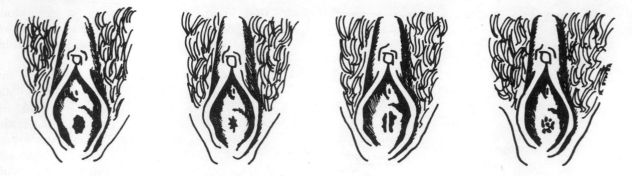

Hymens come in a variety of shapes. These are four of the many possibilities.

the hymen. This condition is called *imperforate hymen* and requires surgical correction before the menstrual flow can escape. Again, this condition is quite rare and is usually discovered early in life during a pediatric examination.

The *vaginal opening* is the point connecting your external and internal genitals. If you wish to probe beyond the opening (many girls can insert one finger without discomfort), you can feel the moist, elastic walls of your vagina, a canal that stretches from the vaginal opening to the *cervix,* or neck of the uterus.

If you reach as far back as you can into your vagina, you may be able to feel your cervix. Pressing on it gently, you may find that the cervix feels like an enlarged version of the tip of your nose—with a small dimple in the center.

This dimple is the opening—also called the *os*—of the cervix. The menstrual flow passes out of the uterus, through the os, down the vaginal canal, and out the vaginal opening. The cervix, though it feels firm, can be moved around a little and the os, although it is tiny, can open (or dilate) wide enough to permit a baby to pass through. The os is usually very tiny, however, and the cervix seems to close off the upper end of the vagina.

This fact may give some comfort to those who fear

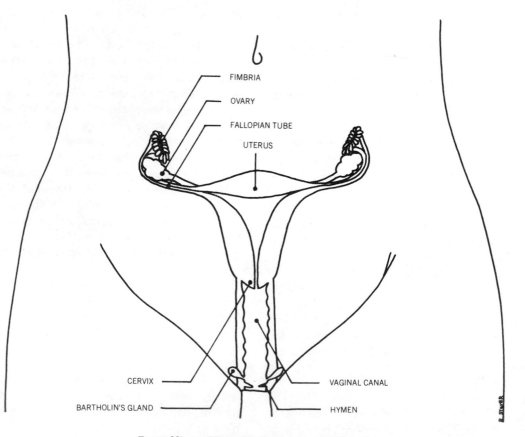

FIMBRIA
OVARY
FALLOPIAN TUBE
UTERUS

CERVIX
BARTHOLIN'S GLAND
VAGINAL CANAL
HYMEN

Front View of Female Reproductive System

that tampons and other objects can get lost inside them. These objects *can't* get lost. They have nowhere to go unless you remove or expel them from your vaginal opening!

The *uterus* is small, muscular, and pear-shaped. Ninety percent of the nonpregnant uterus is muscle tissue with the cavity of the uterus generally the size of a small slit. This organ is remarkable for its elasticity, however, since it is able to expand to many times its original size in pregnancy—and then become quite small again after the baby is born.

At the upper portion of the uterus are the *Fallopian tubes,* passageways from the uterus to the *ovaries* where the egg cells are found. Each month, an egg cell is released from one of the two ovaries in a process called *ovulation* and then begins its journey to the uterus. If met by male sperm and fertilized (conception), this is the beginning of a new human being. This tiny collection of cells will travel on through the tubes to the uterus where it will attach itself to the rich *endometrial walls* (lining of the uterus) to grow and develop.

The unfertilized egg, on the other hand, disintegrates as does the endometrial tissue that has been building up in anticipation of a fertilized egg to nourish. It is this material that comprises the menstrual flow.

We have been describing, of course, the anatomy and monthly cycle of a mature or maturing female. Much of adolescence is spent in transit to maturity and it is the progress of this journey that seems to worry so many young women.

PHYSICAL DEVELOPMENT

I'm 14 and flat as a board! Help!

Flatsy

Everyone but me has their period and I'm feeling pretty scared and out of it!

Fifteen and Out of It

I have a terrible problem: no pubic hair! I'm so embarrassed in PE class! What should I do? Please don't tell me I should talk with my mother or see a doctor. Just answer my question. I bet it isn't every day you get a letter like this!

Anxious Fourteen

We've had letters, notes, phone calls, and conferences with young women who worry about their physical development. So if you're feeling anxious about whether your development—including breast growth, pubic hair, genital appearance, and menstruation—is

following a "normal" course, you're far from alone.

"What is the *normal* age for . . ." is the most common preface to questions about the changes adolescence brings.

It would be nice if we could give you definite easy answers—like saying that a girl's breasts should start budding at the exact age of 11 years, 3 months, and 7 days, occurring in systematic harmony with all other body changes, or that a normal girl should start her first menstrual period *(menarche)* at exactly 2:05 P.M. on her thirteenth birthday and be stabilized in a regular cycle by the age of 14.9!

We can't give you easy answers but we *can* give you a better understanding of how your body grows and develops.

Your body, part of you, the individual, has its own special time clock. We can tell you *how* the changes of adolescence begin and what age spans for these changes are *average.* Note, we say *average* instead of "normal" because there are so many variations of normal!

However, we can't tell you exactly when you will experience specific changes of adolescence or, since you are probably already well into adolescence, when this process of physical change will be complete. That's for your body to decide.

How does this time clock work?

While a baby girl is born with thousands of immature eggs *(ova)* in her ovaries, it isn't until she is about eight (this is an *average* age) that the first preparations for puberty begin. The exquisite timing of this is a miracle that is not yet fully understood.

We do know, however, that the process begins in the brain and involves the glands under the direct control of the *forebrain*. The *pituitary gland,* the master gland of the body, plays a major role here, stimulating the ovaries with a special hormone known as Follicle-Stimulating Hormone, or FSH. This hormone triggers action in the long-dormant ovaries and the essential hormone *estrogen* begins to be produced, then released into the bloodstream.

Now noticeable changes begin to occur.

The girl's hips may broaden as early as eight to ten years of age.

The first signs of breast development may occur about this time, too. These initial changes are very subtle. First, the tissue just under the nipple elevates slightly. The nipple itself may then begin to change.

About this time, too, the girl may experience the beginning of a growth spurt.

Pubic hair generally follows later—somewhat before menstruation.

Less obvious changes are happening around this time, too.

The uterus is growing and its lining is thickening.

Female Breast Development
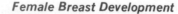

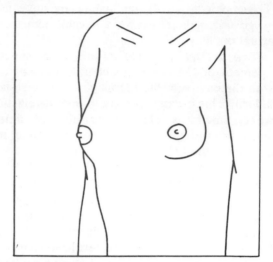

1. Breast buds begin.

2. Breast and areola grow.

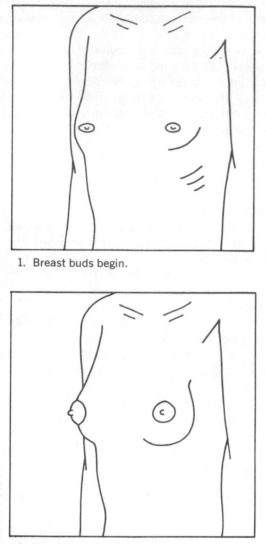

3. Nipple and areola form separate mound, protruding from breast.

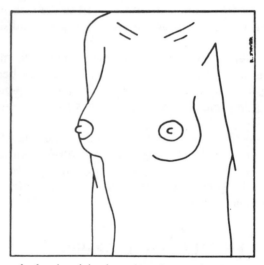

4. Areola rejoins breast contour and development is complete.

Vaginal secretions change from alkaline to acid and a girl may notice a clear, whitish discharge some time before menstruation occurs.

The bones are also affected by hormones. As hormone concentration increases in the body, growth of the long bones decreases. A girl usually grows to within a half inch of her maximum height after beginning to menstruate.

There are many normal variations within this timetable, which may begin as early as 8 and continue to age 19 or beyond, covering many stages.

Breasts, pubic hair, and menstruation are, perhaps, the most visible manifestations of your progress toward adulthood and seem to cause the most concern among teen-agers. Each one of these aspects of development involves several stages.

The breasts, for example, begin as small buds—between the *average* ages of 8 and 13. The *areola* (the area around the nipple, or papilla) widens. In the next stage, the breast itself grows larger, followed by further enlargement of the areola. Next, the nipple and surrounding areola form a small, separate mound that protrudes from the breast. Then, in the fifth or final stage, which may happen—on the average—anywhere from age 12 to 19, the areola becomes, once again, part of the contour of the breast. (See illustrations.)

Pubic hair, too, follows a definite pattern.

Usually, it will appear somewhat after breast development has begun, starting its first stage between the ages of 9 and 15. This initial pubic hair is usually straight and fine. We've had a number of letters from young people alarmed at their *straight* pubic hair. We hasten to reassure them that they are only in stage one—and completely normal!

In stage two, the pubic hair coarsens, darkens, and spreads over a wider area of the genital region.

In stage three, the hair looks like an adult's but may be more limited in area.

In the fourth stage, the inverted triangular pattern of hair distribution is established. This last stage may occur between the ages of 12 and 19.

Also, during these stages of pubic hair development, leg and underarm hair will begin to appear.

Although we give age ranges here, it is the ongoing process of development that is most important.

Breast development is the most reliable indication that puberty is well under way. Some breast development *always* precedes menstruation. This development may not be dramatic, but it will always be present before menarche.

Studies have shown that menstruation often follows the beginning of breast development by two or three years. Some girls, particularly those who begin to develop in the younger range of normal, may experience a shorter waiting time between breast growth and menstruation.

A number of young people will tend to start maturing earlier than others. There is some indication that heredity may be a factor. Some may be duplicating their mother's maturation pattern. Others may begin puberty long before the average age range because they may have special conditions of the pituitary gland affecting hormone function. For reasons not yet fully understood, blind girls show signs of growing up physically earlier than their average sighted counterparts, some studies show.

In short, there are many factors affecting your personal growth timetable. You may find yourself probably very much within the realm of average.

But even an average rate of growth may be only a partial reassurance.

The *fact* of dramatic physical change can be difficult to live with and grow with.

Many girls worry, not only about the timing of their physical changes, but also about

- Size of breasts
- General appearance of breasts
- Menstruation, including menstrual irregularities
- Vaginal discharges
- Changing feelings about those around them
- An increase in sexual feelings and fantasies.

We will deal with your changing feelings primarily in Chapter Four and your growing sexuality in Chapter Ten.

Right now, let's concentrate on your physical con-

Female Pubic Hair Development

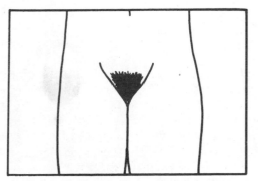

1. Initial pubic hair is straight and fine.

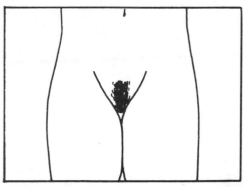

2. Pubic hair coarsens, darkens, and spreads.

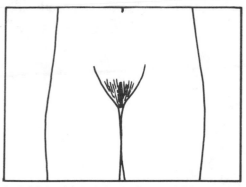

3. Hair looks like adults' but limited in area.

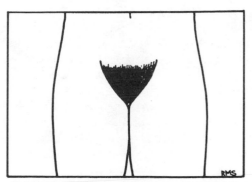

4. Inverted triangular pattern is established.

cerns about your breasts, menstruation, and vaginal discharges—concerns that ALL women have.

BREASTS

I have an awful problem! I'm ashamed of my breasts because they are pointed instead of rounded like those of the girls I see in the showers at gym. My best friend told me that everyone's are like that until they start really growing, but another friend said I'm just deformed. Who is right?

Desperate

"Desperate" 's best friend is right.

She is going through a normal stage: the fourth phase of breast development, albeit a bit later than some of her classmates.

As the letter from "Desperate" illustrates, breast *appearance* may be of crucial concern for a young woman, particularly if she has to shower or dress with classmates after gym. There, comparisons seem inevitable. This, coupled with society's veneration of the perfect breast, can cause a lot of anguish if you happen to be a bit different from the ideal. You may be relatively flat—and get teased. You may get teased about large breasts. You may worry about breasts that just don't seem to match, or that seem unusual in any way.

I'm 15 and wonder whether my breasts are normal. They are not rounded like my 18-year-old sister's. And is it normal for the circle around the nipple to be brown instead of pink? What is inside my breasts? Do the breasts have muscles?

Wondering

"Wondering" has come up with several often-asked questions.

Let's consider her question about breast structure first.

On the outside of the breast, there is the *areola*, the circular skin area around the nipple. The size of your areola—like the size of your breasts in general—tends to be an inherited characteristic. (If your breast size and appearance differs from your mother's, remember that you may have inherited your breast characteristics from your father's family's genes instead.) The areola may vary in color from *very* light pink to dark brown, depending on your complexion. If you have been pregnant, you may notice that your areola has darkened. This is a normal change of pregnancy and is often permanent.

There are several openings—one large and several small—in the nipple. These connect to the openings of the milk ducts. There is a milk duct for each of the approximately 20 lobes that make up the breast. These contain many small glands. As well as glands, there are nerves, arteries, veins, lymph channels, and some amount of fat in the breast. Connective fibers help to

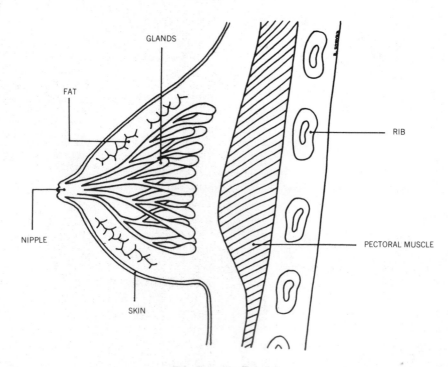

The Female Breast

give the breast its rounded shape. However, the breast may not have this rounded shape until late adolescence. There are no muscles in the breast itself, but there are pectoral muscles just beneath the breast on the chest wall.

I'm 14 and flat-chested. All my friends are bigger than I am. I'm so upset because they make fun of me!
Flats

I'm 15, 5 feet 1, and skinny. My bust measurement is 32. I think this is small. Don't you?
Skinny

Normal bust size is a relative term. Heredity—as we pointed out—plays a major role in determining what your size will be.

Time is also a factor. "Flats" may still be in the process of developing. Studies have shown that the *average* American female Caucasian does not reach a final stage of breast growth and development until the age of 17—or beyond. For reasons as yet undetermined, some black and Oriental teens may reach this stage a year or so earlier.

Weight, too, may influence the size of your breasts. "Skinny," for example, may find that gaining some weight just *might* increase the size of her breasts.

It is heredity more than weight, however, that is the major determining factor in breast size. You have undoubtedly seen small women with large breasts and obese women who seemed fairly flat-chested.

In the case of an obese girl who seems to be flat-chested, it could be that the fat *surrounding* her breasts is masking their true size. If she were to lose weight, she might discover whole new contours.

Flat-chested underweight women, too, may achieve a new breast size with weight gain, since a small amount of fat padding the breast's glandular tissues gives the breasts a great deal of their roundness.

I'm superflat and was wondering about bust developer devices. How safe and effective are they? Can I do exercises or take a pill to make my breasts grow? Something's gotta work! Help!
Pam

Generally, no devices or exercises can help increase bust size. Exercises will affect only pectoral muscles underneath the breast, not the breast tissue itself. There is nothing that can be done with mechanical devices to enlarge the breasts. (More about this in Chapter Six.) While some women may notice a slight breast swelling while taking birth control pills, this increase is quite small and few women would be willing to take the risks involved in taking the Pill only to

achieve such slight changes. In most cases, small breasts are the result of heredity, not hormone deficiency, so hormone therapy has little to offer.

Padded bras may offer temporary comfort, but long-term contentment can only come from accepting and learning to love the uniqueness of your own body, whether you are small or large—or somewhere in between!

I'm overweight and my breasts are too big! How can I make them smaller?
Busty

I desperately want to decrease my bustline because I'm an athlete and need a smaller bust. Help!
Bothered

Breast reduction may be easier for "Busty" than for "Bothered." Many obese adolescent girls may find that the surest way to decrease their bust size is to lose weight. It is advisable, however, to lose weight on a sensible diet plan geared for gradual and steady weight loss. Not only is this a good idea for your general health (see Chapter Five), but also it may help lessen the chance of stretch marks. These stretch marks happen when the elastic fibers of the skin—stretched by rapid growth or increase or decrease in weight—lose their elasticity and ability to contract. The resulting stretch marks are permanent and are best avoided by gradual weight loss. (Many teens, of course, develop these in the course of breast growth without being overweight. While stretch marks do not go away entirely, they may become less obvious with time.)

"Bothered" may find that she will have to adjust to her size. A number of noted female athletes are far from flat and have simply learned to adapt to their bust size.

A good, well-fitting bra, fitted by an expert saleswoman at your local department store, may help increase comfort a great deal.

However, the girl who finds, in late adolescence or young adulthood, that her breasts are *unusually* large may wish to consult a plastic surgeon regarding reduction surgery.

Although this surgery can offer considerable relief to the woman who suffers physically because of unusually large breasts, it is not painless nor inexpensive. It is also a procedure that, except in very rare instances, a reputable surgeon would not perform on an adolescent girl.

Plastic surgery—either to make breasts larger or smaller—is generally not performed until full adolescent development has been attained. Many surgeons prefer not to perform such surgery on young women until they reach the age of 20—or beyond. (Read more about plastic surgery in Chapter Six.)

My breasts are a different size. My left breast is quite a bit smaller than my right one. I feel like a lopsided freak and am very embarrassed. Will they ever be the same?

Lopsided

Many young women complain of asymmetrical, or uneven, breast development. It is not uncommon in adolescence for one breast to develop at a faster rate than the other. Generally, the slower breast will catch up with the other one. Breasts are rarely a perfect match, however. In most women, one breast may always be *slightly* larger than the other.

In rare exceptions, due to a congenital defect, one breast will remain undeveloped. In such instances, after the young woman has reached full maturity, she may choose to have plastic surgery to increase the size of the undeveloped breast.

We can't emphasize too strongly, however, that generally breast surgery is *not* done during adolescence while one or both breasts are still in the process of development.

HELP! Instead of having nipples, it looks like there are cuts or the nipples are pointing in. I'm scared to talk to my doctor about it. Is there something wrong with me?

Scared

I'm 14 and have ingrown nipples. A lady came to my school, showing how to examine your breasts. I think that she said that ingrown nipples can be a sign of cancer. But my nipples have always been like this. Could I still have cancer?

Worried

I'm 16 and one of my nipples is inverted. When I was born, both nipples were inverted, but, gradually, my left nipple changed. I went to a doctor two years ago and he didn't seem to be concerned about it. My mother says I was born with this and not to worry about it because it just means I could never breast-feed my babies. Is this true? She also told me that a lot of girls have this problem, but I still feel like a weirdo. If my right nipple never changes, could something be done surgically to correct it?

Jacquie

Inverted nipples—nipples that turn inward instead of outward—are not uncommon and can appear in male or female breasts. This condition is usually caused by foreshortening of the milk ducts with fibrous tissue strands binding the nipple down. This is usually present at birth, but becomes most noticeable later in life.

If, on the other hand, the nipples are normal and then invert in later life, this can be a sign of an underlying tumor and medical help should be sought immediately!

The three letters here, however, indicate that "Scared," "Worried," and Jacquie have probably grown up having inverted nipples.

Sometimes—as in Jacquie's case—the enlargement of breast tissue during puberty will cause one or both of the nipples to turn out. This may happen, too, during further engorgement of breasts during pregnancy, making it possible for some women to breast-feed their infants.

This isn't always the case, however. Nipples that continue to be inverted can interfere with breast-feeding, but now there are special shields made for women with inverted nipples that make it possible to breast-feed.

Inverted nipples *may* present a hygiene problem. Secretions may dry and cake in the nipple crevices. Infections, too, are common in women with inverted nipples due to the abnormal development of the milk duct lining. There may be abscesses and/or drainage of pus from such infections.

Although some physicians will recommend massage to help correct inverted nipples, this treatment is usually not effective.

Even surgery is not always completely successful in making the nipple entirely normal. In the surgical procedure, the nipple is put in its normal position, but, in the process, vital nerve fibers may have to be severed. Because of this, the nipple may be cosmetically more pleasing, but may not be able to erect.

I have some dark hairs around my nipple. My mom said that pulling them out will cause cancer. How can I get rid of this hair?

Sue

Many women, like Sue, have hair on their breasts, often around the nipple. Hair growth may be influenced by ethnic origin and hormonal balance. Such hair growth does not necessarily signal abnormality. The only cause for some concern would be if the sudden appearance of this hair were also accompanied by a number of masculine traits. Otherwise, your main concern will be cosmetic. (For more information about hair removal, see Chapter Six.).

My nipples are not really developed yet. The only

times they seem to be is when I am cold or turned on sexually. Is this an unusual problem?

Barbara

Barbara has described normal breast changes. Sometimes the nipples are relatively flat. But during stimulation, sexual or otherwise (cold, contact with clothing, and so forth), they become erect.

My boyfriend bites my breasts and often bruises them. Can biting or pinching breasts injure them? Can this cause cancer?

Bruised

While breast injuries do not necessarily cause cancer and while gentle bites, squeezing, and pinching may not be harmful, excessive biting and too vigorous pinching or squeezing may cause a breast infection or inflammation. Extremely hard pinching may cause some hemorrhage into the tissues and chronic and repeated irritation of breast tissue (over a period of years) *may* result in cancerous changes.

I'm 16 and scared to death. I may have breast cancer. I have a discharge from both my breasts. Sometimes it looks like water and other times like milk. What do you think this could be?

Evie

Most women have a small amount of nipple discharge.

This discharge is the secreting fluid that keeps the nipple ducts open.

Usually the amount of this discharge is so small that it isn't noticeable, but some women secrete more than others, particularly, it seems, if they have been taking oral contraceptives for a long period of time. This discharge may be milky or clear or green, gray, or yellow and is generally no reason for alarm, especially if it comes from both nipples. Some studies have linked a clear or straw-colored nipple discharge with menstruation in some young women.

When can a breast discharge indicate a problem?

If it contains pus: This is the sign of an underlying infection. Consult a physician.

If the discharge is bloody or pinkish: A doctor should examine the breasts for possible disorders. However, if one is pregnant, a blood discharge may not be the sign of an underlying breast disease.

A brownish discharge: Especially with a lump present, this may indicate a sebaceous cyst with some infection. A physician should be consulted.

Nipple discharge may also be caused by *intraductal papilloma,* a warty growth in a major breast duct, or

by cystic disease of the breast, which we will discuss a little later on in this chapter.

While breast cancer is quite rare in teen-age women, it is important to be aware of any changes occurring in your breasts.

Most changes that you see at this point, of course, will be connected with your continuing development.

I have a lump under my nipple that is really sore! I can't stand to touch my nipple even. Is this some kind of disease?

Sharon

Sharon's problem sounds like an "adolescent nodule."

This is a common occurrence during puberty. This enlargement and swelling, usually under the nipple, makes the nipple very tender and can thoroughly alarm the adolescent girl *or* boy who is experiencing this.

What causes the nodules? Nobody knows for sure, but there is a theory that it may be due to the increased production of hormones at puberty. Usually this nodule will disappear in a short time. It is important to know this. Reputable physicians will never operate on a young teen girl's breast to remove such a nodule, since such surgery is unnecessary and may interfere with future breast development.

I have sore, lumpy breasts. If this isn't cancer, what could it possibly be? Help! I'm too scared to tell anyone about this!

Janelle

Breast cancer is not especially common (but can occur) in teen-agers. Furthermore, breast lumps that are tender and sore are *usually* benign (noncancerous).

Women have learned to be alert when they feel a breast lump and, we hope, more and more are feeling free about seeking medical attention.

This new awareness is good.

There is, however, some needless alarm about breast lumps and cancer, especially among teen-agers.

Every lump is *not* cancer. In most cases, it will be benign.

Still, it is important to check with your physician if you discover a lump in your breast.

It may be that the lump you have discovered tends to disappear and then reappear at another stage of your menstrual cycle. This is quite common and it is for this reason that your doctor may ask you to come back for another breast examination at another point in your cycle.

What could a benign breast lump mean? There are a number of possibilities. The following are some of the more common disorders of the breast.

Fibrocystic Disease is, perhaps, the most common of these disorders.

While the exact causes of fibrocystic disease are unknown, we *do* know that this disorder tends to appear most in women in their childbearing years (from puberty to menopause). Production of the hormone estrogen, then, may have something to do with the growth of cysts within the breast tissue. Some physicians believe that cystic disease happens as the result of hormone imbalance.

These cysts may grow in one part of the breast or throughout the breast. They may be microscopic or egg-sized.

There are, generally, three kinds of fibrocystic disease. First, there is the type involving only *one, large cyst* that is *usually* not painful. Second, there can be *multiple small cysts* that do tend to be tender or painful. Third, there is *adenosis* or proliferation of ductal cells, which is sometimes, though not always, painful.

Fibrocystic disease may be most noticeable when the breasts swell just prior to menstruation. The breasts may be especially tender at this time and the cysts themselves more easily felt.

Although these cysts are benign, a young woman with fibrocystic disease, especially the adenosis type, may be more prone to develop breast cancer in later life. That is why regular breast examinations and medical checkups are advisable.

In the meantime, what can be done to help alleviate fibrocystic disease? At the present time, relatively little.

Surgery and removal of one or more cysts may be helpful for diagnostic purposes (to make absolutely sure that the cysts are benign) and to remove a troublesome cyst. But since cystic disease seems to be hormonally caused, surgery cannot necessarily cure it.

Another aid to accurately diagnosing benign cysts is an X ray of the breasts called a *mammogram*. The complete safety of this procedure is controversial at the present time, however, and it is used sparingly on women who have not yet reached middle age.

Some doctors give patients suffering from fibrocystic disease diuretic drugs (water pills) to help lessen premenstrual water retention and subsequent swelling of the breast. This can help some painful symptoms, but is not recommended as a long-term treatment.

Other doctors try aspiration of a cyst by inserting a needle into the breast and extracting fluid from the cyst. While this method of treatment can be helpful, especially in making sure that there are *not* malignant cells present, it cannot be called a cure.

Despite the lack of a definite cure, fibrocystic disease does not fall into the grim, incurable disease stereotype. Many women, especially those with a mild form, will have no symptoms at all. Others will have considerable discomfort, but generally this tends to happen just before the menstrual flow each month and the pain is not constant.

The most significant fact to know about cystic disease is one we mentioned a little earlier: Women who have this disorder *may* be more likely to develop breast cancer later on. While this is *not* an inevitability, it is reason for caution.

All women should examine their breasts regularly, but for the woman with fibrocystic disease, regular examinations are *especially* important.

Fibro-Adenomas are tumors that occur most often in younger women (teens to the mid-thirties). They may be tiny *or* fairly large and are composed of gland and fibrous tissues. These tumors are round, firm, and not painful. While their cause is not known, their treatment is fairly simple. The physician will remove the tumor in a simple and fast surgical procedure.

Cystosarcoma Phyllodes is a relatively rare, fast-growing, and generally benign tumor that occurs most often in teens and young women. Since it grows fast and since about 10 percent of these tumors may be malignant rather than benign, a woman with sudden, large breast lumps should see her physician immediately. This tumor or tumors must be removed, generally in a simple operation that—in the case of benign tumors—does not deform the breast.

Moles commonly occur on the breasts. These should be watched, and if they begin to change in color, increase in size, or bleed, they should be surgically removed.

As we stated earlier, most breast lumps are *not* cancerous.

But it's important to begin the habit of lifelong health vigilance. Learn what your breasts feel like now and how they may change with your monthly cycle, so that if anything unusual occurs later on you'll notice right away.

As well as feeling for lumps, look for unusual changes. If you notice a dimple or pucker in the breast, if a previously normal nipple suddenly becomes inverted, or there is a change in your breasts' contour or skin texture, do consult your physician immediately!

About once a month—perhaps about a week after you expect your menstrual period to begin—it is a good idea to examine your breasts.

This is easy to do and takes relatively little time.

How do you do it?

Check the illustrations and then read the following:

Breast Self-Examination

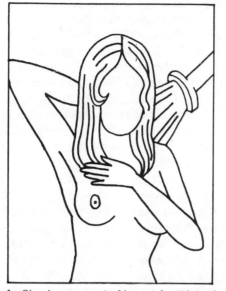

1. Check every part of breast for thickening or lumps.

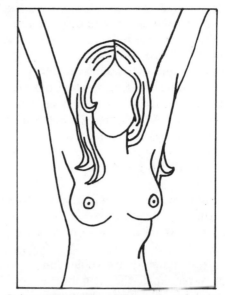

2. Raise your arms, look in the mirror for changes in contour, skin texture or color.

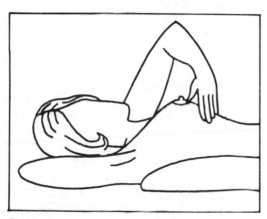

3. Lie down and repeat examination.

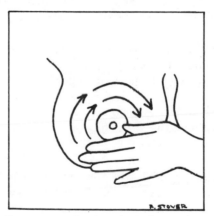

4. Always use a circular, clockwise motion.

1. First, as you shower, touch every part of your breast, probing gently in a circular, clockwise motion for any thickening of breast tissue or for lumps.

2. After you get out of the shower, raise your arms over your head and look at the contours of your breasts in the bathroom mirror. Note any changes of contour, skin texture, and the like.

3. With alternate arms extended over your head, lie down and repeat the circular check of your breasts.

4. Remember to feel ALL parts of the breast, working from outer contours to the nipple area in a gentle, circular motion.

If you do notice anything unusual during your regular self-examinations, do check with your physician. It will probably be a minor problem, but only your doctor can confirm this.

Breast self-examination is a vital part of a good health maintenance program. Although you may be less likely in these years to have any serious problems with your breasts, self-examination is a good habit to get into—one that could someday save your life!

MENSTRUATION

Some call menstruation "the curse." Others call it an illness. Still others consider it too shameful—and dirty—to mention.

Menstruation is none of the above. It is not a curse, not an illness, not a shameful, unclean monthly phenomenon.

Basically, menstruation is a very positive happening in your life. It is, perhaps, one of the best barometers you have to show that your body is healthy and functioning normally.

However, it's easy to see how the myths and mis-information about menstruation could thrive, since until quite recently medical science and women them-selves had very little accurate information about men-struation as a biological process.

Even now, some of the myths survive.

How many of the menstrual myths and old wives' tales do YOU believe?

Take the following true-false quiz to see if you have innocently fallen for some of them!

True or False?

1. Women should not bathe, swim, or wash their hair while menstruating.

2. It's important to avoid exercise during your pe-riod.

3. Stay away from your plants while you're men-struating. If you water them, they'll wilt.

4. Teen-age girls should not use tampons.

5. A woman is unclean and should douche regularly.

6. It's unhealthy to have sex during your period.

7. It's impossible to get pregnant during your pe-riod.

8. Women make poor executives because of pre-menstrual mood fluctuations and because they get run down from loss of blood and can't maintain a stable level of energy.

9. Cramps are all in the head.

10. Menstrual blood is "bad blood" and therefore dirty.

These ten statements are ALL false and reflect some of the inaccurate information that abounds about menstruation.

Let's go back over some of these myths, point by point, and correct them.

1. Bathing and washing your hair during menstrua-tion is not only permissible, but desirable! A daily bath or shower is a good idea, whether or not you are men-struating. Washing your hair when the need arises is also practical—no matter what day of the month it may be. If swimming is part of your life-style, men-struation does not have to keep you on the sidelines several days a month. Go ahead and swim! Some women find that tampons are most practical and com-fortable for swimming.

2. If you lead an active life, there's no need to crawl under the covers and stop living during your period! Active teens seem to have less trouble with cramps. In fact, there is some evidence that exercise can ac-tually *help* if you do suffer from cramps. (More about this later.)

3. The plant myth is so ridiculous, it's hardly worth

mentioning. We just included it to show you how far-fetched some of the old wives' tales really are!

4. Teen-age girls *can* use tampons—and a number do, from the first day of their very first menstrual pe-riod. (We will be talking about tampons—and pads—later on in this chapter.)

5. While we will also be talking about douching later on in the chapter, perhaps the most important point we'd like to make about this feminine hygiene process is this: The vagina is self-cleansing under normal con-ditions, and unless a medicinal douche is prescribed by a physician for the treatment of a specific vaginal infection, douching is an option, not a necessity.

6. Some women find that their sexual desires are stronger just before and during menstruation. With others, this may not be the case. Sex during menstrua-tion is *not* unhealthy. It's an option many people choose. Some women prefer to wear a diaphragm (see Chapter Twelve) for sexual intercourse during men-struation. As well as acting as a reliable method of birth control (conception is *not* impossible during menstruation), the diaphragm catches and holds the menstrual flow.

7. As we said in number 6, conception during men-struation is not impossible. It has happened, although it is less likely at this time. It is always wise—what-ever time of the month it may be—to use a reliable form of birth control.

8. This myth about the basic instability of women due to premenstrual tension or hormonal influences has done a lot of damage to the cause of working women in years past. These old prejudices are fading, however, as we understand more about the menstrual cycle and, indeed, ALL human life cycles. While a rise in her hormone levels during ovulation may give a woman an energy boost and heightened sense of well-being and a drop in these levels just before men-struation can cause some depression and a variety of other symptons. These are predictable fluctuations that can be dealt with. Some Olympic athletes have given top performances during menstruation. So do thousands of other women, in all walks of life. Recent studies have revealed that, among working women, absenteeism due to so-called female complaints is at an all-time low. This old myth is being disproved in so many ways every day. Most successful women have simply come to know themselves and their bodies well and have learned to pace themselves so that they can get the most out of both their high- and low-energy days. Studies are also showing that ALL of us, male and female, are subject to cyclical rhythms. You've probably heard about biorhythms and the fact that, during any given day, you will have high- and low-energy periods. Although women experience an addi-tional cycle—menstruation—that men don't have, the

hormones that regulate this extra cycle (most notably estrogen) protect women from some common ailments suffered by men—like heart attacks and strokes. While some younger women may suffer from these disorders, they are much less likely to do so than their male counterparts. So physiologically, women may be at an advantage!

9. Cramps are *not* "all in the head." This is something that frustrated and angry women have been trying to tell male doctors for years. Now medical research has discovered some of the real causes for cramps—which we will discuss in detail later on in this chapter.

10. The menstrual flow is not dirty and it isn't all blood. It is a mixture of blood, mucus, and degenerated cells that are fragments of the lining of the uterus. This lining, called the *endometrium,* is built up and shed monthly.

Now that we've examined some of the prevailing myths about menstruation and have discussed what menstruation *isn't,* let's take a look at what it *is.*

Could you tell me the difference between the menstrual period and the menstrual cycle? Are they the same? What is the normal time between periods? Is it ever normal to skip a period—without being pregnant? There's so much I need to know!

Sheri A.

While most women equate menstruation with the actual menstrual period—the once-a-month bloody discharge—the menstrual *cycle* is a continuous process involving ovulation, changes in the tissue lining of the uterus, and, finally, shedding of that lining via the menstrual flow.

Menstruation involves the entire body, not just the

The Menstrual Cycle

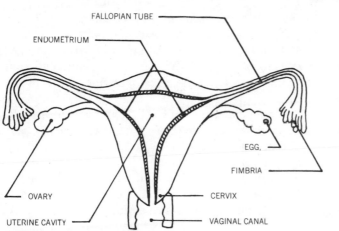

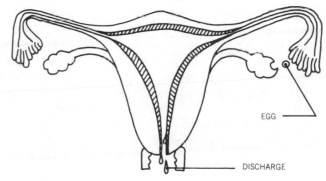

1. Hormonal levels rise and the uterine lining is prepared to receive a fertilized egg.

2. Around mid-cycle the ripened egg leaves the ovary and travels through the fallopian tube.

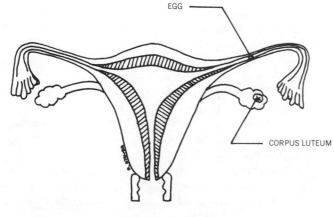

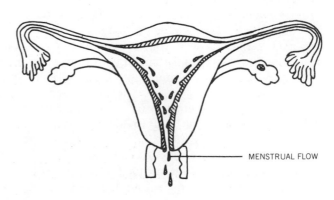

3. The egg approaches the uterine lining.

4. If conception has not taken place, the egg disintegrates and the lining is shed as menstruation.

uterus. The entire monthly cycle is controlled by a part of the brain known as the *hypothalamus* and by the pituitary gland. These control the ebb and flow of hormones—estrogen and progesterone—that cause women to develop and to have regular menstrual cycles.

A regular cycle may vary widely from individual to individual. While a 28-day cycle might be considered *average,* a 21-, 30-, or even 60-day cycle may be normal for you.

How do you calculate your cycle length?

Day one is the first day of your menstrual period. Start counting there. You may have your period for an *average* of three to seven days. At this time, your estrogen level is low and you may feel a little short on energy.

When your period ends, keep counting. Now your estrogen level is rising once more, preparing the lining of your uterus to receive and nourish a fertilized egg. With this surge in your hormonal level, you may feel a sharp rise in energy and a sense of well-being.

Around mid-cycle—perhaps day 14 or 15—your cycle will begin to reach its peak. A second hormone—progesterone—joins estrogen in preparing the lush uterine lining for a fertilized egg. The egg itself has ripened and now receives the hormonal signal to leave the ovaries and begin its journey through the Fallopian tubes to the uterus. It is during the egg's four- to six-day journey to the uterus that it is most likely to be fertilized. If you have sexual intercourse during this time, you are much more likely to get pregnant than at other times. Relying on calculation of your "safe" times (called the rhythm method of birth control) is risky, however. While the release of the egg (ovulation) is most likely to happen at mid-cycle, the exact timing is very difficult to calculate. And while pregnancy is most likely to happen at mid-cycle, it can occur at any time!

At this mid-cycle time, with two hormones at top levels, you may feel unusually good. These hormones will reach a high level about day 20 and then start to drop if your egg has not been fertilized by the male sperm. The egg itself will begin to disintegrate and the lining of the uterus will start to break down. About day 28, this will start to pass from your uterus, through your cervix and down your vagina, as the menstrual flow.

How does a cycle countdown look on a calender?

Let's say that your next-to-last period began on April 1 and the period after that (your last one) started on April 29. You have a 28-day cycle.

Since your cycle is controlled by a part of your brain, it can be affected by a number of factors.

Joyce, for example, stopped menstruating entirely for three months after her mother's death.

Cathy skipped one period during her first month away at college and another one during the first-semester finals.

A bad cold delayed Mary's period for three days, and worry about the possibility of pregnancy may have caused Tina to be several days late.

There are many more factors, as we will see, that may cause your cycle and your periods to be irregular.

I'm 14 and had my first period over three months ago, but haven't had a period since. My mother says not to worry, but I'm worried!

Pamela R.

I went on a diet and lost 25 pounds. That's great and I'm so happy. The only problem is, I haven't had a period since losing all that weight. Is something wrong with me?

Puzzled in Pa.

Both of these letters show common irregularities.

In Pamela's case, the irregularity is not at all unusual. In fact, it is quite common in early puberty for cycles to be irregular. The exquisite, individual timing of your biological time clock may not be set for some time.

At the menarche, your estrogen levels may be fluctuating more than usual. You may have a heavy period and then no period at all for a few months. Also, you may not yet be ovulating.

How do you have a period without ovulation?

Early in puberty, you may be producing plenty of estrogen, but it may take a while before the second hormone, progesterone, is manufactured in sufficient quantity to assume its task of triggering ovulation. The rise and fall of the estrogen level, which signals the shedding of the uterine lining, may begin some months before your body is mature enough to produce progesterone on a regular basis. It is possible, then, to have some periods without ovulation. However, some girls have regular, ovulatory cycles from the menarche on . . . and it's impossible for you to tell for sure whether or not you *are* ovulating. So girls who have recently started menstruation and who may be sexually active should be just as careful about birth control as those who are more mature.

On the average, most girls have regular cycles by the time they have reached the age of 18 OR have been menstruating for several years.

After this time, irregular periods, no periods, and bleeding between periods may be symptoms that something is wrong and should be brought to the attention of a physician.

Irregular Periods, for example, may be the result of

emotional stress, jet lag, or an undisclosed physical problem.

Spotting Between Periods may be a common side effect from an IUD or the Pill (see Birth Control chapter) or may be due to emotional stress, diet, an ovarian cyst, or uterine fibroid or polyp. It may also be—but seldom *is* at this age—a symptom of uterine cancer.

What If You Suddenly Cease to Have Periods?

If there is no possibility of pregnancy or if your pregnancy test was negative, you and your physician may explore the causes of absence of menstruation (called secondary amenorrhea) by considering a number of possibilities. Your physician may ask you if any of the following has occurred.

Unusual Amount of Stress in Your Life.

The death of someone close to you or the loss, through a breakup or divorce, of a boyfriend or husband can play havoc with your cycle. So can a new experience like college. It is very common for freshmen women to skip one or more periods as they adjust to the demands of college life and, perhaps, to the joy and pain of being away from home for the first time.

A Major Weight Change.

If you have lost—or gained—10 to 15 percent of your total body weight, your menstrual cycle may be affected. This is particularly likely to be the case if you lost weight via a fad diet or by compulsive self-imposed starvation called *anorexia nervosa* (we will discuss this condition further in Chapters Five and Eight). An iron deficiency and malnutrition can also cause menstruation to cease.

Use of Drugs.

If you use tranquilizers (downers) heavily, they may have a "down" effect on your menstrual cycle as well, repressing it along with other body functions.

Birth control pills can cause you to get lighter than normal periods, and in some women, their periods actually become nonexistent!

If you have had no unusual emotional stresses, significant weight fluctuations, or possible drug influences on your cycle and there is no possibility of pregnancy, your physician may wish to explore other possibilities—tumors, polyps, and other disorders in your reproductive system.

What Are Some of These Disorders? There are *uterine fibroids*—most common in older women, but not an impossibility in the teen years. These benign tumors vary in size and location and may cause an alteration in menstrual bleeding. Surgical removal is in order if a fibroid causes unusual bleeding and/or pain.

There are *ovarian cysts* or *tumors*. These vary in size and type. Some need to be surgically removed; others will simply disappear in time.

Endometriosis—or the overgrowth of uterine lining tissue outside the uterine cavity—is not uncommon in teen-agers and may be caused by irregular ovarian function. *Endometrial hyperplasia* often causes menstrual irregularity and may also cause cramps and heavy bleeding. This condition may be helped by temporary interruption of ovulation—such as pregnancy, taking birth control pills or other hormone therapy. In extreme cases, surgery may be in order. When possible, surgeons tend to prefer the conservative approach—removing only the overgrowth of tissue. Only in rare instances of unusually stubborn and troublesome cases will a surgeon consider removing the uterus and/or ovaries—and this would rarely be done when the woman is young.

Various *chronic diseases* (see Chapter Nine) may also affect your menstrual cycles.

Another uncommon—but not impossible—cause of irregular menses in teen-agers is cancer. While most cancers involving the reproductive tract occur among older women, recent studies have shown that teen girls whose mothers were treated during pregnancy with the synthetic estrogen *diethylstilbestrol* (DES), which was used until the early sixties to prevent miscarriages, may be at a risk of developing a rare form of vaginal cancer. While *relatively few* of the many thousands of girls who were exposed to this drug while still in the womb have developed this cancer, it is a good idea to have regular gynecological checkups if your mother did take this drug while carrying you. You can get further information about DES and a free pamphlet, "From One DES Teenager to Another," by writing to: DES Action, P.O. Box 1977, Plainview, N.Y. 11803 or by calling (516) 433-7070.

PREMENSTRUAL BLUES AND MENSTRUAL PAIN

A few days before my period starts, I feel really awful. My breasts hurt and I gain weight. Why does this happen and what can I do about it?

Sally G.

Mood changes, headaches, weight gain, water retention, and tender breasts are common premenstrual symptoms. A large percentage of women experience one or more of these.

Are YOU—at times—a victim of the premenstrual blues?

Do you cry for no reason at all as your period nears?

Are you tense and irritable just before menstruation?

Do your clothes suddenly seem tighter?

Does the scale say you're up a few pounds (even though you've been super strict on your diet)?

Do your rings become incredibly tight?

Are you plagued with diarrhea? Constipation?

Do you feel unusually tired or depressed?

Is your head pounding?

If you've answered yes to one or more of these questions, you could be suffering from the premenstrual syndrome.

If you're feeling miserable at this time, blame it on hormones!

Water retention, which can give you a heavy, bloated feeling, headaches, tight rings and clothes, and a general feeling of malaise, can happen in response to shifting hormone levels. The higher your estrogen level, the lower the amount of water and salt that will filter through your kidneys. Instead of being passed out of your body as urine, the excess water is retained in your body tissues.

Some researchers feel, too, that hormonal imbalances can contribute to mood fluctuations.

If premenstrual problems, especially water retention, plague you, what can you do?

You may try a few changes in diet during this time. It is especially important to restrict your salt intake in the week before menstruation if you tend to have a water retention problem.

"But I *don't* eat that much salt!" you may be saying.

Be aware of the *hidden* salt in your food! There is salt in diet drinks, hot dogs, ham, lunch meats, and crunchy snack foods, as well as a lot of canned foods, including soups.

If a change of diet doesn't help, your physician may prescribe diuretics (water pills) to help alleviate your water retention problem and, ideally, the uncomfortable symptoms that go with it.

If your premenstrual problems are unusually difficult, you and your doctor might discuss some form of hormone therapy. There are several types that might help.

For some women, however, genuine distress doesn't begin until the actual menstrual period starts.

This distress is *real*.

While your feelings about your body and about men-

struation may influence your perceptions of it as a normal or negative experience, cramps are *not* "all in the head."

Every month on the first day of my period I get almost unbearable cramps that even shoot down my legs. Sometimes my legs shake! I've had my period for five years, since I was 11. I'm scared to talk to my doctor for fear he'll say that it's all in my mind. I know it's not and I'm scared to death!

Melanie B.

As Melanie illustrates, cramps may mean more than that dull ache in the abdomen. You may have pains in your legs and back. You may have chills, feel shaky and sweaty. You may faint or feel nauseated. You may feel a dull ache or painful spasms. You may be inconvenienced—or practically immobilized.

The causes—and cures—for cramps are still being investigated.

At the present time, however, physicians tend to classify cramps—also called painful menstruation or dysmenorrhea—into two categories.

The rarest type is *secondary dysmenorrhea*, which has as its cause some sort of anatomical disorder or dysfunction (for example, an infection, an ovarian tumor, or endometriosis).

The most common category is *primary dysmenorrhea*, which is *not* caused by any identifiable disorder. It is estimated that nine out of ten women will suffer from this kind of cramping at some point in their lives and many of these will be young women in their teens or twenties.

What causes these cramps?

The most-often cited causes are muscular contracttions of the uterus and changes in the blood circulation of the uterus, resulting in spasms of the arteries within the uterine wall.

There are causes behind these causes, however.

Some medical researchers suggest that these cramps, which are not always consistent from month to month, may be due to an imbalance of the hormones estrogen and progesterone.

The newest research findings are attempting to link menstrual cramps with the production of substances known as *prostaglandins*. These fatty acids come in many varieties and are produced by organs of the body, including the uterus. They have not yet been classified, but they closely resemble hormones.

The two prostaglandins produced in the uterus are F_2 (alpha), which causes uterine contractions, and E_2, which relaxes the uterine muscles. Some researchers theorize that a clash between and imbalance of these prostaglandins—resulting in the dominance of F_2 over E_2—may be a major cause of cramping.

Further evidence that cramps may be linked to hormones and hormonelike substances is the fact that cramps—like premenstrual symptoms—usually occur in women who are ovulating. Very young teens who are not yet ovulating (due to a low level of the hormone progesterone) tend to have painless periods. It is only when they begin to produce higher levels of hormones and prostaglandins and to ovulate that they experience cramps. Some physicians have found that using birth control pills, which prevent ovulation, for a few months may help alleviate the cramps.

A few months' respite from painful cramps can do wonders. Having several painless periods (after a siege of painful ones) may change a girl's attitude about menstruation. She may stop dreading it so much and stop tensing at the mere suggestion of pain. She may find, then, when she stops taking birth control pills, that the old misery doesn't automatically return.

In that sense, what is in your head—how you feel—about menstruation can influence, though not necessarily cause, your cramps. If you're feeling unusually tense one month, you may experience cramps. If you tense at the first hint of a mild cramp, you may find your pain intensified. Also, if you feel that menstruation makes you ill and take to your bed automatically at first evidence of your period every month, your fears may be fulfilled. The feeling of pelvic congestion may increase with inactivity.

Generally, cramps seem to plague young women more often than older women. Doctors are still investigating reasons for this, questioning whether it is time or the experience of pregnancy and childbirth (which a majority of women still share) that helps lessen the pain.

For years, physicians believed that cramps might be caused by a narrow cervical canal, which makes it necessary for the uterus to contract harder to expel the menstrual flow. This theory assumed that the stretching of the cervical canal, through childbirth, solved the problem. This may be true in some instances, but relatively few women have been found to have true cervical *stenosis* (another name for narrowing of the cervical canal). In years past, doctors would often surgically dilate (or stretch) the cervical canal. Today, this procedure has generally given way to drug treatment in severe cases of cramps.

What drugs can help cramps?

Some women find relief with aspirin or aspirin substitutes like Tylenol. Apart from its pain-relieving function, aspirin has been found to have antiprostaglandin properties, which may be why it is generally quite effective in helping to reduce the pain of cramps.

Other nonprescription remedies—like Midol and Pamprin—are combinations of pain-relievers and diuretics that may help both the pain and the bloated feeling caused by water retention. If these prove ineffective, there are a variety of prescription pain remedies.

What else can help ease cramps?

Heat—in moderate doses—via a warm heating pad or tub bath may help.

Exercise—believe it or not—can also help to ease your pain. A recent study shows that 70 percent of the teens in that study who had suffered from cramps and who subsequently followed a regular exercise routine found definite relief after a reasonable amount of time. The greatest benefit, researchers found, occurred after several months of regular daily workouts.

Any number of exercise methods may help: a brisk walk, dancing, a team sport you particularly enjoy, bicycling, or a regimen of specific exercises. Some of the latter may be particularly helpful in reducing the pain of your cramps *over a period of time*.

What are some of these exercises?

Total Body Relaxer.

Lying on your back, relax every part of your body, part by part, from the toes up. Tell your toes, then your ankles to relax. Take deep breaths. When you get to the pelvic area, take an extra amount of time to relax. If you are having a lot of problems with tensions there, try panting for a few minutes, then relax. Continue relaxing each part of your body, up to and including your forehead. Lie in this state of relaxation for several minutes.

Abdominal Push.

Still lying on your back, put your hands at your sides and bend your knees (keeping your feet on the floor). As you inhale, push your abdomen out. Hold your breath and then exhale, flattening your abdomen as much as possible. Relax for a few minutes. Then repeat the exercise up to ten times.

Toe Touch.

Stand up. Put your feet together and extend your arms to the sides. Twist to your right side and try to touch your right foot with your left hand. Then repeat this on the other side. Try this exercise ten times on each side.

Arm and Leg Stretch.

Still standing, put your hands at your sides. Then move your arms up and forward while extending your left leg as far backward as possible (while keeping your toes on the floor). Count to five while holding this position and then return your left leg to the starting position and repeat the exercise with your right leg. Do this exercise five times with each leg.

If exercise, heat treatments, and nonprescription remedies do not help your cramps, and particularly if these cramps are severe and debilitating each month, do check with your physician. He or she will examine you to see if there is any disorder that may be causing the cramps. In most cases, however, your discomfort will be due to primary dysmenorrhea. A physician may then prescribe stronger pain-killers or analgesics. Physicians generally prefer to try these prescription drugs first. Then, if your discomfort persists, your doctor may suggest that you try taking birth control pills for a few months.

No matter how severe your cramps, help is generally available. You do not have to retire from the human race once a month. You *do* have alternatives. And doctors today—as they learn more and more about the causes of cramps—are much less likely to dismiss your cramps as "all in your head."

Sanitary Products

I've had my period for three years now and I simply dread it. It interferes with everything and I hate having to wear those pads. My mom uses tampons and she told me that when I start using them, I won't want to use anything else ever again. The problem is, I'm afraid that I might have a difficult time starting to use them. Do you know an easy way to start out? I hate wearing pads because they seem to stop me from doing the things I'd like to do.

Isolated

All my friends use tampons, but my mother won't let me because she says they're not safe. Are they— or not?

Zoe N.

My friend and I are wondering if it's true that if you wear tampons, you won't be a virgin anymore?

Kimberly S.

What is better and safer to use—tampons or pads? I think I'd like to use tampons, but not if it would hurt my body in any way. What should I do?

Uncertain

The issue of tampons versus pads sparks much debate among teen girls and between these girls and their mothers.

There are several myths and misunderstandings about tampons that make some girls—and a number of mothers—wary of tampon use.

A Tampon Will Take Your Virginity.

Untrue! You are a virgin unless you have had sexual intercourse—period! The presence—or absence—of a hymen is *not* definitive proof of virginity. Some girls, in fact, are *born* without hymens. In most girls, the hymen is elastic and stretches easily, allowing use of a tampon. Also, tampons are available in a number of sizes, including a junior size. If you feel comfortable wearing a tampon, there is no medical reason why you shouldn't—from your very first menstrual period!

Tampons Are Dangerous Because They Can "Get Lost" Inside You.

Untrue! The vaginal opening is the only one large enough to admit a tampon. The cervical *os* (the opening which leads to the uterus) is much too tiny to permit the passage of a tampon. So a tampon remains in your vagina until you take it out. Generally, the string will remain outside your body. If it does get pushed up into the vagina, you can still easily reach it and/or the tampon with your fingers.

Tampons Cause Vaginal Infections.

Untrue! Tampons come wrapped and are certainly as safe as pads. They do not usually cause infections. In some cases, a woman may forget to remove the last tampon she inserted during her last menstrual period, though this is rare. After a few days, she may notice a foul-smelling discharge, due to bacterial growth on the tampon. This discharge, however, can generally be stopped simply by removing the tampon.

What form of sanitary protection is most popular?

These days, studies show, it's about 50–50—and on the rise in favor of tampons. This is a marked change from the past. Only five years ago, only 16 percent of menstruating women used tampons. Now the percentage is roughly 50 percent and climbing.

As women become more aware of their bodies and of alternatives available to them in all areas, many are transcending the traditional taboos and learning the truth behind the old tampon myths. An increasing number of teen-agers are using tampons from the menarche on.

Yet tampons may not be right for *you*. Much depends on your personal feelings and choices.

Some young women who feel nervous as yet about anything inserted in the vagina may prefer pads. So may girls who have uncommonly rigid, nonelastic hymens.

Pads are a perfectly safe method of sanitary protection. There may be some problems connected with their use, but nothing you can't deal with.

What are some possible problems?

Pads may show under your clothes. This is not in itself a problem since menstruation is *not* a shameful secret. However, some girls feel self-conscious about boys knowing that they are menstruating (and teasing them about it). This is particularly true of younger teens who are still in the process of adjusting emotionally to their body changes. Fortunately, there is an effective solution to this, if this might be a problem for you. The newer adhesive-backed maxi- and mini-pads—giving you freedom from the old belts (which showed more than the pad)—offer the advantage of fewer bulges and more comfort.

Pads may inhibit you in some activities (like swimming) and the problem of odor may exist, particularly if the pad is not changed often. (The menstrual flow is not odorous until it interacts with normal vaginal flora bacteria and is exposed to the air. Since tampons are worn internally and are not exposed to air, the problem of odor is minimized.)

It is only fair to point out that tampons, too, may present some problems—especially for the first-time user—as the following letters illustrate.

Help! I read the instructions on the tampon box very carefully, but I still seem to have a lot of trouble inserting tampons. I've tried time and time again, but inserting them is still painful. I've been using the kind without the applicator. Can you tell me what I might be doing wrong?

Anonymous, Please!

My friend and I have a problem with tampons. We want to use them, but we can't get them in. What could we be doing wrong? What is the best brand to start with?

No Napkins Again!

Problems with tampons may be caused by several factors.

Lack of Information About Your Body. If you don't know your body, placing a tampon correctly may be difficult if not impossible!

Some girls, for example, aren't sure exactly where the vagina is located. One girl, who complained about painful and unsuccessful insertion attempts, was trying to squeeze a tampon into the urethral opening above her vagina. Still another, whose hymen covered a part of the upper portion of the vaginal opening, never tried

moving the tampon down a little. Others have inserted tampons into the rectum and still others have failed to insert the tampon farther up in the vagina, past the muscles near the opening. (Unless the tampon is past these muscles, it will be uncomfortable.)

If your vagina seems to close up suddenly as you try to insert a tampon, this could be a matter of nerves—not anatomy!

Nervousness. When you're nervous, the muscles around your vaginal opening may tighten, making insertion of the tampon difficult and painful. When experimenting with tampons, choose a time when you're not in a hurry and when family members aren't likely to line up urgently outside the bathroom door. You might even consider experimenting with tampons on a day when you don't have your period. A bit of Vaseline or K-Y Jelly on the tampon or tampon applicator will help ease the insertion. Relax and take your time! Many girls think when they experience difficulty learning to insert a tampon, "I'll *never* be able to do this! There's something wrong with *me!* I'm one of the few women in this world who will *never* be able to wear a tampon!"

Take heart. Relax and say "I can!" Millions of women wear tampons and most of them could readily

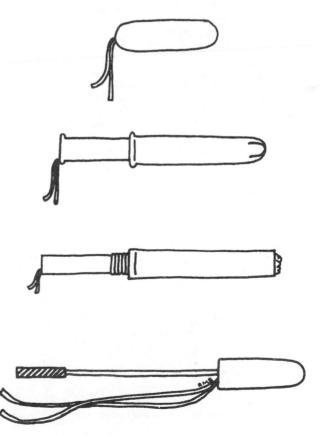

Four Different Types of Tampons

identify with your initial struggle. Once you learn how to insert a tampon, it's easy, fast, and painless. So have patience—and persevere!

The Wrong Kind of Tampon—For You. There are several kinds of tampons (see illustration). There are those with cardboard applicators, those with blunt or rounded plastic applicators, those with applicator sticks, and those with no applicators at all. The best tampon for *you* is a very personal decision, one you may make through a lot of trial, error—and frustration!

Many girls assume that those without applicators are easier to use, but this is not always the case. Al-though some ads may extol the virtues of tampons "without bulky applicators," applicators are rarely bulky and some women may find that an applicator helps them to place the tampon correctly—and with no discomfort. (Most applicators are smooth and pre-lubricated for easy insertion.)

A tampon without an applicator is compact, easy to carry and to insert for the woman who knows her body well and doesn't mind using her finger to insert the tampon into her vagina. However, a tampon without an applicator may be hard and dry—and not as easy to insert if you are a beginner at it.

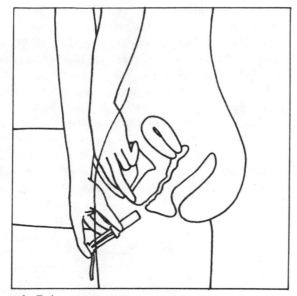

1. To insert a tampon, grasp tube with one hand and spread labia with other.

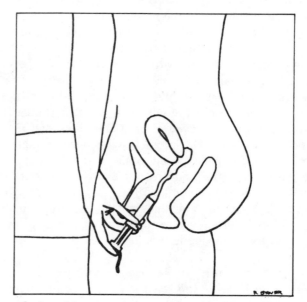

2. Insert tampon, aiming at the small of the back.

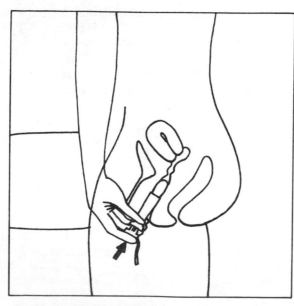

3. Gently press inner tube into outer tube.

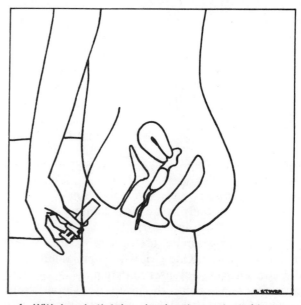

4. Withdraw both tubes, leaving the cord outside the body.

For women who are hesitant to insert a finger into the vagina, a tampon with an applicator or applicator stick may be best.

All of these types of tampons are safe and effective. Which type and brand you use is entirely a matter of personal preference.

Lack of understanding about correct insertion. Most tampons come with detailed instructions. Read these carefully before you even start trying to insert the tampon.

You can insert a tampon from a standing position—with one foot on a chair or on the toilet—by squatting slightly with legs apart, or by sitting on the toilet with legs apart. For those who elect the sitting position, it may help to thrust the hips forward and lean back.

Now that you're in position to insert the tampon, what next?

Let's assume that you're inserting a tampon with an applicator. (However, the basic technique for insertion is pretty much the same no matter what kind of tampon you choose.)

It may help to refer to the accompanying illustrations as you read these instructions:

a) Grasp the middle of the insertion tube with one hand and spread the labia (if need be) with your other hand, to make your vaginal opening accessible.

b) Relax!

c) Put the end of the insertion tube at your vaginal opening. Remember that the tampon must be inserted at an angle—not straight up! Aiming at the small of your back may help you to get the correct angle of insertion.

d) Start inserting the tampon applicator (without pushing on the plunger!) *in a twisting, circular motion* until your thumb touches your body.

e) Now, with the forefinger of the hand holding the applicator, gently push in the tube's plunger until it disappears into the outer tube. When these two ends meet—with your thumb touching the outside of your vaginal opening—the tampon is in place. (Some girls make the mistake of pushing the plunger before the first half of the applicator is inserted into the body. Others insert it only part way and then push. In each instance, the tampon will be placed too low and will feel uncomfortable. A properly placed tampon should cause no discomfort.)

f) Making sure not to pull the tampon string, remove the applicator tubes.

g) If your flow is extra-heavy and even a super-size tampon isn't enough, you may want to combine use of a tampon with a mini- or maxi-pad or you can use two tampons at once. How? Simply insert the first tampon. Then, holding on to the string of the first

tampon, insert the second and tie the strings together for easy removal.

h) To remove a tampon, simply pull on the string. If the string is not immediately visible, don't panic. It may be curled up in your labia and is easy to find. If, for some reason, it is pushed up into your vagina (rare—since most strings are too long to get lost in this way), it is still easy to retrieve. The string and the tampon itself are always within reach of your fingers.

I'm confused about so many things. Can a tampon fall out? How often should it be changed? And what about deodorant tampons? Are they better?

Gina P.

Once it is placed correctly, a tampon will not fall out. The muscles around your vaginal opening will hold it in place.

How often do you change it? About as often as you would change a pad (at least every three to four hours, even if your flow is light). As you become more experienced in tampon use, you will recognize the subtle signs of a tampon that needs to be changed.

Deodorant tampons are the newest in a series of feminine hygiene marketing campaigns. With tampons generally, odor is not a problem since they are worn internally. Some women find that they like the new deodorant tampons. If they can be worn without irritation, deodorant tampons represent simply another choice in the great variety of tampons available. But keep in mind two important facts:

1. Deodorants are not necessary on tampons.

2. Deodorant tampons may cause irritation in your vagina, particularly if you have a history of allergies. A warning to this effect is printed on each package of deodorant tampons. What kind of tampon you use is up to you, but many physicians suggest that a deodorant tampon has no advantages over a traditional tampon and *may* have the disadvantage of irritating vaginal tissues. Many doctors feel that the risk of irritation makes the use of these tampons inadvisable.

VAGINAL HEALTH—AND INFECTIONS

What is all this I hear about feminine hygiene? What can I do to prevent odor? Should I use a spray or douche? Why do women douche? Should I be doing it?

Wondering

Simple soap and water—bath or shower—cleanliness is the best possible safeguard against odor.

Body odors, including odors in the genital area, may be caused by bacteria acting on perspiration and other normal secretions. Since the vaginal area is warm and moist—an ideal environment for bacterial growth—it is important to wash the area regularly to reduce the number of these odor-causing bacteria.

Garments causing perspiration—nylon underwear, pantyhose, tight jeans—can increase the possibility of bacterial growth and odor. To help alleviate this problem, many pantyhose now come with ventilated crotches and many nylon panties have cotton crotches. (Cotton is absorbent while nylon is not.)

Daily baths or showers and avoiding—as much as possible—nonventilated, nonabsorbent, perspiration-causing clothes are the greatest aids to maintaining vaginal health.

What about douches and sprays?

Feminine hygiene sprays—once heralded as the key to "daintiness, security, and femininity"—have long since been questioned as effective hygiene aids. At best, they have proved unnecessary; at worst, they are another source of irritation to delicate tissues of the vagina and vulva.

Douching is the cleansing of the vagina by expressing a solution of water and vinegar or a commercial douche preparation into the vagina from a douche bag or squeeze bottle. In the normal, healthy woman, however, there is generally no medical necessity for douching. The healthy vagina is, essentially, self-cleansing.

Some women like to douche after sexual intercourse to wash away any remaining secretions. (However, a bath or shower can also do this!) There is a myth among some women, especially among teens, that douching is a form of birth control. It isn't! Douching immediately after intercourse is a useless birth control gesture since the sperm are already well on their way to the uterus and Fallopian tubes.

Some women like to douche after their menstrual periods. This, too, is not necessary, but an option. However, good sense must prevail. Daily douching is *not* advisable! A once-a-week douche is the safe maximum.

Why can douching be unsafe? A recent study at Yale revealed that excessive douching may be a factor in pelvic inflammatory disease, or PID (a serious pelvic disorder we will discuss in detail in the VD and Birth Control chapters), and inflammation of the Fallopian tubes (salpingitis). Of the women studied who were afflicted with one of these disorders, 90 percent douched frequently (more than once a week). Fewer than half the disease-free women douched frequently. The physicians conducting this study suspect that frequent douching may carry disease organisms that may exist in the vagina to the Fallopian tubes. Frequent

douching, too, may alter the normal acidic balance of the vagina, making vaginal infections more likely to happen.

For women who do choose to douche occasionally, one tablespoon white vinegar mixed with one quart of warm water or a premixed commercial douche may not do any harm unless you are allergic to some of the ingredients.

Sometimes a douche is advisable. For women who suffer from some varieties of vaginal infections, a physician may prescribe a medicinal douche. This is, generally, the only instance where a douche is advisable rather than optional.

I have this discharge of clear, slightly white mucus from my vagina. What's wrong with me?
                                          Suzanne R.

A clear, whitish, nonirritating discharge is normal. It is a mixture of mucus from the cervical glands, bacteria, and discarded vaginal cells. It may turn from white or clear to pale yellow as it is exposed to air. There are a number of entirely normal secretions in the vagina, from the Bartholin's glands and the vaginal walls as well as the cervix.

Several factors may increase the amount of these normal secretions.

Hormonal Changes such as increased estrogen level during ovulation can cause an increase in the clear mucus discharge. This can also occur in women who are taking birth control pills, since these elevate hormone levels.

Sexual Excitement can cause an amazing increase in vaginal secretions, enough in some cases to soak your underwear. This, too, is entirely normal and is part of the female's sexual response.

Other Factors that may make vaginal discharges more profuse are diabetes, antibiotics, IUDs, and emotional stress.

When does a discharge become abnormal? What kind of infections can happen and why do they happen?
                                          Julie P.

A discharge is abnormal if:

- It causes irritation
- It is mixed with blood (nonmenstrual)
- It has a foul odor
- It has a color different from your normal discharge
- It causes itching.

Such a discharge is usually a symptom of a vaginal infection (called *vaginitis*) and is a sign that you should consult a physician.

There are several kinds of vaginitis and the discharges may vary.

Yeast infection (also called *monilia, fungus,* or *Candida*) has as its symptoms a thick, white discharge the consistency of cottage cheese. Other symptoms include itching of the vulva and vagina and white patches of fungus over reddish, raw areas.

This condition is usually caused by an imbalance of the natural bacteria which help maintain the proper acidic, antifungal environment of the vagina and monilia fungus that thrive in a moist, unventilated place. Tight clothes, nylon underwear, and pantyhose can help yeast organisms to grow. The vaginal balance may also be upset by antibiotics such as tetracycline, which can destroy the beneficial vaginal bacteria; birth control pills; and even menstruation, which can alter the vagina's acidic environment. Women with diabetes tend to be particularly susceptible to monilia.

Yeast infections are rarely—if ever—sexually transmitted.

How is a yeast infection treated?

A one- to two-week (or longer) regimen of antifungal medication (vaginal suppositories and creams such as Nystatin and Monistat) may help. If yours is a particularly stubborn case and seems to be due to the use of antibiotics or birth control pills, your doctor may suggest stopping the use of these, if at all possible. Also, if you are sexually active and subject to recurrent attacks of monilia, your physician may consider examining your sex partner just in case yours may be one of the rare instances where the partner may carry the fungus.

Trichomonas usually produces a frothy, greenish-yellow, foul-smelling discharge. Other symptoms may include itching and inflammation of the vulva, frequent, painful urination and, in some cases, severe lower abdominal pain.

Trichomonas is caused by a protozoan organism and, unlike yeast infections, is—in most cases—sexually transmitted. It can also be spread via washcloths, towels, toilet seats, and wet bathing suits. To help prevent Trichomonas from happening to you, *do not* use a towel, washcloth, or wet bathing suit that someone else has used.

The most common treatment for Trichomonas is the medication Flagyl. Although this is usually given in pill form, there are also Flagyl vaginal suppositories, both available only by prescription. Flagyl seems to be effective in the majority of Trichomonas cases. If you are sexually active, of course, your sex partner must also be treated.

Hemophilus vaginalis will manifest itself in a white or gray, smelly discharge. Here, the discharge may be copious and irritating. You may have cramps and pelvic pain as well. Once diagnosed, this condition is usually treated with oral and/or vaginal antibiotics. Please refer to Chapter Eleven for more information about this particular discharge.

Nonspecific vaginitis will often produce a white or yellow discharge, possibly streaked with blood. This is vaginitis that is *not* caused by the organisms discussed above. Here, too, your vulva may be inflamed and you may have painful urination and, possibly, cramps and vaginal discomfort. However, you will not have the intense itching that is characteristic of monilia or Trichomonas.

Nonspecific vaginitis may be caused by a sudden multiplication of bacteria in your vagina and can be triggered by various drugs, possible irritation of the vagina during intercourse, tight, nonventilated clothes (nylon underwear, jeans), or even exhaustion!

Sulfa drugs are generally used to treat nonspecific vaginitis and are usually available in the form of a vaginal suppository.

Painful urination may also be the sign of a urinary tract infection or bladder infection *(cystitis),* which may occur when these bacteria invade the urethra and/or bladder. In some women, this can be a chronic condition. If you're having such symptoms, consult your physician. For more information about urinary tract infections, please see Chapter Nine. If you are sexually active, urination as soon as possible after intercourse and general cleanliness of your external genitalia may help to keep bacteria out of the urinary tract.

Allergic vaginitis—with either inflammation or a discharge or both as symptoms—can result from an allergic reaction to bubble baths, perfumed douches, deodorant tampons, colored toilet paper, and the like. Usually, removing the source of irritation will solve the problem.

Although the various types of vaginitis *may* be identified by a specific discharge, tests by a physician are usually required to *make sure* that you have that specific infection.

Since treatments may vary widely from one type of vaginitis to the next, an accurate diagnosis is extremely important!

A WORD ABOUT VD: Some discharges may be due to venereal diseases. Accurate diagnosis and prompt treatment are *especially* important if you think you might have some form of VD. We will be discussing venereal diseases, including gonorrhea, syphilis, herpes simplex, crabs, pubic lice, and venereal warts in Chapter Eleven. If you suspect that you have—or have been exposed to—a venereal disease, get help at a clinic or from a private physician immediately. Untreated venereal disease—especially gonorrhea and syphilis—can have serious consequences.

Questions—And More Questions!

I have so many questions to ask about my body! Where can I go for help—in my own area?

Leah Y.

I have fears about being examined by a gynecologist! What does a pelvic exam entail and does it hurt? What is a Pap test? Help!

Nancy W.

I'm 15 and feel different. It's hard to explain, but I just don't feel good about my body. I can't figure out whether it's beautiful or bad. Guys don't seem to take a great interest in me and I wonder sometimes if they ever will. I feel like something is wrong, but I'm not sure what. Any suggestions?

Rhonda K.

You will probably always have some questions about your body—and self-doubts as well.

If you have questions about your physical growth or functioning, consult with a physician, adolescent clinic, women's health center, or any of the other sources of help listed in the Appendix of this book.

For information about common examination procedures (including pelvic exams and Pap tests), communicating with and choosing a health care professional, please see Chapter Fourteen.

As well as having questions about your body's development and functioning, you may also have questions—like Rhonda does—about your feelings and attitudes about your body. Like Rhonda, you may have trouble expressing these.

How you feel about your body is very much tied in with how you feel about yourself as a woman.

Some young women try to deny the fact that they are growing toward womanhood by slouching to hide developing breasts.

Others welcome such signs that maturity is on the way.

Some women calculate their own worth by their bra size and by conventional attractiveness in general.

Some young women may be so busy putting themselves down for not looking like a fashion model that they may miss seeing their own unique beauty—which has nothing to do with bra size or other measurements.

To know ourselves is to know our own unique, individual beauty.

Yet, many of us may be reluctant to explore who we are—physically and psychologically. We may be waiting for a man to tell us what we so want to hear—and to believe—that we are wonderful, that we are beautiful, beloved individuals.

But there is a funny and sad twist to this waiting game.

When a man finally does say that we are beautiful—in many ways—we won't hear his words *or* believe them unless we have grown to discover, accept, and understand the beauty of our bodies and of ourselves!

CHAPTER THREE

Man's Body / Man's Experience

Masculinity is . . .

"Being one of the guys!"

"Surviving."

"Athletic skill."

"Independence, being your own person."

"Scoring!"

"Hard to define."

When I first began to mature, I felt . . .

"Why can't it all just happen overnight?"

"Curious about what was happening."

"Uncomfortable."

"Embarrassed. The other guys hadn't started maturing yet."

"Happy! I enjoy my body and I always have."

When I think about looking at or touching my penis, I feel . . .

"GOOD!"

"Guilty (but it feels good anyway!)."

"I'm afraid I may be smaller than average. I'm not sure."

"I'm interested. I'm interested in all the changes in my body—even those I don't really understand. . . ."

The changes of adolescence are dramatic and not always easy to understand.

A boy's journey toward manhood is just as dramatic and perhaps even more perplexing than a girl's growth toward womanhood.

There are several reasons for this.

There is a much greater variation in male physical development—from start to finish. One 14-year-old boy may be, indeed, still a boy. A 6-feet-2, bearded, baritone classmate may be, indisputably, a man—at least physically. Even when maturation is completed, there tends to be a larger variation in height and physical build among men than there may be among women.

Along with this wide variation of normal comes the ever-present peer comparison and physical competitiveness that tends to be more *direct* among guys. You compete, fight, and need each other. With a gang of friends, you can make it. Alone, the going can be really rough. Being one of the guys, however, involves proving that you're one of them. As you grow, you grapple for power. Fights, competition of all kinds, and constant comparisons are part of this power struggle as each guy secretly wonders "Am *I* OK?" In many circles, being *really* OK means being a jock, being a stud, being well-built.

But not everybody is a well-built athlete. Some guys are hairier than others. Practically no one is a so-called stud. But everyone worries: about penis size, about sexual prowess, about being accepted by the gang, about his own masculinity. These worries can translate into competition, too: circle jerking and speed contests to see who can "come" fastest and shoot the farthest.

Many guys worry about their feelings, too. You may feel a bit uncomfortable at times with the urgency of your sexual desires or with the presence of so-called feminine feelings like tenderness, gentleness, and sensitivity. Sometimes you are quite justifiably afraid. Sometimes you may feel like crying, but do you dare? Will admitting your fears or letting your tears fall make you less of a man?

If you have grappled with some of these uncertainties, you're far from alone. There are so many prevailing definitions of what a man is—what he does and what he doesn't do.

And this traditional role of a man, the strong, ambitious, tough provider and protector, may weigh heavily on you. It is, perhaps, this vision of manhood that makes many boys reluctant to grow into men. You may wonder if you're strong enough or smart enough to take on such awesome responsibilities. You may resent the fact that you feel you have to. You may fear that, in becoming a man, you may have to give up important parts of yourself. You may wonder, too, how you can cope when you may feel strong only *sometimes*—and scared and unsure a lot of the other times!

Becoming a man is, in essence, a complicated process. The better you understand the changes that your body is experiencing and what is normal, the better you will begin to understand and accept yourself—as a man and as a human being.

I'm almost 15 and not too sure about the way sperm are made. My friend says they come from the balls,

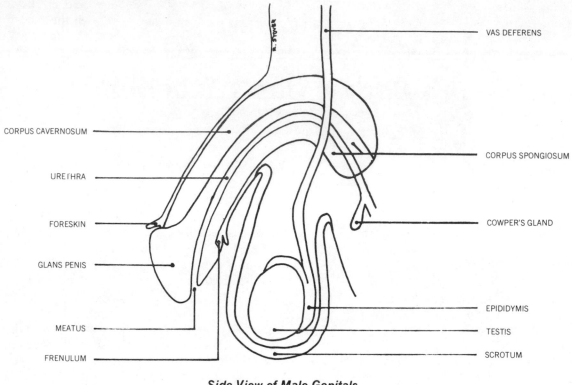

CORPUS CAVERNOSUM

URETHRA

FORESKIN

GLANS PENIS

MEATUS

FRENULUM

VAS DEFERENS

CORPUS SPONGIOSUM

COWPER'S GLAND

EPIDIDYMIS

TESTIS

SCROTUM

Side View of Male Genitals

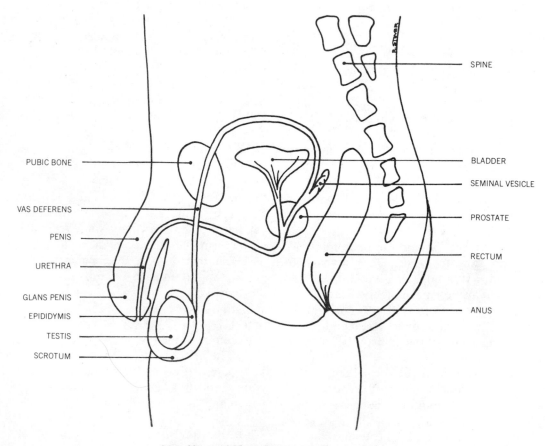

PUBIC BONE

VAS DEFERENS

PENIS

URETHRA

GLANS PENIS

EPIDIDYMIS

TESTIS

SCROTUM

SPINE

BLADDER

SEMINAL VESICLE

PROSTATE

RECTUM

ANUS

Side View of Male Reproductive System

but it doesn't feel like there's fluid down there. Where does the fluid come from? I know that there are parts of me involved in this besides the parts I can see, but what are they exactly?

Dennis W.

Dennis has voiced several frequently asked questions that all add up to one very important question: "What are the parts of the male reproductive system and how does it work?"

GENITALIA

There are, basically, three parts to the male reproductive system.

First, there are the *organs of production*—the testicles.

At the beginning of puberty, on a chain reaction signal from the hypothalamus, pituitary, and pineal glands, the testicles begin to produce the male hormone *testosterone*. This hormone triggers the common changes of adolescence such as the enlargement of genital organs, growth of pubic hair, and deepening of the voice. As puberty progresses, the testicles also begin to mature the sperm cells that are present—in an inactive state—from birth and that, if united with the female's ovum—or egg—will produce a baby.

The two *testicles* are encased in the *scrotum*, which hangs under the penis. It is quite common—and normal—for one testicle to hang somewhat lower than the other.

The sperm cells are produced in a series of tiny chambers within the testicles, and as they mature, they begin a long journey through the second part of the male reproductive system: *the ducts for storage and transportation of the sperm.*

First, is the *epididymis*, a long, tightly coiled canal (uncoiled, it would stretch about twenty feet) that lies over each testicle.

Next, the sperm travel to the *vas deferens,* a shorter continuation of the epididymis. This brings the sperm from the scrotum to the abdominal cavity, passing to the back of the bladder and joining the *seminal vesicles* forming the *ejaculatory duct* where the sperm is stored.

The *prostate gland,* which lies against the bottom of the bladder, secretes much of the *seminal fluid* that, combined with fluids from the seminal vesicles, carries the sperm from the body. The prostate gland enlarges dramatically when you reach your teens.

Other secretions come from the *bulbourethral glands* (also called Cowper's glands), two tiny structures on either side of the *urethra,* the passageway through which both urine and seminal fluid pass out of the penis. During sexual excitement, these bulbourethral glands produce a clear, sticky fluid that is thought to coat the urethra for the safe passage of the sperm. This Cowper's gland fluid is *not* seminal fluid, *but* it may contain a few stray sperm.

The third part of the male reproductive system is the *penis.*

When a mature or maturing man is sexually excited, he may ejaculate his seminal fluid out of the penis in a series of throbbing spurts. The total volume of this sticky, white ejaculate is, on the average, about one

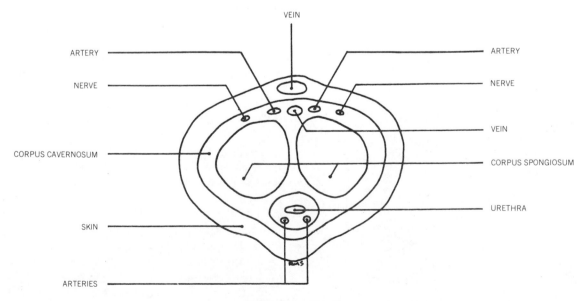

Penis Cross Section

teaspoon and is mostly made up of secretions from the prostate gland and seminal vesicles. Although sperm comprise only a small part of the total ejaculate, they are impressive in number. There may be about *400 million* sperm in one ejaculate! Obviously, the sperm cells are tiny, so small, in fact, that 400 million could fit on the head of a pin!

The penis, though obviously in view, may seem mysterious in its construction and its ability to transform from soft to hard in a matter of seconds.

A lot of people think that the penis is a skin-covered cylinder. This isn't so. The penis is made up of spongy tissues interlaced with large blood vessels (see crosssection illustration). There is a constant flow of blood in and out of the penis, which, despite a wide normal variation in size between men, *averages* three to four inches long and one and one-quarter inches in diameter (in the flaccid state) in the *mature* male.

When a man becomes sexually excited, however, this even blood flow stops. The blood vessels expand, bringing more blood into the penis. Valves in these veins retain this blood under pressure, causing the spongy walls of the penis to expand and become hard. This is called an *erection*.

The skin of the penis is loose to allow for expansion

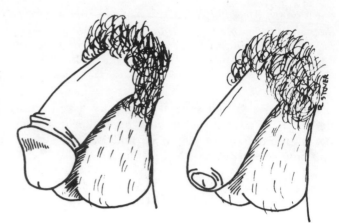

Circumcised Penis   **Uncircumcised Penis**

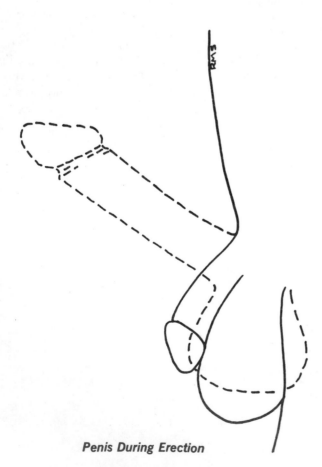

Penis During Erection

during erection. In some males, there is the *prepuce*, or *foreskin*, which covers the *head*, or *glans*, of the penis in its flaccid state. Although all males are born with this foreskin, many have it surgically removed, usually soon after birth, in a minor operation called *circumcision*. All Jewish males are circumcised for religious reasons, but it has been common practice in this country for the majority of hospital-born male infants to be circumcised. The practice today is becoming somewhat controversial, with some doctors questioning the automatic nature of this procedure and calling circumcision an option rather than a necessity.

The circumcised and uncircumcised penis may look a bit different in the flaccid state. Otherwise, each functions normally and there is no concrete evidence that circumcision—or lack of it—sharpens sexual response.

The uncircumcised male, however, must take special care to keep his penis clean, since a foul-smelling substance called *smegma* may collect under the foreskin if the penis is not washed daily.

Circumcised males don't experience this accumulation of smegma, and according to some medical studies, have a lower incidence of cancer of the penis.

Circumcision, as we said before, is usually done in the first few days of life. However, some teen-age boys and adult men elect to have this done, often due to a particularly tight foreskin—a problem we will discuss a little later on in this chapter.

What we have just been describing in the chapter so far is the reproductive system of the *mature* male.

It is important to know how your body is working—or will work—and it's also vital to know how you reach this point of maturity. For some, it is this journey, not the destination, that is of most concern.

PHYSICAL DEVELOPMENT

I'm 13 and don't seem to have grown as much in the penis or developed as much pubic hair as the other guys I know. I feel really out of it!

S.D.

Males, as well as females, are subject to the highly individual rhythms of their own biological time clocks. The changes of puberty in the male may begin as early as 8 or as late as 15. Puberty may finish between the ages of 14 and 18. Therefore, some very normal 14-year-olds appear to be grown men when some of their equally normal classmates still look like little boys!

Slow development—often a genetic characteristic—may be even more worrisome for a boy than for a girl. First, because girls tend to start puberty about a year earlier than their male classmates and then the other guys start to grow and develop, the late bloomer may really feel left behind. In most cases, however, the so-called late bloomer is entirely within the range of normal.

What are some of the age ranges for the boy's development into a man—and what sequence do these changes follow? There are many variations, of course, but the major changes—triggered by the male hormone testosterone—may follow a basic pattern, shown in the following text and in our accompanying illustrations and charts.

1. The testes begin to grow. This may occur between the ages of 8 and 15, with an *average* age of 13 for this stage of development.

2. The first, fine, downy traces of pubic hair will appear between the ages of 10 and 15, with an *average* age of 12 to 13.

3. There is a rapid growth spurt, where a boy may seem to increase in height very rapidly! This will generally occur between the ages of 11 and 16, with 12 to 13 as an average age range for the beginning of this growth spurt.

4. With this growth comes rapid growth of the penis

Male Pubic Hair Development

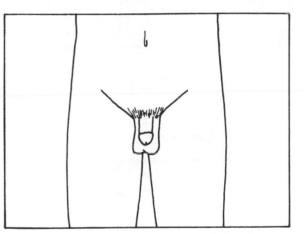

1. Straight hair appears at penis base.

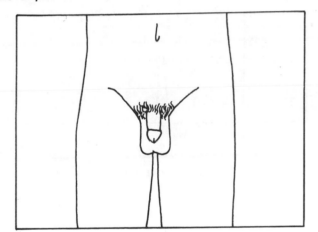

2. Hair becomes curly and coarse.

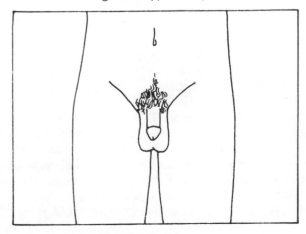

3. Hair is full, limited in area.

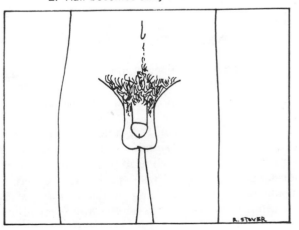

4. Full development.

Male Genital Development

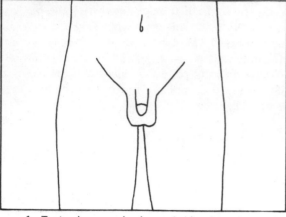

1. Testes increase in size and skin of scrotum reddens.

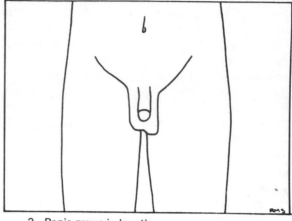

2. Penis grows in length.

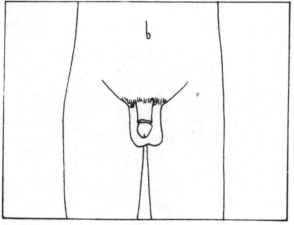

3. Penis grows in width.

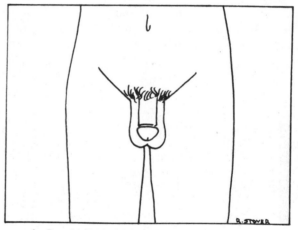

4. Development is complete.

and testicles. This will occur between 12 and 15 *on the average*.

5. The area around the nipples may become enlarged and, in some cases, slightly raised. This may occur around the age of 13.

6. Pubic hair is becoming coarser, thicker, and covers the triangular pubic area. This may happen between the ages of 11 and 16, with 14 as an average age.

7. Next, the voice deepens and hair appears in the armpits and above the upper lip. The average age for this is about 14 or 15, with normal variations from 12 to 18.

8. The prostate gland enlarges and sperm production begins. A boy may ejaculate semen, either during sleep ("wet dreams"), while masturbating, or during other sexual activities. These sperm may or may not be viable (capable of fertilizing an ovum). Studies have shown that the *average* age for the first ejaculation is about 13 or 14, but, again, there is much *normal* variation.

9. Facial hair and other body hair appears sometime between the ages of 14 and 18, with 17 as an average age. Some guys have a great deal of hair on the chest, arms, legs and even the back, while others are relatively hairless. This, like your rate of development, may be genetic. It may also be a racial characteristic. In general, blacks and Orientals tend to have less body hair than Caucasians. But lack of chest hair does *not* mean that you are hormonally deficient in any way or any less a man. Among your peers, however, body hair and pubic hair may be a big deal.

During the development years, pubic hair, especially, is often used as a measure of manhood. Few guys feel secure enough about their own anatomy or sexuality to tease anyone else about penis size (and those who *do* feel secure are not likely to tease!), but pubic hair—or lack of it—is fair game.

For the early maturing male, this can be a problem. In many instances, the 11- or 12-year-old with a considerable amount of pubic hair may even shave it off to look more like his classmates. It can feel very threatening to look too different from the rest of the gang.

Life can be especially rough for late bloomers. They may worry a great deal about their manhood and these fears may be reinforced by the shower-room jeers of their more hairy and developed classmates.

Some boys try to avoid such incidents by avoiding gym. During a 1973 study of adolescent boys at a Los Angeles area junior high school, a number of boys came in pleading for a medical gym excuse because they were embarrassed to appear before the other guys with what they considered to be a smaller-than-average penis.

Normal penis size covers a wide range, has nothing to do with a man's masculinity, and the differences are most apparent in the flaccid—or soft—state. Often, as we mentioned earlier, a smaller penis increases proportionately in size more when erect than a larger one will. So the differences are not as great as they may seem. Size of the penis is not an indication of one's sexual prowess—or lack of it. Many teens and their parents may wonder, especially if a boy is a late bloomer whose penis hasn't grown appreciably, if something is wrong "in the glands."

Except in rare, isolated cases in which a pituitary gland disease does retard normal sexual development, there is usually nothing wrong with the glands. The late bloomer is, most commonly, simply a normal guy whose often genetically determined biological time clock is simply a bit slower. An examination by a physician may help to reassure everyone that all is well.

In other instances, overweight may be the culprit when a penis looks unusually small. Fat padding can very effectively hide the penis, making it appear much smaller than it really is. Loss of weight (see Chapter Five) will generally reveal a very normal-size penis.

SPECIAL PROBLEMS

I'm shorter than the other guys and so I get picked on a lot. I'm sick of it! I'm 14 and 5 feet 2 tall and haven't had much physical development yet either. My father is 6 feet 2 and my mom is 5 feet 8. Do you think I'll grow any more?

Tired of Fighting

I'm 15 and am shaving already, but there's one problem: I'm pretty short (5 feet 5) and some kids at my school give me a lot of guff about it. My family is fairly short, too. My dad is 5 feet 6 and Mom is 5 feet 1. Does this mean I'll always be short, too?

Shorty

Among 14- and 15-year-old boys, there is a very wide range of normal height—from 4 feet 7 to 6 feet 2! For guys on the lower portion of this normal range, the label "normal" may be scant consolation. The shorter guy may wonder "Is this it? Aren't I going to grow any more? Am I doomed to be short?"

Whether or not you are to be short for life depends on a number of factors.

First, there is heredity. If you appear to be a late bloomer and have tall parents, you will probably grow a great deal more, once puberty gets under way.

Can anything speed up this process?

Most physicians are reluctant to tamper with the natural process of puberty, but several steps can be taken. First, a doctor may do a complete physical, including thyroid, blood and urine analyses, and X rays to determine bone age, as well as interview the parents and try to get a complete family history of pubertal development. It may be that delayed adolescence is a family trait. (Parents may not remember, until their memories are prodded, that they, too, were late bloomers.) After this thorough investigation, the boy and his family may be reassured that he is, indeed, quite normal.

If reassurance doesn't help and it appears that the boy will suffer serious psychological damage due to the fact that he is different, a physician may elect—in some cases—to accelerate the process of puberty by administering male hormones. This will cause rapid development of male sexual characteristics as well as a growth spurt. There are side effects to the hormone therapy, however, and, in some cases, accelerating the growth process may cause the boy to be shorter as an adult than he would have been had nature been allowed to take its course.

For this reason, many physicians do prefer to let natural development take place in its own time and give the boy a lot of reassurance and, if necessary, counseling and therapy to deal with some of the hassles of being different.

Society tends to put a premium on size in males. However, like a number of other societal expectations, this "tall, dark, and handsome" measure of desirable manhood is a myth. There are many very loving—and loved—very masculine men who are short, blond, and quite ordinary-looking.

Help! I'm a guy and I've got breasts! No kidding! The other guys make fun of me and call me a sissy. I'm 13 and miserable. What's wrong with me?

Miserable

There are several conditions that may cause breast swelling in the adolescent male.

First, there is the *adolescent nodule,* already noted in the preceding chapter. This small, firm swelling under the nipple may occur in one or both breasts and has been linked to the increased secretion of the male sex hormones just before puberty begins. Although this nodule may be tender and cause some concern, it does not require treatment. Most of these nodules subside within a year.

Second, and perhaps most common (occurring in 50 to 85 percent of all adolescent males), is a condition known as *adolescent gynecomastia.* This breast enlargement, which looks much like female breast development (gynecomastia means "female breast"), seems to be caused most frequently by an increase and, perhaps, a slight imbalance in the amount of hormones during early puberty.

Less common types of this condition are found in boys with undescended testicles, perhaps as a result of too *few* male hormones in the bloodstream, and in boys with certain birth defects. It has also been linked with prolonged and heavy use of amphetamines (uppers).

Gynecomastia, in its most common form, tends to subside as the teen boy progresses in his physical development.

Although males with this disorder may be teased about it relentlessly, it may be comforting to know that, first, it tends to be a temporary condition and, second, it is no negative reflection on your manhood. A guy with gynecomastia or, for that matter, with an adolescent nodule, is *not* turning into a woman. He is just as masculine as the next guy.

I get hard-on's in the strangest places—like when I'm riding on a bus or even in class at school. It's embarrassing! Why does this happen?

Steve H.

Erections, which occur when the spongy tissues of the penis become engorged with blood, can happen in infancy and childhood, but seem to become more frequent—and certainly more noticeable—in adolescence. As Steve notes, it doesn't take much to bring one on. There is always that hard-on that hits twenty feet before you get to your bus stop (and you're sitting in the middle of the bus!) or the one that hits, as if on cue, just as you're getting up in front of your class to give a ten-minute social studies report! Silently cursing the strange ways of nature, you may wonder "Why now? Why me?"

As you probably already know, sexual feelings and fantasies can cause erections. But so can vibrations on a bus, tight clothing, exposure to cold, fear, and other stimuli.

Many men wake up in the morning with an erection.

While some doctors believe that this may be caused by the pressure of a full bladder, others contend that it is the result of waking during a certain part of the sleep cycle, the part where dreams occur. Dream researchers have long since pointed out that all people show some measure of sexual response—erection in the male, lubrication in the female—during this REM (Rapid Eye Movement) or dream stage of sleep. Research has also shown a rise in the level of the male hormone testosterone during this active stage of sleep.

Although an ill-timed erection may be embarrassing, it is not usually as noticeable as it *feels!*

I'm 19 and have ugly white bumps (like pimples) on my penis. I've had them for three years. Could this be a long-lasting form of VD?

Wondering

Not every bump on the penis is VD, although it's certainly good to be aware of the possibility of VD, symptoms of the various venereal diseases and, to seek prompt treatment when you seem to have such a symptom.

The white bumps that are bothering "Wondering" may simply be blocked oil glands on the skin of the penis and don't really mean anything. Many guys worry about bumps, scars, or birthmarks on the penis. However, these do not impair the penis's function and may be most apparent to the man himself.

The last two days, I've had pain in my penis and something that looks like milk comes out. I'm scared. I know it can't be VD because I haven't had sex, but what could it be?

Marty S.

Marty's problem is seen frequently in adolescent males. His penis pain and milky discharge may be caused by *retrograde ejaculation.*

What causes this phenomenon?

It occurs when an ejaculation (release of semen) is incomplete or prevented from happening. This may happen when a guy is masturbating, but reluctant, for any number of reasons, to ejaculate. So, as he feels ejaculation about to occur, he places a thumb over the head of his penis to prevent the ejaculate from escaping. Or he may be ready to ejaculate while kissing or petting with a partner, but the semen is held back by tight pants or, again, a thumb over the opening of the penis.

In any case, the ejaculate may go backward into the prostate gland, causing engorgement and, at times, infection of the prostate, called *prostatitis.* In this condition, the symptoms may include pain that may be felt at the base of the penis or in the testicles and also, perhaps, a small amount of clear or milky discharge from the penis.

If you have symptoms similar to Marty's, you should consult your physician. You may feel embarrassed about the sexual practice that helped to cause this condition, but you really have no cause for embarrassment or fear. This is a common practice and/or occurrence in young males and most physicians are very understanding about this. Your doctor will be able to help you best, however, if you level with him, giving him all the facts. This condition can be treated medically by one of several available methods. The best method of preventing retrograde ejaculation and its complications is stopping the practice of inhibiting ejaculation of semen from the penis.

However, if, unlike Marty, you are sexually active and have a discharge from your penis, this may be a sign of venereal disease. (See Chapter Eleven.)

My penis is swollen and painful and I can't pull back the foreskin. What could this be and what could I do about it? I hate to go to the doctor. I'm afraid he might say I have to be circumcised and that scares me a lot! Is it a bad operation?

Wayne G.

What Wayne is describing could be a condition known as *paraphimosis,* which occurs in an uncircumcised male when the foreskin is tight and cannot be fully retracted. The painful swelling that this condition causes is best remedied by circumcision. Our advice to Wayne—and anyone else who might have this complaint—would be to seek medical help immediately.

There is another problem that may beset the uncircumcised male. *Phimosis* is the diagnosis when the foreskin adheres to the head of the penis and cannot be pulled back at all. In this case, too, circumcision is the usual method of treatment.

Although circumcision in the adolescent or adult male may be more involved than it is for an infant, it is still a safe and minor surgical procedure, usually requiring only an overnight hospital stay.

I have pain in my groin and I'm not too hot on going to the doctor. Could you tell me what this could be?

Bob T.

Bob's letter is much too vague for us to make a possible diagnosis. Besides, if you do have a pain in your groin, it is important, in most instances, to consult your physician for an examination.

What *could* pain in the groin mean?

Hernia, which occurs when abdominal contents bulge through a spot in the abdominal wall, could be causing the pain. It may mean that the blood supply to this area has been reduced and this could be serious. Seek medical help immediately. Surgery is the usual method of treatment.

Swollen glands could be another cause of pain in the groin. There are lymph glands in the groin region and if these become infected, they may swell painfully. Treatment with antibiotics will usually alleviate this problem.

Twisted testicles can be yet another cause of pain and this condition usually occurs when a testicle has not fully descended into the scrotum and its blood-supply cord becomes twisted. Although this is not particularly common (since most boys with undescended testicles are treated surgically before puberty), it is serious when it does happen and requires immediate surgery.

"Blue balls": This last reason for an ache in the groin, you may be relieved to hear, does *not* require surgery or, indeed, medical treatment. It simply takes time—perhaps a few hours—to go away. This pain, which may also be felt in the sex organs, may happen when a boy has had a prolonged erection without ejaculation, for example, in a heavy petting session. Blue balls is caused by prolonged engorgement of blood in the penis and pubic area.

I'm 15 and sometimes when I wake up in the morning I find that I've had what is called a "wet dream," I guess. My pajama bottoms are sticky with "come." Is there something the matter with me or am I normal? My mom says that if I were more of a man, I could control myself. It makes me so embarrassed. Am I in any way abnormal?

Allen K.

"Wet dreams" or "nocturnal emissions" are not only normal, but involuntary (that is, you have no conscious control over them). These wet dreams are the release of semen during sleep and are most likely to happen with boys who don't masturbate a great deal or have regular sexual intercourse. Some are embarrassed and try to hide any evidence from their mother (who might notice a stain on the sheets or pajamas). Most mothers, however, are a lot more understanding than Allen's mother. If wet dreams *are* a matter of concern, it may help to realize that these nocturnal emissions are completely normal. A man produces sperm cells constantly and this is simply nature's way of releasing the stored semen.

Often, a male's first ejaculation may come during a wet dream. Many other boys experience this during masturbation. Still others experience their first ejaculations during some form of sex play or intercourse.

I masturbate about once a day and enjoy it. I wonder, though, how much is too much? Could I use up all my sperm now and not have any left when I'm married?

John L.

Although we will be discussing masturbation—both male and female—in detail in Chapter Ten, we have received *so* many questions from guys about it in reference to their body that a few comments here might be in order.

First, masturbation is a normal, almost universal practice. Contrary to old wives' tales, masturbation will *not* make you sterile, blind, insane, or give you acne.

Guilt can be one side effect, particularly if you belong to a religion—or a family—that strongly frowns on the practice. Some people see masturbation as immoral. Others consider it a matter of personal choice. What's important is how you feel about it.

Can you masturbate too often? Again, it is impossible—and not really constructive—to set any rules. The only cautionary note we might add is this: Masturbation is not meant to take the place of other things in your life. If you find yourself using masturbation as a crutch to avoid encounters with others or if it is causing you to turn inward and become less able to share and to function in other ways, you may want to reevaluate its place in your life and make some changes.

Can you ever use up your sperm supply—and thus become sterile in later life? No. Fortunately, if you do happen to be concerned about your future fertility, sperm are being manufactured in the testes on a continuous basis and you are not likely to run out of them now or in the future.

The gang I run around with camps out at a nearby park at least twice a month. Sometimes, during our camp-outs, we play sex games like feeling each other's dick and circle jerking. I enjoy this at the time, but feel very bad about this the next day. Is this kind of thing normal or does it mean that I'm going to be a homosexual? If age matters, we're all 13 and 14.

Joe L.

Group masturbation is a very common practice in adolescence, particularly among males. This type of masturbation may take several forms. These include: circle jerking (group masturbation while sitting in a circle or in close proximity. The participants may even have a contest to see who can ejaculate first and farthest), masturbation in the presence of a friend or friends without touching one another and, finally, mutual masturbation where friends sexually stimulate one another.

Intense curiosity about one another is quite normal, especially in the early teens when so many changes are taking place. It is really not so unusual that you would be interested in comparing yourself to other males. Seeing how your friends are developing may be a way of reinforcing your feelings about your own development.

Group masturbation has similar motives. Your sexual feelings, your ability to have an erection and to ejaculate are reinforced when you see other young males having the same experiences. Testing your ability to function sexually and, in some instances, to give pleasure to another person *may* be less threatening in the early teens with people of your own sex.

This is not always the case, of course. There are some boys who have never had such experiences—and that's normal, too!

Whether or not you *do* participate in group masturbation is very much a matter of personal choice and is no reflection of your present or future sexual preference.

Most guys who participate in these adolescent sex games are not—and do not become—homosexuals. It is normal for these boys to have such experiences and then to go on to have sex with women.

A certain percentage of males (and females, too), however, will find that they always prefer their own sex and, for them, this, too, is normal. Their adolescent experiences did not *make* them homosexual. They simply *are* homosexual. (For more information about homosexuality, turn to Chapter Ten.)

I'm 17 and am always thinking about sex. I wonder if I might be oversexed. My girl friend doesn't seem to share these sexual feelings. Are women less interested in sex than men? Also, when we're petting, I come close to coming, but control myself and only come maybe hours later when I'm home and can masturbate. Could this holding back harm me?

Phillip R.

A delayed ejaculation or no ejaculation at all after petting should not cause problems beyond a possible attack of "blue balls." (Of course, if an actual ejaculation is suppressed, it may lead to prostatitis. Please refer back to our earlier comments on retrograde ejaculations and prostatitis in this chapter.) Controlling ejaculation is much like controlling other body functions and is not, in itself, harmful.

It is quite normal for both men and women to think about sex often. Although most women do tend to take more time to become fully aroused sexually, most have the capacity to enjoy sex as much as men do. A woman is not physically less of a sexual being than you are. She is just subject to more societal restrictions even in these so-called liberated times. There is also fear of pregnancy, which is a fear based on reality, even in this age of readily available contraception. There is the fear that she will become just another conquest to you and that she will garner a bad reputation. Even though the old double standard seems to be on the way out, vestiges of it still cling.

This conditioning isn't something that can be banished overnight by either of you. And it isn't universally shared. Some women come from families where sexuality is considered a positive thing—for men and for women. Whatever your family background or feelings, it's important to talk, to understand your differences, and to empathize with one another's feelings. Most important, don't put yourself or the other person down.

At my high school, where I'm a senior, just about everyone seems to be having sex—the "in" people at least. A lot of the guys joke that if you don't make it with a girl, you're a fag. So I say I have sex, but I don't. Not yet. I think about it a lot and enjoy kissing, etc., but even though my body says yes to sex now, my mind says no, because I'd like to go to medical school eventually and if I got some girl pregnant that would go out the window. What it adds up to, I guess, is that I just don't feel ready to have sex right now. Yet I like girls a lot, so I'm not a homosexual. Am I weird?

John W.

Peer pressure to have sex is an ever-present reality in the lives of some teen-agers, especially boys. Some guys do have sex and still others do a lot of bragging about it.

However, if you are a guy who doesn't feel ready to have sex at this time, you're not weird at all. Knowing what is right for you—and what isn't—at any given time is an important part of maturity. Choice is a major element of responsible sexuality.

At this time, you may choose to enjoy sexual fantasies, kissing, petting, and/or masturbation and choose *not* to have intercourse. That's perfectly OK. How you express your sexuality is very much up to you. People who are quick to apply labels like "weird" or hurtful ones like "fag" (which hurts no matter what your sexual persuasion may be!) may not realize that *no* two people are exactly alike. We shouldn't judge others by what *we* think, feel, and do. We should also not necessarily pattern our behavior after what the other kids do—or say they do—if that would not really be our choice. Being your own person is, perhaps, one of the most exciting aspects of becoming a man.

Becoming a man can mean combating a lot of pressures and a myriad of stereotypes: the real he-man who is big, strong, tough, and always in charge; the king of the castle, who rules over his family as a benevolent despot; the super-jock who wins all the time; the bright young man whose confidence never falters; the sexual superman who always scores and leaves them begging for more.

In many instances, these stereotypes have been even more hurtful to men than they have been to women. No mere mortal could possibly measure up to all of these, for these are not real men, but myth men. Discovering this can be a relief. Then you know that being a man does *not* mean:

• Always having to be strong and tough and in charge. The men who are most secure in their masculinity are able to express tender feelings, to admit it when they are wrong, and to share responsibilities with others. Secure men know, too, that real men come in all sizes.

• Being king of the castle. The king is, more frequently these days, abdicating in favor of the young man who sees new freedom in a marriage where problems, decisions, joys, and sorrows are shared equally.

• Having confidence that doesn't quit. A young man, especially if he is bright, may mix confidence with a fair assessment of his limitations. Knowing yourself means being aware of your strengths and your limitations—and learning to live with both.

• Being a sexual superman. This mythical being never really existed except in the minds of boys who wonder about themselves. Some sexual experiences will be pleasurable; others, you'd rather forget. Your masculinity is not contingent on your sexual performance, the number of sex partners you have, or the size of your penis.

Being a man means being your own person—and this person will have a variety of unique and universal qualities.

You may be assertive sometimes and quite legitimately afraid at other times. You may be tough and tender, strong and gentle. To be a man is to give yourself permission to experience the whole range of your emotions—to laugh and to cry.

To be a man is to enjoy both your strong body and your soft feelings and to realize that being a *real* man means simply being you!

CHAPTER FOUR

Your Changing Feelings

I feel . . .
"Scared!"
"Like I hate myself!"
"SHY!"
"Confused."
"Lots of pressure."
"Torn between my parents and my friends."
"NERVOUS!"
"That I want to be part of the crowd, but my own person, too."
"My parents treat me like a baby."
"Guilty."
"Like crying half the time."
"Lots of love around me."
"That I need someone special."
"Lonely."
"Depressed."
"Bored."
"Hopeful."
"Excited about the future!"
"Like I'm just starting to know myself."
"Feel? Wow, I'm not sure. I feel so many things . . ."

Feelings abound in the adolescent years.

You may feel bored and excited, depressed and elated, nervous, rebellious and needy.

You may find yourself loving—and hating—intensely, crying a lot and feeling new fears about all kinds of things, including the fact that you're growing up.

I'm 14 and wish I could be four and Mommy's little girl again. I start crying when I think of me as a child when my mother used to sing to me. I can't stand the thought of me and my parents getting older. I know that everyone gets older and eventually dies, but it makes me cry. I'm worried about myself. There is nothing I look forward to anymore. I used to dream of what I would do when I grew up, but I can't even think of that anymore. I look back and I cry. I'm fighting my feelings constantly!

Barbi

Barbi is contending with a barrage of feelings right now.

There is nostalgia for her past, a past that may seem better and more carefree in retrospect. As a child, she dreamed of adulthood and the independence she would someday have. Now, as she stands on the threshold of autonomy, Barbi feels too frightened to face it.

Why is she frightened? Because growing means change and change can be scary. In changing, you lose some things while gaining others. Barbi seems to be experiencing a great deal of grief over these present and anticipated losses. While she fears the eventual loss of her youth and the loss of her parents—and the love and security they represent—by death, she may be mourning a partial loss of them now. Perhaps she may feel that she and her mother are growing apart. There are no more bedtime lullabies, not the kissing and cuddling she once enjoyed. She knows that she must grow up to become independent. She wants to. Yet, growing away from her mother is sad as well as exciting. It seems, perhaps, that there are two distinct Barbis: the safe, secure child cradled in her mother's arms and the adult-to-be, completely on her own. No wonder the present Barbi—caught between these two images—is feeling so frightened.

Life will never be quite the same for Barbi and for countless other adolescents who may share her feelings at times. We are constantly growing and changing in many ways. We experience inevitable losses: the loss of youth, of childhood security, of our parents as protectors, even of specific dreams as we turn these into reality. We have much to gain, of course: the wisdom of life experience in place of youth; the satisfaction of making our own security, gaining new friends in our parents and a new family of friends as well as, perhaps, a family of our own; and the exhilaration of reaching a goal and finding new dreams to replace the old ones.

At times, though, we may all grieve for the past. When we do, we shouldn't fight these feelings. Whether one copes by crying, writing long, sad passages in a diary, talking with parents or friends, or just *thinking* about it all, it's vital to keep in mind that these feelings are valid and need to be aired in some way. In letting these feelings out, by expressing grief, you can start letting go of the past and, eventually, embrace the present and the future.

You might be able to do this alone or might need help—from a parent, friend, favorite teacher or school counselor, clergyman, or doctor—in facing your grief at the losses that inevitable changes bring into your life and in dealing with the pressures and insights that may come with the changes.

What kind of changes can affect your feelings? All the changes of adolescence, of course, but some changes more than others. Some changes are emotional ones, ones that cannot be seen, but are certainly felt. As you grow, for example, you become increasingly aware of a need for a separate identity. You may begin to ask "Who am I—really?"

THE "WHO AM I?" QUANDARY

I'm having a difficult time trying to be me because I don't know yet who ME is! But I'm trying some exercises in self-awareness. I asked myself just a minute ago, before starting to write this letter: "Which stationery would I rather use?" Instead of "Which must I use up first?" That's a start, isn't it?
Lori H.

Yes, it *is* a start! A choice of stationery may seem trivial, but it is one of countless ways of asking "What do *I* want?" What you want, what you feel, and what you do are all part of who you are.

Sometimes, it may be hard to see yourself as separate, let alone unique. In some ways, you may feel like a human patchwork quilt. You've been told (too many times) that you have your father's coloring, your mother's hand gestures, your grandfather's nose, and a temperament like Great-Aunt Harriet's. Terrific, right?

If you've been hearing this over and over, you'd probably do anything to be different; yet, even as you rebel, try to change your manner, your hair color, and even, perhaps, fantasize about changing your name, your family is still very much a part of you. You do have a genetic legacy from them as well as learned behavior picked up from living with them for years. You also have qualities shared and/or influenced by your friends and other people you admire. Sometimes you may wonder if there's anything original about you at all!

The fact is, of course, that no one on earth has exactly the same collection of physical and emotional traits that you have. Even if you're an identical twin, there will be personality and life experience differences. What you do with your genetic legacy, how you develop—or don't develop—your special talents and skills, how you choose to be, now and in the future, what values you take from your family and friends and which ones you reject, all this and more adds up to a thoroughly unique you. The combination is, ultimately, largely your choice and nobody puts himself or herself together in quite the same way.

According to New York psychologists Mildred Newman and Dr. Bernard Berkowitz, authors of *How to Be Your Own Best Friend* and, most recently, *How to Take Charge of Your Life,* you find yourself not by *reacting* (rebelling or taking a different stance from your family just to be different from them), but by *acting,* by developing your own point of view, which you choose and which may or may not agree with your parents'.

Developing your own point of view about yourself can help you to discover who you are in many ways.

Making observations about yourself—even about some of your habits (an important part of you)—may be a good beginning to developing this personal point of view. Even the seemingly mundane may be important.

"For example, you might say 'I'm the kind of person who likes to take showers instead of baths!' or 'I'm the kind of person who likes to rest before doing my homework!' " says Ms. Newman. "This kind of self-affirmation, talking to yourself about yourself, builds your self-image."

What you *like,* the things you enjoy, can be significant.

Asking yourself what kind of a person you would *like* to be can aid self-discovery, too.

"Perhaps if you ask yourself 'What would I like to see happen?' it might be easier," says Ms. Newman. "Then it's not such a big step from what you would like to see happen to what you want. This can ultimately prepare you for the big question: 'What can I *do* to make it happen?' "

Other finding-yourself questions that Newman and Berkowitz suggest are:

• What turns me on? When was the last time I really felt excited about something?
• What flashes through my mind just before I go to sleep at night?
• When I'm free to choose, how do I spend my time?

This latter question may be particularly significant, especially if you discover that you are spending much of your time in passive pursuits—like watching TV. If you are passive—despite active dreams—it could mean that you are dissatisfied with things as they are, but lack the energy or motivation or conviction to change.

Since YOU are largely responsible for choosing the unique combination of qualities you have, you can also choose to change what you don't like. This is an important fact to know, something that can lessen that terrible feeling of "What's the use?" when things aren't going the way you'd like.

There are always going to be things you don't like. As you grow, you gain new insight not only into what you can do, but also into what you can't do, what your limitations are. Becoming aware of your shortcomings—possibly for the first time now—can be a real shock. While you probably tend to be quite tolerant of faults you see in your friends, you may be relentless in your criticisms of yourself, feeling that if several things are wrong with you, then nothing may be *right!*

LOW SELF-ESTEEM AND SELF-HATE

I hate myself. I feel like I can't do anything right. I get embarrassed over stupid things. There's a guy I like and my friends say he wants to get to know me better. I think he'd like me if I could talk more, but I don't know what to say to him. Help!

Untalkative

I'm a loser. I'm 16 and never had a date. I flunked swimming lessons last summer and have only one friend. I took my driver's test today and flunked that, too. Everyone makes fun of me. I'm fat, ugly and all the kids at school can't stand me and ignore me. Even my own mother hates me!

Desperate

I'm so shy, don't have any friends. People say I must think I'm terrific because I won't speak to them, but they don't listen to me when I try. I feel so lonely. One reason I don't say anything is that I don't want anyone to know how stupid I am because I have a low vocabulary and can't express my feelings well. I try to hold my feelings back, but they often burst out at my mother when she tries to help me and that makes me feel worse about myself. I hate myself for being so shy and dumb!

Dummy

I wonder how it feels to be beautiful. I try to be— inside and out—maybe that's why they say life is a constant struggle. I'm struggling to be a beautiful person so that when I die, I'll be remembered as a piece of the sun. Sometimes I think I'm on the right road and my sunshine is peeking out. Then I shout at my mother and then all my selfishness and hate pour out—and the sunshine retreats.

Martha

Self-hate is an all-too-common reaction in teens in the process of discovering themselves. However, because it involves an unrealistic emphasis on your liabilities while denying your positive qualities, it is an obstacle to finding yourself. You can get hung up on a fault—real or imagined—and convince yourself that what you dislike about yourself automatically cancels out anything good about you. You may feel that you don't have anything to offer. That, of course, is never true!

Let's look back for a moment and examine the people behind the letters you have just read.

In the first letter, "Untalkative" puts herself down for making mistakes and getting embarrassed. Yet, we all make mistakes. Often, this is how we learn best. A mistake, then, can be a learning opportunity, not a tragic flaw, and is certainly not an occasion for a putdown. "Untalkative" also doesn't seem to realize the very positive fact that she has good friends and a guy who likes her. Only her own feelings of inadequacy keep her from communicating with him. She feels, perhaps, that if he knew what she was *really* like (that she makes mistakes, isn't perfect, is afraid sometimes) he wouldn't like her. The opposite, in fact, may be true. Paragons of perfection—if they exist at all— would be hard to identify with and to love. We often love our friends most for their very human qualities. Yet, we put ourselves down for being just as human.

"Desperate," the writer of the second letter, has made a very hurtful habit of accenting the negative and of making assumptions about other people's feelings. Since "Desperate" was a patient who *told* us her sad tale (rather than simply writing to us), we can tell you about the other side of this girl who says that everyone hates her, she fails constantly, and is fat, ugly, and alone. First, "Desperate" is only ten pounds overweight and would be very attractive if she took care of herself. She is a kind and talented person who is very good at art and has a knack for growing gorgeous plants. She assumes that the kids at school hate and ignore her. The fact is, she is so quiet that her classmates, caught up in their own problems and activities, just don't notice her that much. Their indifference, however, does not come from actively ignoring her, but from not knowing her. Most people do tend to be relatively indifferent to others until they get to know one another.

"Desperate" is also making assumptions about her mother's feelings of hate for her. The fact is, her mother is having serious marital problems and is contending with so many feelings of her own that she doesn't have the time or energy to be as concerned with her daughter's feelings as she might ordinarily be.

"Desperate" is correct is some observations about herself. She is not a talented athlete. She needs more instruction (and experience) before she can become a good driver. She isn't making the most of her assets. But she can change all this. She can learn to become an adequate swimmer and a good driver if she so chooses. She can also discover her good qualities if she can grow past her self-hate to self-realization. Especially at first, "Desperate" may need special help and support from various people in her life—from her physician, school counselor, and close relatives—to begin to see herself in a more positive way.

The guy who labels himself "Dummy" is, in reality, far from dumb and, despite his protestation to the contrary, expresses himself beautifully in his letter. He is not only not being realistic about his faults, but also not being realistic about dealing with his feelings. Trying to deny feelings and hold them in only makes a person hurt more. It is inevitable that these feelings will burst out in ways that will only reinforce his self-hate, unless he learns how to accept and to deal with these feelings constructively.

Martha, in her desire to mirror the sunshine, has a lovely idea. However, her expectations may be a bit unrealistic. We can't always be beautiful inside and out. We all have faults. We all have impatient moments, say things we wish we hadn't, and have feelings we'd never tell. This just makes us human. Being beautiful sometimes—maybe even most of the time—is a commendable goal, but just *being* is OK. Recognizing your right to be is the first step away from self-hate.

Dr. Theodore Isaac Rubin, a noted New York psychiatrist who has written an excellent book called *Compassion and Self-Hate: An Alternative to Despair*, points out that there are two parts to your recognition of your right to be.

"First you realize 'I am because I am,' " he says. "You don't need any justification for your existence—like prizes or special accomplishments. These may give you some satisfaction, but they in no way justify your existence. You would *be* without these things and you are infinitely more important than these things. This realization may help to free you from the self-hating need to be universally loved or admired, unfailingly sweet, helpful, giving, or wise. In short, the best. And any other unreal expectations you may put on yourself."

The second important thing to be able to say to yourself is "I am I," Dr. Rubin points out.

This means accepting all of you—assets, liabilities, feelings, moods, and actions, none of which, you may discover, exist in pure form, but in endless and fascinating combination. You can be funny *and* grumpy. Sometimes you're really bright and with it. Other times you make mistakes. Everyone does.

"You must learn to love and accept the fool in you

as well as the wise person," says Dr. Rubin. "This doesn't mean that you close your eyes to the possibility of changing some of the things you don't like about yourself, but it does mean that you don't put yourself down for those things. You choose to change because you want to. Changes and variation in moods, feelings, desires, and goals are part of the human condition, especially when a person has a great deal of aliveness!"

Many young people—and older people, too—have trouble accepting some of the feelings in themselves that are part of being alive: feelings like jealousy, anger, selfishness, a need for privacy, and shyness.

JEALOUSY

I'm a jealous person and can't seem to help it. I hate myself for being jealous of my friends because they may be smarter or more popular than me. How can I stop being jealous?

Les

This feeling, often called the "green-eyed monster," isn't a monster at all. It just *is*—and it strikes everyone at times.

It may strike when your best friend makes the cheerleading squad or wins a scholarship. You may feel pangs of jealousy for a stranger who seems to have everything. Or you may find yourself grappling with the green-eyed monster when your girl friend (or boyfriend) spends some time with someone else.

Although people are prone to put themselves down for jealousy, it is a very human feeling and the causes behind this feeling are many.

Although Les says that he hates himself for feeling jealous, chances are, his feelings of jealousy stem from his own self-hate. Jealousy is often the result of having a low opinion of yourself, so much so that you feel cheated and deprived, as if everyone has more than you do.

Jealousy may also come from fear of loss. With self-hatred or low self-esteem, you may feel that you have so little to offer that it wouldn't take much—even a brief conversation with someone else—to prompt your boyfriend or girl friend to leave you.

Realizing that we're all jealous at times, that it's just another human feeling, may help to alleviate some of the pain or guilt you may feel over envying a friend or not trusting a loved one. Growing to appreciate your own special qualities and possibilities can help a great deal, too. You may discover that you're *not* a have-not. You're pretty much like anyone else—and very special in your own way.

However, since no one is perfect and we will always

have flashes of insecurity, even a good, accurate self-image will not make you totally immune to jealousy attacks.

What do you do when you're suffering from an acute attack of jealousy?

First, recognize what is happening, without putting yourself down.

Next, you may want to share your feelings with someone who may point out that you have a lot going for you, too, and/or reassure you that everyone has jealous fits.

An attack of jealousy can also give you a great opportunity for positive action, whether you decide to confide your feelings to someone or keep them to yourself. Ask yourself a few questions like:

- What do you envy in this other person?
- What do you feel that you—specifically—lack?
- Is this something you can change?

If, for example, you find yourself jealous of someone else's figure or grades or circle of friends, start thinking about how you might improve your looks, make your grades more acceptable to you, or how you might reach out to others more effectively.

ANGER

I have a problem with my temper. I manage to control myself sometimes, but at other times, I explode! Sometimes I take my anger out on people who had nothing to do with making me mad in the first place! How can I get over this?

Paul J.

In my family, we're not allowed to argue or answer back or even talk about how we feel. Sometimes I get so mad, I'm ready to burst! But I don't say anything. I have a problem with headaches and stomachaches pretty regularly. I wonder if these could have anything to do with the fact that I'm not allowed to express myself. I read somewhere that this could happen. I also feel depressed a lot. Help!

Cynthia G.

Anger is another inevitable human emotion. Anyone who says "I never get angry!" is either lying or completely out of touch with his or her feelings.

Of all the emotions, however, it is anger that is most often denied and left unexpressed. Unexpressed anger is still very much with you, though, and it seeps out in strange ways. A backlog of unexpressed rage can make you fly off the handle at some minor annoyance or displace your anger onto an innocent (and safe)

victim. It can cause you to lose control of your behavior and throw a tantrum to release everything you've pent up. It can make you turn on yourself. Depression, many mental health experts believe, is really anger turned inward. Your unexpressed rage may even turn on you in physical ways—with the stomachaches or headaches that Cynthia mentions. (More about these "Mind Over Body" problems in Chapter Eight!)

Women can have particular problems with anger, since, traditionally, little boys are allowed to fight and show their anger while little girls are supposed to be "nice."

Anger, however, happens to nice people. You cannot avoid getting angry. Feelings just happen. What you *can* control is how you *express* your anger. We are responsible for our actions, not our feelings. This distinction between feelings and actions may save you a lot of guilt.

Michael, for example, found himself in a difficult situation last year. Amid the pressures and activities of his senior year, he was helping his mother care for his terminally ill father, an ill-tempered, lifelong alcoholic. Frightened of death, jealous of Michael's youth, and angry at his own growing inability to care for himself, Michael's father raged and complained continually. Sometimes it was so bad that Michael thought to himself: "I hate him! He's a terrible person! I wish he'd just go ahead and die!"

However, when Michael's father did die, Michael almost went to pieces with grief and remorse, hating himself for ever being angry at such a sick, helpless man and feeling somehow responsible for his death because he had, in anger, wished him dead.

A perceptive school counselor helped Michael work through his grief and anger, pointing out that we all have all kinds of feelings and may, for a moment, wish a loved one dead. These feelings are neither terrible nor unusual. It's what you *do* about them that matters. Michael came to realize that he had not brought on his father's death. He had helped his mother to take excellent care of his father. His actions, then, were kind and helpful.

Not all situations involving anger, of course, are as dramatic as Michael's. Maybe a friend makes a cutting remark and you get mad. Or your parents say you can't go to an unchaperoned boy/girl party and that's that! You find yourself steaming over with rage. What can you do?

If a peer says something cutting, you might let him or her know that you're angry. A simple "I" statement like: "I feel angry about what you just said . . ." is, perhaps, a better approach than "Well, you're a creep, too, and I hate you!"

When you simply report how you feel, instead of

instantly attacking the other person, the other may be better able to listen to your feelings instead of getting defensive and hurling more abuse your way. A reasonable, level-headed approach often commands respect and is more effective than an explosion.

While the "I" statement can be valuable in conflicts with parents and older people as well, there may be times when you can't air your anger at the person who has stirred these feelings in you. A parent may have said ". . . and that's that. Case closed!" A teacher may not give you any room to argue. A friend may have said something crummy to you last week just before leaving on a month-long study tour of Europe.

However, you can still ventilate your anger, thereby possibly avoiding depression or distressing physical symptoms that may come in the wake of unexpressed anger.

What can you do?

• Physical exercise can be a great anger release! Try a vigorous game of tennis—or any sport with hitting. Or jog or run until you're exhausted!

• Take a long walk to let off steam—and to notice beautiful things along the way.

• Pound your bed pillows and scream into them if you feel like it.

• Write a letter expressing exactly how you feel. Then tear it up.

• Try some hard physical work—like gardening, mowing the lawn, or scrubbing the kitchen floor.

• Talk about your feelings with someone who will listen and keep your feelings in strict confidence.

• Cry. Crying can be very therapeutic—for women *and* men!

You may find other nondestructive ways to help dispel your anger, but the important thing to know is this: It is harmful to sit and simmer in your anger without expressing it in some way. Unexpressed anger will not only cause depression, headaches, stomachaches, or other physical symptoms, but it may also consume you and block out all kinds of happy feelings. Working through your anger—in some way appropriate for you—will help clear the air for joy.

SELFISHNESS

I'm 19, a college student, and planning for a career I hope will last a lifetime. I'm finding out a lot about myself including the fact that I don't want to have children. I'm not even sure I want to get married unless I find someone who is as independent as I am and can live with my independence. My roommate says that my whole attitude is really screwed up and

that people who don't want children are extremely selfish. Now I feel bad. Am I selfish?

Jill N.

I'm a guy, 17, and don't want to go to college. I want to go into carpentry. I was never that great a student anyway, but my parents have this thing about me going to college and making something of myself. I think as long as I do what I love, I'll be somebody, but they say I'm selfish to not do this one thing for them. I say it's my life, but I still feel kind of guilty.

Ken R.

Jason and I have been going together for about a year. We're both 16. I love him, but I want to be a virgin when I marry. He says that if I really loved him, I wouldn't be so selfish. Is standing up for my own values (even if they're kind of different) selfish?

Wondering

Selfish tends to be an overused label. When people call others—or themselves—selfish they probably mean "too concerned with self." But it is vital to be concerned with yourself—and how much is too much is open to debate.

Some might say that, as long as you don't hurt others by doing what you need to do, you're not selfish. Yet there are times when you must hurt others, even though your intentions may be the best—like when you're breaking up with a boyfriend or girl friend you don't—and can never—love.

Sometimes the *selfish* label may be earned. At those times, though, you would be the first to know it. You know when you're being a creep or mean, insensitive or uncaring. Your conscience will nag you nonstop!

At times, though, our consciences may work overtime—with a generous assist from parents, friends, and lovers.

In Jill's case, for example, her roommate is labeling her selfish simply because Jill's values and dreams for the future differ from her own. But the roommate can't be blamed too much. She is merely echoing a prevalent societal attitude.

However, this notion that childless (or childfree) people are, invariably, selfish is a myth. Some very warm, generous people have no children—for a variety of reasons. Some parents, on the other hand, have babies for very selfish reasons.

If Jill feels that she cannot successfully and happily combine a career with motherhood and opts for a career, that may be the right choice for her. Having a baby she really doesn't want—just to avoid criticism—would be selfish, indeed!

Ken, too, is in the middle of making a choice that may be right for him, yet controversial. While we owe our parents respect, we don't owe them the rest of our lives. Therefore, just because what he wants for himself and what his parents want for him are in conflict, Ken isn't necessarily selfish.

It might help Ken—and others in his position—to ask "Whose problem is this—really?"

If he loves carpentry and would be happiest in that trade, it would be better for him to pursue it than to spend several listless years drifting through (or struggling to stay in) college.

Why are his parents so adamant about his going to college? Do they want him to do what he does best *or* do they want the vicarious pleasure of saying "My son, the college graduate . . ."? In this case, they may be the selfish ones. With his best interest in mind, they might be just as happy to say "My son, the carpenter" or "My son."

It could be, too, that Ken's parents may *not* be selfish. They may be worried and deeply concerned for his future. Will he be able to earn a living and survive? Will he be happy? It may be up to Ken to help them to see that he can be happy—and succeed—in his own way and on his own terms. Maybe they'll never understand. But Ken owes it to himself to follow his talents and dreams and to make his own life. This is not selfish. It's necessary.

It is also necessary to prevent the *selfish* label from coercing you to go against your own values. If you are or have been in a situation like "Wondering," standing up for your own values and beliefs (even if they are different) is *not* selfish! It's part of knowing who you are, and someone who loves who you are will, ultimately, accept your right to be you!

NEED FOR PRIVACY

My mom wants to know everything that happens at school every day. I used to tell her everything, but now it bugs me. I don't have anything to hide, but I just don't feel like telling her everything. What's the matter with me?

Casey T.

I don't have any privacy—none at all! My mother snoops through my drawers, reads my diary, and opens every piece of mail that comes in this house! My conscience is clear, but it sure burns me up when she does this. I'm 15 and feel like I'm living with the FBI!

Mary Y.

I'm a 15-year-old boy and I'm in a sort of jam with my folks. It's because I've started locking the bathroom door. We have one bathroom in the house and

I can't stand it when I'm in there and everyone (parents, sister, brother, dog, neighbor kids—you get the idea!) tramps in and out. They don't seem to need the privacy I do. My folks say the bathroom belongs to everyone and the door should stay open. I don't hog the bathroom—honest. I try to be considerate. I just want to take a bath alone! I ask you, is this abnormal?

Steve C.

The need for privacy is a very normal part of growing up.

In the adolescent years, you are really beginning to see yourself as a separate person with your own thoughts and your own life. Most parents love their children deeply and want the best for them, but, still, it's difficult for some to accept—and live with—your growing separateness and independence.

As Casey points out, part of your growing independence may involve keeping some things to yourself. These thoughts or events may be innocuous *or* controversial. The point is, they are *yours,* and you may feel that you don't want to share all of these with your parents or friends. Or even if you do want to share them eventually, you may want to do so when you choose (rather than when they ask).

Choosing what you will share and what you will keep private is part of becoming your own person. It's difficult at times to reinforce your right to privacy without sounding rude or like you have something horrendous to hide. This is particularly true if your mother (or brother, sister, and so forth) is inclined to snoop through your drawers, diary, mail, or anything else that isn't under lock and key. Siblings may do this to tease. Mothers may snoop, with all the best intentions, because they feel they're losing touch with their teens. This can be a vicious cycle, however, with you needing privacy, what little privacy you might have being violated, and then your further withdrawal into your private self.

Some semblance of privacy is possible for everyone, but it's easier for some to achieve than others. If you share a room with two younger siblings, you won't have the privacy you would have if you had your own room. If your house has only one bathroom, the luxury of settling into a long, leisurely bath—undisturbed—may not be possible too often (if at all). But you can still make your own privacy by realizing that it is OK—even necessary—to have your own private thoughts and dreams.

If your parents are inclined to overstep your private boundaries, it may help to talk with them—calmly. Make no impassioned accusations. Explain that you're trying to find out who you are as a separate individual and that, while you love and respect your parents very much, you need to have your own life, even in little ways. You might reassure them that you value their opinions about big decisions and important happenings in your life, but still you need to have some space, some privacy . . . *not* to hide anything from them, but to grow as an individual.

When you approach the matter reasonably, your parents may listen and be willing to compromise. They may agree to respect the privacy of your diary and/or letters if you try to keep lines of communication open and not shut them completely out of your life. They may respect your right to lock the bathroom door IF you are considerate about not tying up the bathroom for long periods of time.

But perhaps your parents are very touchy on the matter of privacy. Some parents feel that they have an absolute right to know everything—no matter how trivial—or feel very insecure when you assert your individuality. This is a problem for them that, hopefully, they will work out in time.

In the meantime, you might reinforce your need for privacy by taking a long walk when you need to be alone or by enjoying your private thoughts and dreams, accepting these as normal evidence of your separateness.

Someday soon you will be on your own. By nurturing your individuality now, you may gradually help your parents to accept your separateness. It may take time. This kind of transition isn't easy. Having a child grow up and leave home can be a shattering experience for some parents. By showing gradual separateness, you may ease this transition and help to make it less painful for your parents—and for yourself.

SHYNESS

I'm terribly, terribly shy! I'm pretty good-looking and my grades are OK, but I hate speaking up in class because I'm afraid of making a mistake and having people laugh at me. I'm really worried about saying the wrong thing to people, too. This fear keeps me from making friends. I feel trapped by my shyness and very alone!

Penny Anne

I'm shy about talking to other people. I want them to like me so much, but I can never think of anything to say that seems very witty. It seems like to have friends you have to come on strong and I'm not sure I have that in me. Now I hear that people think I'm a snob because I don't talk much. I can't win! What can I do?

Jeff G.

Penny and Jeff are far from alone. Eighty percent of people polled in a recent survey (3,200 out of 4,000) said that shyness had been a problem for them at some time in their life. Forty percent still considered themselves shy!

Shyness can afflict people in many different ways.

Some people are socially isolated and have trouble talking with anyone. Others are particularly shy with the opposite sex and still others are confident in personal relationships, but find it hard to deal with strangers.

One guy who calls himself shy says that he gets weak in the knees when, as a school officer, he has to get up and speak at a school assembly. Another teen who reports being shy is afraid to call movie theaters to listen to prerecorded messages about showtimes—just in case a live person might answer for a change!

What causes some people to be shy?

While some counselors feel that shyness *can* mean that you're so preoccupied with yourself that you lose contact with others, many feel that the roots of shyness may be found in childhood. Many shy teen-agers and adults seem to come from homes where a lot has been expected of them. Held to impossibly high standards, the child may have developed a habit of hanging back, afraid to try, afraid to reach out. Fear of making a mistake and/or of being rejected because of this may be at the core of shyness.

If this sounds like your life story, keep in mind that you cannot change the past. However, you *can* change the present and the future if shyness seems to be a problem for you.

For a start, try to see risk in a different way.

You may make a mistake. All of us do at times. However, in most cases, a mistake is neither a failure nor a catastrophe. It can be a learning experience. Viewing possible mistakes as opportunities to learn may help diffuse some of your fear of failure and enable you to take some risks.

It's OK *not* to take risks all the time. For a start, try taking only ones you feel relatively comfortable taking. For example, you may or may not want to talk with someone right now. If you want to be quiet, OK. But if you feel like talking, yet don't know quite how to begin, try a little risk-taking.

The old "keep-your-mind-on-the-other-person-and-take-an-interest-in-him-or-her" advice may sound trite, but it does have a ring of truth. If you really listen to another, you can usually find something on which to comment or something you can relate to feelings and experiences of your own. If you are busy worrying about the impression you're making, however, you're stuck. You aren't hearing the other person and may have little to offer to keep the conversation going.

But what if you've made yourself so invisible for so long that people don't seem to realize you're alive?

Then you'll have to take the risk of asserting yourself a little.

Sit down and think about what you'd like to do. Maybe you'd like to reach out and make some friends. If you wait for people to come to you, you may wait forever, so an action plan is in order.

First, decide what is possible for you right now. Maybe you're not ready—and never will be—to speak before a lot of people. You'd just like to be able to have a one-to-one conversation with a classmate, perhaps. Think about the person, or people, you'd like to talk with. What is his or her range of interests? What are this person's main attractive qualities? Think about this person as a kind person who is likely to respond to you in a positive way.

Next, set a goal—and a deadline. You might want to start off by saying "hello" to five people this week. Just "hello."

The next week, add a simple, sincere compliment or observation to the greeting.

These may sound like very small beginnings, but they are beginnings. They will help get you in contact with others and will help you to start feeling good about yourself because you tried something that was difficult for you.

If others' responses to your efforts aren't exactly overwhelming, don't despair. It takes many people time to get past indifference and to the point of wanting to know one another. Also, if someone is in a bad mood and doesn't respond in kind to your friendly "hello" this may have nothing to do with you. You are not responsible for his or her black mood. Since you determine your own behavior, you can still be friendly, no matter what the response. One slight doesn't have to spoil your day.

There are some times, however, when others' unresponsiveness *may* have something to do with you.

Mary, now 22 and a college senior, remembers the time during her junior year of high school when she decided to take the risk of saying "hi" to everyone she encountered in the school corridor.

"I spent days greeting everyone and nobody responded," she says. "It was like I was invisible. Finally, I got desperate enough to say 'hi' a little louder to this girl Liza who was pretty nice. Liza looked surprised and came closer to me. 'What? What did you say? I can hardly hear you!' she said to me. I realized then that I was greeting people so softly that no one could hear me! When I finally spoke up, it was a whole different story. People all said 'hi' back and many of them smiled. It was amazing to see the difference. I'm so glad I didn't just decide that everyone was naturally unfriendly—or that I was a social failure—and give up trying."

Mary's story is a testimonial to the value of trying—

and trying again. Anything that will put you in touch with others—a new hobby or sport or special interest—is worth trying. Even if you're just a beginner at something and are bound to make mistakes, it's OK. Learning something new is an opportunity to pursue an interest of your own and to meet others with the same interest. Some may be better at whatever it is than you are. That's fine. You don't always have to be the best. Some people may find pleasure in helping you. Most will respect you for trying.

Often those of us who are shy are afraid to take a risk because we have extremely high—and unfair—expectations of ourselves. You may expect not only to go to a dance, but also to be the life of the party. Such turnabouts rarely happen overnight, if ever! You may feel that, in order to have people notice you and like you, you have to come on strong. This isn't so. You can be quiet and sensitive and listen a lot—and be considered an interesting, fun friend.

Family counselor Norma Waters is fond of telling shy clients an old fable about a contest between the wind and the sun over which was more powerful.

"The wind and the sun debated over which could induce the traveler along the way to remove his coat," she says. "The wind blew furiously, but the traveler only wrapped his coat more tightly around him. Then the sun shone warmly on him. Before long, the traveler removed his coat. This fable points up the fact that pushing too hard to relate to others, being too *on,* may make people wrap themselves more tightly in their shells, so to speak, but genuine warmth seems to get through to most people. Warmth is something you don't always have to express verbally. Other people can generally feel it. As a sensitive person, you may be uniquely able to cultivate this sense of warmth and caring about others."

Accepting yourself as a normal and unique person, who is bound to make mistakes at times, and extending your warmth to others can involve risk, joy, and learning.

At worst—which isn't so bad—you'll *not* fail, but learn. At best, you'll learn *and* feel the joy of getting in touch with others. So the risks aren't really so terrifying. As you come to realize this, you'll get a new sense of control of your life. You can choose to live in isolation or to reach out. You can bring change into your life. Adolescence, of course, brings many changes to your life and, as you grow, so do the expectations, pressures, and . . .

STRESS

I feel like the weight of the world is on my shoulders! My dad expects me to be a great athlete now (I'm not!) and a doctor later. I'm fairly bright, but I don't know if I could get into medical school or whether I even want to try. My parents are so grade-conscious that I'm really scared to bring home a B, and before an exam—any exam—my stomach is in knots and I feel so nervous all the time. I'm only 16.

Ken J.

When I was little, I was always full of life and ready to do anything and didn't care what other people thought. I was fun to be around. Now all I have to say seems to be a sarcastic remark and I always just sit around rather than do something fun and crazy because I'm afraid of what people will think of me. Why have I changed so much?

A Bore

I'm 15 and I get nervous a lot about all kinds of things, like calling someone or going to the store. It seems that everything has become too much for me. Is there anything I can do to calm myself down? And am I crazy??

Almost Crazy(?)

I never knew it would be so hard to grow up. I have so many worries. Does every kid go through this?

Julie B.

Dealing with the stress of changes in your life can cause an explosion of feelings. You may cry or laugh at seemingly inappropriate times. You may feel nervous about a whole range of things. You may feel angry, confused, and upset. Whatever you feel, you feel it intensely.

There are a lot of pressures connected with adolescence. There may be pressures from your parents to measure up to their expectations for you. There may be pressures from your peers. The greatest pressures, however, often come from within. There are the pressures that come with change, trying to reconcile in your own mind the fact that you seem to both love and hate your parents; love, yet compete with your friends; and the fact that while you're trying to be part of the crowd, you're also trying to become your own person and to define your own values. You're trying to find out who you are and make important decisions that may influence who you will become. You begin to see, with new clarity, your limitations as well as your possibilities.

Sometimes it may seem as if your life is in a period of suspension. All you seem to do is wait for the things you want. You're hungry for independence, yet in many ways you are still dependent on your parents. And they may have trouble interpreting your drive for

independence as a positive part of your growth rather than as a personal rejection. There are demands made on you from all sides, it seems. If you are in college, this pressure may be intensified. Even if you are several thousand miles away from home, there are tangible ties with your parents. Sometimes you may feel that you're in a shadow world of increasing responsibility for yourself without some of the compensations of total freedom. You may feel responsible to yourself, to your parents, to your friends, and to your school.

It's no wonder, then, that, in a recent survey, stress and nervousness emerged as the number-one problem voiced by those in the 14- to 21-year-old age group!

People deal with stresses in a myriad of ways.

A teen we'll call Ellen was the youngest in a family of four high-achievers. When she started high school, she studied hard and signed up for drama. She had great hopes of being accepted on her own merits, but this, unfortunately, was not to be. Her teachers and some upperclassmen couldn't seem to forget the three brilliant siblings who had gone before her. Whatever Ellen did couldn't possibly measure up to the legends of her sisters and brother. "How does it feel to be the sister of ———?" was a question she came to dread.

One day, Ellen simply stopped going to school. She started sleeping 14 hours a day and refused to compete in any way. Paralyzed by stress and deep depression, she was totally unable to function until she began going to a therapist and came to discover her own unique worth as a human being.

Bob, on the other hand, deals with stress by plunging into a steady stream of activities. He has very few moments to be alone and think about his feelings, and that's just fine with him. When he was in bed with a mild case of the flu, however, he felt extremely nervous and agitated. Stripped of his method of escaping his feelings, he almost fell apart.

Joanna copes with stress by overeating, while her sister Karen has the opposite reaction: She can't eat a thing! Both worry about their weight—for different reasons—and wish they could find more constructive ways to deal with stress.

Marty, a college freshman, says that he handles stress by concentrating on what's really important to him and just ignoring the rest. Right now, his biggest concern is doing well in chemistry. So he spends a lot of time studying and, as yet, doesn't date much. "I like to take one thing at a time," he says. "After I get more accustomed to the academic pressures, then I'll start to deal with the social pressures. But right now—in my first quarter—I just couldn't handle both."

Marty's method of dealing with stress may seem a bit extreme to you, but an important point emerges from his example: It may help a great deal in stress situations to be able to identify how much is *too* much for you.

Kelly, for example, is able to juggle a full academic load, extracurricular interests, and an active social life quite well, but she manages this because she is in touch with her feelings. She knows when she's getting in over her head. "When things cease to be challenging or fun and start to look like problems or chores, I see that as a warning to slow down," she says. "If I find myself dreading something I would usually enjoy, that is like a warning buzzer in my head to slow down and take it easy."

John finds that his "warning buzzer" is a tendency to pick fights with his 14-year-old brother. "When I feel myself on the verge of another attack on Josh, I stop and say to myself 'Hey, wait! What's *really* bugging you?' I usually find that I'm worried about school or something, and slugging Josh won't help that in the long run!"

How can you cope with stress?

Be Aware.   Being aware of the sources of stress in your life—and your feelings about these—is a vital first step to coping with the inevitable stresses in your life.

Do you find yourself worrying about a lot of things? Can you break these down into specific worries? Which of these can be changed? Which can't? Which can you do something about right now?

Making a mental priority list of things you can do to reduce stress now can help a lot. It is not helpful to chew your nails about doing well on your SATs next year, but it may be helpful to keep up in your classes now, for example.

Taking your life stresses in moderate doses, trying to be concerned only with what you can cope with (or change) right now can cut down a lot on your anxieties and banish that feeling of helplessness. Nothing is more nerve-racking than a whole list of worries that you can't do anything about yet. Concentrate on what you can deal with now. You can make a difference and you *do* have control over your life in many ways.

Ask Yourself If You Are Being Realistic in Setting Your Goals.   If you hate science and it's consistently your worst subject, medical school may not be a realistic goal.

It's impossible to be liked by everyone and, even if you could be, you might find yourself giving up important parts of yourself, aspects of your personality or personal preferences, to fit in with other people's expectations.

So examine your goals and ask yourself two questions: "Is this a possible, attainable goal?" and "Do I really want it?"

Put Your Stresses in Perspective. Some people see everything as life-and-death matters.

Marilee, who can literally make herself ill during exams, is terrified of failing, in spite of the fact that she always makes top grades. While a little nervousness may be energizing, Marilee's anxiety seems to work the other way, making it more difficult to do well. Fighting her fears as she struggles to study adds up to an incredibly stressful situation for Marilee—a situation that doesn't have to be.

"Many teens have such a terrible—and inaccurate—sense of finality," says counselor Sheridan Kesselman. "A teen might say, for example, 'If I don't pass this test, that's IT!' and I'll ask him or her 'What's *it?*' All too often, young people see things as irrevocable. Life isn't like that. Things can be changed. If you don't get what you want one time, you'll get it another time. Learn to ask yourself 'Is this really worth all the anxiety? What is my nervousness accomplishing?' Put things in proper perspective. If you see one thing—a test, a date, or whatever—as the turning point in your life, of course you'll be nervous and tense. No matter what the outcome of the situation you're nervous about, however, life goes on. It *isn't* the end of the world."

To Gain Control—Start Small! If you feel tensions building about everything, don't try to tackle it all at once. Start small and be specific. Regain control of your life in little things, like improving your work in one class at school. Live in the present and deal with one thing at a time instead of dwelling on and dreading the rest of your worries even as you tackle one of them. If you always try to take on twenty things at once, you may be paralyzed by anxiety and frustration. One at a time, however, your problems can be solved.

Realize That You—and Only You—Can Change Your Life.   Only YOU in any given situation can choose to be nervous or to alleviate some of your stress. Taking responsibility for your own nervousness makes it possible for you to do something about it. If, for example, you can say "I get nervous when I'm with strangers" instead of "Strangers make me nervous!" You, not they, are in control. And you can work to change this uncomfortable situation.

Make Time to Have Fun! If you don't think you have time, *make* time! Fun is a vitally important part of your life. The ability to relax and enjoy life will make you better able to cope with stresses when they come. Renew yourself with a hobby, meditation, a long walk, or exercises—great tension reducers.

Exercise. Physical exercise, as we just mentioned, is an excellent tension reducer—and is good for your body. Any kind of exercise you enjoy will do: sports, dancing, walking, running, or spot exercises. The following are some exercises specifically for reducing tension:

• Rag Doll Exercise. Stand with your legs apart, your back straight, your head erect. Then collapse the upper part of your body, keeping the legs straight. Let your head and arms dangle down. Hold this position for a minute. Then slowly return to an upright position.

• Tension-Release Combo. (Wear loose clothing for this one.) Sit erect in a straight-backed chair. Collapse, rounding your back, letting your head hang down and your hands rest on your knees. Concentrate on your arms feeling heavy. Then, make fists with your hands, and sit up and tense your whole body. Relax after a minute and then collapse again. Repeat this exercise three times.

• Stomach-Breathing Exercise. Lie on your back on the floor with your head on a pillow, your legs bent, feet flat on the floor. With one hand on your stomach and the other on your chest, breathe deeply, inhaling so that your *stomach*— not your *chest*—rises. Breathe in through your nose and out through your mouth. As you exhale, whisper "Hahhhh . . ." Do this exercise for ten minutes.

• Total Relaxation Exercise. Sit in a position that is comfortable for you. Close your eyes and relax all your muscles—from head to toe. Starting with your toes, softly tell each part of your body to relax. Breathe deeply through your nose and exhale through your mouth, relaxing your jaw and saying "Oh . . ." softly and slowly as you exhale. Try this exercise for ten minutes. Then continue to sit with your eyes closed for another ten minutes. Gradually, whenever it feels right, open your eyes.

• Fantasy Relaxation Exercise. Lying on your back with a pillow under your head and your eyes closed, breathe deeply in and out. Shut out what's happening now and, via your imagination, travel to a more peaceful place and time. Maybe you envision yourself on a sunny beach in Hawaii. You walk along the sand, the clear, warm water lapping at your toes. You're alone—and at peace—with only the gentle sound of the surf and the tropical breeze whispering through the palm trees. In the distance you can hear a musical wind chime. You sigh and feel your whole body relax. . . . Maybe your relaxing daydream would be something quite different. Fine . . . whatever works for *you!*

When You Can't Cope Alone—Reach Out!   Don't bottle up your anger, fear, and anxiety—all stress-related—for an eventual explosion. Sharing your feelings with others you trust may help you to get the feelings out and to realize that you're not alone. A friend or family member may help you to explore some of the choices you have in a given stressful situation.

There *are* times, of course, when friends and, especially, parents can be a source of stress.

THE PARENT PERPLEXITY

Is it normal for a person my age (14) to have mixed feelings about her parents? One minute I'll think they're terrific. The next, I can't stand them. They do things like come up from downstairs and tell me I left my coat down there. They couldn't bring it up for me, of course! But they can come to my room and tell me. They drive me crazy!!!

Lost and Alone

I have a teen-aged son, 15, and during an argument over curfew the other day, he said "I hate you, Mom!" Five minutes later, he came back with tears in his eyes and said he didn't mean it. I tried to tell him that it's OK to feel hate at times for the people you love. I'm not sure he really believed me. I do know that I have suffered greatly because no one ever told me when I was young that I could dislike or even hate my mother at times and so the furies were buried, only to engulf me in later life. I think this whole love-hate thing is so important for kids to know about—and feel OK about.

A Loving Mom

Ambivalence (mixed feelings) reaches epidemic proportions in adolescence. You may love and hate your parents, want independence from them, yet need them. You may be struggling to find your own values while feeling influenced by theirs. You may come to the conclusion that growing up means rejecting the values of your parents. Rebellion—in some form or another—is part of every teen's life. It's a way of saying "Hey, I'm a separate person!"

Cathy's parents, for example, are fallen-away Catholics who haven't been to mass in several years. For the past year or so, however, Cathy has been up at dawn to go to daily Mass and is thoroughly alarming her parents by talking of becoming a nun. We don't mean to play down the importance of religion in Cathy's life right now—or in the future—but she herself admits that she probably wouldn't be so devout if her parents shared her beliefs.

Carl asserts his separateness by arguing with his parents on political and social questions. But his separateness is questionable: What they're for, he's against. His opinions still hinge on theirs, if only as a reaction.

Rebellion may be a necessary part of growing up, especially if your parents are reluctant to acknowledge the fact that you are a separate individual.

However, if you can develop your own point of view (an idea that Dr. Bernard Berkowitz and Mildred Newman discussed early in this chapter) rebellion per se may not be inevitable.

Conflict may be an inevitability, however.

There are times when you are very much like an adult and times when you feel like a child. You may fluctuate between fighting for independence and wanting to be taken care of once again. You may find this very confusing.

So do your parents! They may be even more perplexed by the changes they see in you than you are. It may be difficult for them to accept the fact that you don't need them as much as you once did. It may be difficult for *you* to admit that there are times, even now, when you still need them very much.

Realizing that all these feelings are normal and can coexist may help. So can examining closely some of your conflict situations to see who (if anyone) is being unfair.

"Lost and Alone," for example, claims that her parents tell her when she leaves her coat downstairs rather than bringing it up to her. Are her parents *really* being unfair?

It could be that her parents are trying to help her to develop a sense of personal responsibility. And "Lost" may unconsciously be using her misplaced coat as a means of keeping close to her parents (even if it means nagging!). This ambivalence—wanting to be close and needing to take responsibility—can cause conflict. Will her parents picking up after her reduce her to child status? Or will following their suggestion that she pick up her coat rob her of her growing independence? How does she feel about this independence and responsibility? Is her signature, "Lost and Alone," a clue to the fact that she equates responsibility and independence with being very much alone and needs to be connected to her parents, like a child again? It could be. But such a conflict doesn't have to occur.

"She can hang up her coat without sacrificing who she is," Dr. Berkowitz points out. "You don't have to use where you put your coat as a passport to growing up. A teen-ager will do this, actually, to stay connected to his or her parents, to keep from feeling lonely and from being too separate."

Gigi, a happy 15-year-old, feels comfortable in her separateness and yet feels that she can rely on her mother when she needs to without being diminished. She also feels free to express her separate opinions and admits that conflicts do happen, but these are a minor part of her relationship with her mother, a relationship built on love, trust, and mutual respect.

"My mother is my best friend," she says. "Sure we disagree on some things, but they're really silly little things like my mother saying 'The cake should have vanilla icing' and me answering 'No, Ma! It should be chocolate!' or something like my mother saying 'No, Gigi, you can't go swimming. It's only 70 out' and me coming back with 'Oh, Ma, it's warm enough!' and then I go swimming and get a bad cold, but Ma doesn't hold it over me. She trusts me and gives me a lot of responsibility. When she works, I fix supper and do the dishes if my brother doesn't (which is usually the case!). Truthfully, I really enjoy having responsibility. It makes me feel older. My mom is really the greatest!"

Happily, a number of parents are like Gigi's mom, combining loving guidance with growing responsibility and sense of fairness. However, there are some parents who can be unfair, too.

Jody's parents, for example, are recently divorced and try to use Jody as a go-between in their continuing battles.

Kevin's parents have decided that he must become a lawyer—like his dad—and call him "ungrateful" when he talks of becoming an artist or art teacher instead.

In each case, the parents are failing to see Jody and Kevin as separate people rather than as extensions of themselves.

Jody has a right to resent being used by her parents in what is an unfortunate and private battle between them. If they could see the picture from her separate viewpoint, they might see that she already feels a lot of grief over the breakup of her family, and feeling torn between two parents she loves very much only intensifies her anguish.

Kevin, too, is feeling torn right now between what his parents expect of him and what he wants for himself. It is a very frequent and emotion-packed dilemma among teens. "What do I owe my parents?" many young people may ask, along with Kevin.

We owe our parents respect and a listening ear.

You can respect and hear their values and opinions without necessarily agreeing with them. This is an important fact to know.

Another important fact: Just because parents may not see things your way doesn't mean they're being unfair. The reverse is also true. You, too, can disagree with them—without being unfair.

The fact that you may disagree simply means that you—and they—are different people! "And everyone has a right to be different," says Dr. Berkowitz. "If you know you're right about something, you don't have to hear it from them. Give them the same right to their views that you would like for yourself. To be truly separate is to accept and recognize that each person is different."

If you realize this, you can be your own person, even in your parents' house, living by many of your parents' rules. It all depends on developing your own point of view, something that is *not* dependent one way or another on how your parents view things. When you have this sense of separateness, you may even feel free to agree with them at times, to make your own some of the values that they hold. That doesn't make you a dependent child. It makes you a growing young adult who has exercised his or her own choice. Just because a value or a choice happens to coincide with someone else's doesn't mean that it is not your own.

When you feel free to choose your values freely—whether or not they coincide with those of your parents—you will be free to express more positive feelings around your family, whether you agree with them in all things or not.

When you're fighting for separateness, those loving feelings that keep recurring (even as you battle) can be confusing and difficult, if not impossible, to express. You may feel that to say "I love you" to a parent may trap you forever in prolonged childhood. The opposite, in fact, may be true. The more separate and independent you become, the more love you may feel for your parents. This may happen often in the late teens and early twenties, when after a few stormy years, you start to see each other as *people*.

Anger, tears, laughter, and loving are part of all family relationships. In adolescence, these feelings may intensify, but, with good communication, you can cope. Seeing each other as people with highly individual—and valid—viewpoints is what good communication is all about. Ideally, your parents will listen to you and care about your feelings. By listening to and caring about the two *people* behind the parental roles, you can help increase understanding and acceptance of one another, even when you disagree.

In some areas of life, disagreements may be frequent and intense and you'll need all the mutual love and understanding you can give and get!

This is particularly true in the area of sexuality.

PARENTS AND SEX

I have strong sexual feelings, but I don't do anything about them except masturbate sometimes. My mother says feelings like this aren't normal for a girl. Am I strange?

Lorena

My mother believes in being open about sex, talking

about it, I mean. She thinks that since I'm 16, I'll be having sex soon and should get birth control pills. I feel like I'm being pushed to have sex and like she's mingling in my private life too much. Am I wrong?

Diane

I'm a nice girl, but if I'm ten minutes late coming home from a date, my dad calls me a "slut" or a "whore" and says he knows what I've been doing. I haven't!!! How can I make him trust me? Sometimes I think I might as well be doing all he says I'm doing, since I get blamed for it anyway!

Jan K.

My parents are very uptight about sex and it's impossible to talk with them. There are things I need to know. What they do say is confusing—like it's a terrible thing for unmarried people to have sex, but it's beautiful once you're married and it's a mistake for a guy, but a tragedy (and a real trashy thing) for a girl. I think I disagree with them, but I need more information to form my true opinions.

Tim W.

I'm 16 and masturbate. I feel very guilty about this. My parents would never get over it if they knew I did this. They'd be so disappointed in me. I feel bad about it, but I still do it!

Hilary J.

Why is it that you can't talk about sex with your parents? My parents are really super people. They've never said anything bad about sex. They've just never said much one way or another. I'd like to talk with them, but can't seem to bring the subject up. I feel so embarrassed!

Alex B.

Your sexuality, which includes sexual *feelings* as well as actions, is a major part of who you are all your life, from infancy to old age. However, as you emerge as a maturing young adult, your sexuality is in the spotlight. It's evident in your body changes. It's especially evident in your strong new sexual feelings.

These feelings can cause a lot of concern.

You may wonder if it's normal to feel as strongly as you do about sex. You may put yourself down for sexual fantasies, feeling as guilty as if you had actually fulfilled these fantasies! You may feel pulled in several directions in deciding how you will express your sexuality.

Perhaps your religion and/or your parents condemn masturbation or premarital sex. You may disagree in principle, but in fact, you may feel guilty about disagreeing, or about acting in ways counter to your family's values. Perhaps, if you come from a family that assumes you will be sexually active soon, you may feel—as Diane does—that your privacy and right to choose is being violated.

In other instances, you may become aware of society's ambivalence about sex (which may be mirrored in some parental attitudes) and you may wonder how it can be terrible to have sex one day when you're unmarried and beautiful the day after the wedding ceremony. You may hear and wonder about old myths like the one that says that women don't really enjoy sex, they just put up with it as a wifely duty. You may even hear yourself voicing yet another myth: "My parents couldn't possibly understand how it is. . . ."

In the sexual area, many parents seem to have acquired a negative image, often unjustly so. If some parents stereotype teen-agers as wild and amoral, teens often stereotype parents as passionless, asexual types who don't know what it's like to be young or to have sexual feelings. Before laying stereotypes on your parents, it may help to see that they're people (as well as parents) and that, right now, they may be in a tough position.

A minority of parents may have extremely negative feelings about sex. (If you have a parent who has such feelings, it may help to realize that you are separate people. It's important to have compassion and understanding for your parent while quietly keeping your own opinions.)

Some parents may not be negative about sexuality per se, but may simply be uninformed. They may pass on misinformation that they sincerely believe is true—with all the best intentions.

Lorena's mother, for example, grew up during a time when it was assumed that women didn't have strong sexual feelings or desires. The fact is, of course, that until recently women didn't feel as free to accept and express their sexual feelings, to see themselves as sexual beings. This freedom, incidentally, does not necessarily mean having sex. It means accepting the fact of your sexuality, including your sexual feelings, as normal and OK. If Lorena's mother could have—and really hear—such information, she might feel less alarmed about her daughter's feelings and might possibly feel better about herself, too.

Some parents are not sex-negative, only fearful for their teens. Most parents love their teen-agers deeply and want the best for them. As you mature sexually and the possibility of acting on your sexual feelings becomes more likely, your parents may feel afraid in many ways: afraid of losing you, afraid that you'll be hurt, afraid that you'll fail to see the value of their beliefs, afraid that your future may be jeopardized by a mistake now.

There is some basis for these fears. An unwanted or premature pregnancy may scar young lives. You may be hurt. You will grow away from your parents, whatever actions you take (or don't take) sexually.

Some parents, however, may express their fears in hurtful ways.

Jan's father, for example, expresses his fear that she will have sex by labeling her a *slut* and a *whore*. Unfortunately, these labels can be self-fulfilling. Like Jan, many teens feel that, as long as their parents don't trust them anyway, they might as well be wild. What hurts, of course, is the fact that such sexual acting out is not necessarily the teen-ager's positive choice, but rather a reaction against parental labeling and lack of trust. It can be an unhappy situation for both parents and teens.

Some parents, too, can express their fears through newly restrictive rules or by long lectures on the dangers of early sexual experimentation. From their vantage point, they may see that you have a long way to grow even yet and may wonder how ready you are to assume the risks and responsibilities that go with sex. They may fear for you until they learn that you can survive.

Patty, for example, found that her mother had a fit when she discovered that Patty was having sex at 16. After her initial relationship, however, Patty chose not to have sex again until she was 20. Then she found her mother's reaction quite different.

"My first relationship was sort of unfortunate," says Patty. "While it lasted, it was neat, but I thought Bill would love me forever. When we broke up, I was just crushed! It was like a total rejection. I wasn't ready for that. My mother could see this coming, but I couldn't. Four years later, Ted came into my life and then I felt ready to handle intimacy and the fact that I might be loved forever—or rejected. I started taking birth control pills. One day, in front of my mother, my purse tipped over and the pill container fell out. My mom saw them, but didn't make a fuss. She just said she was glad that I was taking responsibility and that she hoped I was happy in this relationship. I know she'd prefer it if I wasn't having sex. I respect her feelings, even though I don't agree with her. I never try to hit her over the head with my lifestyle. We quietly respect each other."

Respecting one anothers views, like Patty and her mother do, may help to take some of the pain out of differences of opinion and life-style.

It may also help to see how you are alike, what values you may have assumed—even unconsciously.

Renee, for example, sees herself as a very free 16-year-old. She has been having sex for about three months now and says that her parents would just *die* if they knew. "They're so uptight," she says. "I believe that sex is natural and beautiful. It's a part of me.''

Although Renee is voicing positive feelings about sex, she has some unconscious reservations about what she is doing. This is demonstrated most, perhaps, by the fact that, despite the fact that she does not want to get pregnant, she refuses to use any form of birth control. "That's planning for sex and I feel that's wrong," she insists. "I mean, sex should just *happen*. . . .''

If Renee *really* felt OK about having sex, taking responsibility and planning for it, in a sense, would not be anathema to her. A certain amount of planning—like taking birth control precautions to avoid an unwanted pregnancy and to help alleviate the fear of this happening—may only make sex more enjoyable. Many of those who feel that it's wrong to plan for sex, however, are really saying that they don't feel right about the fact that they're having sex. Seeking birth control means admitting to yourself and to others that you're having—or will have—sex. Some adolescents feel too guilty to do that. They would rather hide the fact of their sexuality not only from others, but also from themselves.

Even if you can't be honest with others about your sexuality, it's important to be honest with yourself. If you're not as free as you thought, if your actions are violating your true feelings, you may want to reevaluate some of your choices.

We are all products of our society and of our families as well as unique individuals. Much of what we feel about ourselves—sexually and otherwise—is learned at home. In our families, we exert strong influences on one another. For this reason, it is helpful if we can talk about some of our feelings and views. Many sex educators feel that the best possible sex education is one that is centered at home.

But discussing sex with your parents is often easier talked about than done. All too often, communication about sexuality can be short-circuited by embarrassment and fear, fear of being misunderstood or judged, and embarrassment about ourselves—and each other—as sexual beings.

It's important to get past the old stereotypes and assumptions and take the risk of sharing. You might start out in a cautious way, asking your parents' feelings about a specific matter, discussing some sexual information you have heard or read (or even sharing the source—like this book—with them) and asking what your parents think about it, how and why they agree or disagree.

Communication about sex isn't always easy. Sometimes it may be impossible. If your parents don't want to talk about sex or share feelings and ideas with you and have made this clear to you, other people in your life—including older relatives and friends, your physician, nurse practitioner, or sex education counselor or teacher—may be able to help you. (For more information about your sexuality, see Chapter Ten and the Special Needs Resources list in the Appendix.)

It is likely, however, that as you and your parents grow to see each other as people, your communication will improve. You may find that you agree on some things and disagree on others . . . and that's OK. You can disagree. You can live very different lives . . . and still love each other very much.

LOVE

As you struggle to love—and yet gain freedom from—your parents, you may feel new attraction for people outside the immediate family circle—older friends, teachers, role models, peers, and romantic interests—a wealth of new people to know and to love in many different ways . . .

I love my English teacher Miss Watson. I just love the way she looks at life and how she is with people. I'd like to be just like her. People say it's just a stupid crush, but I really do love her. But sometimes I wonder about myself because I'm a girl.

Corine

I think I'm in love with the lady next door. She's 32 and wonderful. She praises me a lot and thinks I have a good sense of humor. She always listens when I talk, which my parents and girl friend don't do a lot. She thinks of me as just a kid, I'm sure. Nothing physical has happened between us and I'm sure it's not likely, since she is happily married and has a baby girl. But I sure have fantasies about her! Am I wrong to feel this way? (Oh, her husband is nice to me, too, but I like her best!)

Art G.

Knowing and loving older people—besides your parents—can be an important part of growing up. You may be looking for role models outside your immediate family. You may be looking for someone "safe" to love and to fantasize about sexually until you feel ready to handle and act out such intimate feelings with a peer. You may just enjoy sharing feelings with someone who understands you and empathizes with you and who just happens to be older than you are.

Corine, for example, loves her English teacher as a friend and as a role model. It is perfectly OK to love and admire a person of your own sex. In fact, it may be a very necessary part of loving yourself. If you reject all other women (or men) as unworthy and unlovable, then you're rejecting yourself, too. On the other hand, feeling love and admiration for an older friend of the same sex can help to affirm your good feelings about yourself and your future. It is unfortunate that love outside the family circle is, all too often—and often unfairly—equated with sexual acting out.

The fact is, however, that you can love someone intensely as a friend and never have sex. On the other hand, many people have sex and yet never touch each other as vulnerable human beings. Love and sex are not necessarily one and the same.

Art's love for his neighbor can be important to his development, too. This neighbor, an attractive woman who feels secure enough about herself to help Art affirm his own good qualities, can help him begin to have confidence in social situations with women.

Loving, *nonexploitative* friendships with older people during adolescence can do a great deal of good. An older friend may be able to offer you something your peers can't. Especially in early adolescence, your peers are also busy coping with their own development and identity searches. Sometimes it helps most of all to share the struggles with them. But there may be times when you need to be with someone who can give you more emotionally and who may have a little more insight into what's happening. Friendships with older people should not replace peer friendships, but they can help to fill in the gap between your family relationships and friendships with people your age. It may really help to have someone listen to you, share feelings with you, and think you're special.

There can be pain in loving someone older, too. Maybe the person you love isn't interested in being a friend or a role model for you. Maybe the other person is seeking to exploit you—sexually or emotionally. Maybe you'd like to translate the relationship into a romantic and/or sexual one, but feel put down when he/she says no, or feel guilty for even having such thoughts!

What if you're rejected—or it looks like you may be exploited?

Strange as it may seem, rejection—while it hurts—can make love and friendship that much sweeter when it does happen with someone else. (And it will!) It's important to realize, too, that some people just aren't capable of generous, giving, nonexploitative relationships. That's a problem for them and it's too bad. But it doesn't mean that you're not worthwhile as a friend or not lovable, or that you have to give yourself sexually in order to be loved. You may realize that you can't change the current situation, but, in getting out and moving on, by looking after yourself as a lovable person, you can be open to other friendships and further growth in developing a positive self-image.

What if you're having sexual fantasies about an older friend?

People have all kinds of sexual fantasies and it isn't so unusual to have them about someone you know and love. Don't put yourself down for your fantasies about a teacher or family friend or whatever. Remember that you are not responsible for your feelings, but your actions do count. Translating or attempting to translate a sexual fantasy into reality requires a lot of soul-searching, including considering what you could gain versus what you might lose. If you feel that a sexual overture to a friend might jeopardize the friendship, you might decide that the risk isn't worth it. Be aware, too, of what the consequences might be for the other person and what choices you might be asking him or her to make. Laws prohibiting sex between adults and minors (usually under 18) are practically universal. There are also other relationships in that person's life and personal convictions the person may have that may be in conflict with what you want. Most adult friends, faced with such choices and who may also have a deep concern for you, may be likely to decline to have sex with you. In many ways, your fantasies may be preferable to reality.

While we may deal with sexual feelings within these friendships and choose whether or not to act on them, seeing and respecting one another as people is most important. Such mutual respect makes friendship—and love—possible.

Too many people, it seems, separate friendship and love. Ideally, the two are complementary. The best friendships have love and commitment. In the most enduring love relationships, the partners see each other—first and foremost—as friends.

I'm in love, but my parents say I'm silly, that it isn't possible to be in love at 14. Is it?

Don P.

I know I'm in love because I can't eat or sleep and I can't stand to be away from Larry, my boyfriend. We're together constantly and when I'm not with him, I'm thinking of him. It's so bad, my grades are slipping and my girl friends are mad because I don't call them anymore. But my life is Larry! My mom says it's a bad case of infatuation. But I think it's the real thing. What do you think?

Leah C.

It's possible to love very intensely at 14—or younger. It's impossible to set an age limit on ability to love. We love in different ways, according to the person and situation, all our lives.

Too many people try to minimize the love young

people may have for one another as "puppy love." But the fact remains that the love younger people feel has much in common with what more mature people feel when they love one another. The excitement and joy are there and the pain, too, if the love is lost. In teens, these feelings may be even more intense.

A vivid illustration of this fact is best-selling poet Peter McWilliams whose first book about love—and loss of love—was published when he was 17. Peter's age, however, was very pointedly omitted from his biography!

"People so often minimize the love and pain young people feel," Peter, now in his mid-twenties, says. "They may say it's just puppy love or 'Oh, how cute!' But I know that some of my most loving and pain-filled poetry was written when I was a teen-ager. After my first book came out, older people wrote to tell me of their own loves and losses. They were really identifying with what I had to say, but, in some cases, I'm sure, this was only because they didn't know my age. If they had known I was 17, they would have read my love poems and said 'Oh, what does *he* know?' Or they might have read my pain-filled poems on loss of love and said 'Oh, you'll get over it . . .' instead of 'I understand . . .' "

Valid—and deep—feelings have no age limits. However, the character of love may change, depending not so much on your chronological age as on your emotional maturity and feelings about yourself.

Infatuation is a term applied to being "in love with love"—when being in love is more important than loving and giving to someone. This can happen often with people (of all ages) who are emotionally immature.

Immature love of this type can take over your life and make you unable to function in other areas. You constantly think and fantasize about the other person. You feel a need to cling to one another and are very needy. Yet your mutual neediness keeps you from finding lasting happiness or fulfillment. You may feel a lot of anger and fear in the relationship because you don't have the security you need (yet only YOU can give yourself this security you are looking for in the other person). People who are emotionally immature concentrate more on getting than giving. They may fall in love with idealized images rather than people, and when the real person doesn't live up to this vision, disillusionment quickly sets in.

"These people have not given much thought to themselves as individuals and how they want to grow individually," says New York psychologist Dr. Howard Newburger. "They have huge gaps in their self-esteem and try to borrow from each other. In a sense, they're like two lame people clinging together. They also idealize each other's strengths, not really seeing each other as people. When one discovers that the other is simply human, it may be cause for great bitterness and hostility."

This is in sharp contrast to a mature, growing love, which is possible only when you love and value yourself and are able to share, and to enjoy life separately and together.

"I see real love as being aware of each other as individuals," says Dr. Newburger. "You are aware of the needs and wants of one another (not just your own). You realize that we all need space to grow. You are kind to one another. Your love is dynamic. You are independent and fulfilled individuals whose lives are worthwhile (and you see them as worthwhile) to begin with. Life together is simply *more* enjoyable, perhaps. Yet, even while together, you see each other as free, unique, and independent people."

In what other ways can we define mature love?

• Mature love is energizing. It means that you have more energy to give in all aspects of your life: your studies, your friendships, your family relationships, your special interests as well as your love relationship. All are enhanced by your good feelings, rather than cease to be important.

• Mature love is accepting. You allow one another space to be yourselves and don't feel compelled to transform one another. You learn to accept yourselves as you are, to recognize that you are responsible for yourselves as individuals, and to forgive what you are not—instead of criticizing and blaming one another.

• Mature love can survive joy and pain. You're strong enough—and trust each other enough—to be vulnerable, to cry together as well as laugh together. You can take the risk of being honest with each other.

• Mature love means that there is more to your relationship than physical attraction. You can get just as excited talking and sharing feelings as you can about sex.

• Mature love is enhanced by time. You know that time will mean growth, that time will only make your relationship better, so who needs to rush into anything?

• Mature love means neither instant fulfillment nor diminishment of who you are. You have found fulfillment in yourself as a distinct individual. You feel that your partner is wonderful, but realize that you're special, too. You have the security of knowing that if, for some reason, your love would die, *you* could survive.

• Mature love means that you're best friends.

A loving friendship of this type hinges on emotional intimacy, on trusting each other enough to be vulnerable.

It isn't easy to reach this stage of trust with another

person. It takes time to build . . . something we often forget in our era of instant everything.

Attraction at first sight is possible. Real love takes time—and growing.

"Intimacy is knowing what you and he (or she) are about," says Dr. Newburger. "This involves trusting one another enough to take a chance of revealing yourself. It takes time to develop that kind of trust where you know that a personal revelation will neither embarrass the other person nor be thrown back at you. The sharing that this intimacy involves provides the opportunity to let your feelings grow into love."

Mutual commitment to each other's growth as independent people is, perhaps, the most important element of this kind of love.

"This love is an overflow of our own fulfillment," says Dr. Newburger. "Love means finding joy in each other's growth and happiness, whether the other person finds this happiness with or without us. . . ."

The possibility exists that those we love may go on to *other* loves. The very real possibility that a deep, caring love relationship can fade away is something we all know. We've all experienced the loss of loves, in many ways, at many times. And so we may all identify with the following letter.

I've just lost what I thought was the love of my life. I feel devastated, angry, grief-stricken, and forlorn. I'm a bright, independent college junior and I can cope by myself, but I cry when I think of what we had together. I feel like a fool for crying so much. I can live without him, but not as happily, that's for sure! There are times when I wonder if I'll ever get over this hurt.

Suzi R.

This letter was written by a woman, but it could just as well have been written by a man. In fact, a recent survey in the *Journal of Social Issues* revealed that men may feel more depressed and lonely in the wake of a breakup than women!

So the shock and the sorrow of losing a love is familiar to all of us—men and women, young and old. What do you *do* with these tumultuous feelings?

Others may try to console you with criticisms of the other person or cheery advice like 'Oh, don't be sad. There will be someone else!' These may deepen your hurt, since you may still feel a need to defend the other person and may resent an attitude that seems to minimize the importance of the love you have lost.

There may be a temptation on your part to anesthetize yourself with drugs, alcohol, frantic activities, or by becoming involved right away with someone else— just to forget. These measures may also deepen your pain eventually, especially if you use another person as an attempt to forget what you can't seem to forget: that you've grieving for a love you feel can never be replaced.

Perhaps the healthiest response to the loss of a love—by breakup, death, or divorce—is to go with your pain and grief. Just let it happen. Rage. Scream. Cry. Let all the pain and anger out. You may fear— like many do—that once you start crying, you'll never stop. You have visions of yourself going absolutely crazy with grief if you let it happen. This is not likely to happen.

"Those who go crazy with grief are the people who try to deny it," says poet Peter McWilliams who, with psychologist Dr. Melba Colgrove and psychiatrist Dr. Harold H. Bloomfield, has written the excellent book *How to Survive the Loss of a Love.* "Even if it's awful, I think it's important to sit down and *feel* the pain, really feel it. It's OK to grieve. We have to keep telling people that. It's OK to feel terrible and angry and to take time to heal. A physical injury takes time to heal. So does an emotional wound."

Part of the healing process is feeling angry and hurt as you grow past your grief. Forgiveness, which will be possible in time, is also vital.

"It's important to forgive the person you have lost," says Dr. Colgrove. "Whenever there is bitterness, there will be ties. Forgiving is vital to your freedom."

This forgiving—and this new freedom—can bring you a renewed sense of joy.

"This joy comes from finding yourself and seeing this loss as part of your personal growth," says Peter. "When you forgive the other person, you will be able to look back and be happy for the *good* aspects of that lost relationship."

Sad and wistful moments may come—again and again—perhaps years from now, when you hear a song on the radio or smell a hint of that special perfume she used to wear or see a spectacular sunset that he would have enjoyed. But, if you have grown with your grief, your sadness will be mixed with joy—joy not only because you survived the loss of a special love, but also joy in the fact that you were able to love then and will, either now or someday, love again.

DEPRESSION

I'm feeling very depressed because my boyfriend just broke up with me and my best girl friend said something real snotty to me today. I feel bad. How can I get out of this depression?

Cammie

I'm writing this about my sister Carol who is 15 and very depressed. This has been going on for about three months and in this time, her grades have dropped off at school and she doesn't seem to want to do anything. This past week, it got worse. She won't even get out of bed to go to school. She'll hardly eat and when she talks it's about how hopeless everything is. My mother thinks she ought to see our doctor, but Dad thinks she's just trying to get attention and get out of school. I agree with Mom that this is serious. Until recently, Carol was a good student and liked school. She can't seem to help herself. Can we help her?

Mike H.

One of my football teammates says that eating junk food can make you depressed. My girl friend says that she gets depressed for no psychological reason before her period. Can you get depressed for reasons that have nothing directly to do with your feelings?

Ted N.

I'm feeling depressed, but my aunt says that's dumb, that a kid my age (14) can't really get depressed. If not, what is this I feel?

Sally J.

Until two months ago, I was happy and active. Now every time I get a chance to do something, I'm too tired to. I'm miserable and my temper is so short, I don't know how anyone can stand me. I've gained ten pounds and never had a weight problem before. I feel like I'm about 90 years old. I miss the old me so much! I'd do anything to get her back!

Desperate

Depression, according to an estimate from the National Institute of Mental Health, is widespread, hitting all age groups. It will strike between 4 and 8 million Americans severely this year and appear, in milder forms, in another 10 to 15 million.

Although depression is common, it tends to be an elusive disorder, difficult to pinpoint. For example, there may be those who claim to be depressed, but who are, on closer examination, suffering from disappointment. And there are people who don't realize on a conscious level that they are depressed, but who complain about all kinds of vague physical pains or who feel bored all the time.

There are a myriad of possible factors that may be linked to depression. Depression, in fact, may simply be an umbrella term covering a wide range of possibilities.

We often imagine that depression follows a traumatic loss: the death of a loved one, a romantic breakup, a significant failure, or a parental divorce, for example. This may well be so. However, there are a number of less obvious depression triggers as well. The following are only a sampling of these.

- Many women feel low during the drop in hormonal levels just before the menstrual period.
- Although their findings are still controversial, some researchers believe that there may be a link between excessive consumption of so-called junk food, especially the sugar-laden varieties, and depression.
- Certain drugs, including alcohol (yes, it is a drug), amphetamines (uppers), and barbiturates, may trigger depression. (In a recent study of suicide victims, one third were found to have alcohol-related problems.)
- Subtle losses can cause depression.

At first glance, it may be difficult to equate the word "loss" with attaining a goal or becoming independent. Yet, there are significant losses connected with these.

When you attain a goal—winning a prize, getting a job you've always wanted, acquiring a car, your own apartment, or getting into the college of your choice—your joy may be mixed with a touch of sadness. You may start thinking "What now?" The fact is that, in achieving a goal, you have lost it and may feel the need to find new goals.

Growing independence can also bring subtle losses. You may feel the loss of parental protection and support. You may also feel the loss of unlimited opportunity. Your options are narrowing. In choosing some of these options, you lose others. There are some dreams that must be let go.

You are newly aware of your limitations as well as your possibilities. You may now realize, for example, that while you enjoy dancing, you may not have the talent or the discipline to become a luminary in the American Ballet Theater or to dazzle audiences as a cast member of *A Chorus Line*. If you do have the talent, discipline, drive, and opportunity to achieve these goals, you may realize that these may not be compatible—at least for now—with others, like marriage, a family, and work toward a Ph.D. in physics. In making some choices, we lose others forever, and postpone still others. So along with the excitement of making our life choices, there can be a sense of loss—loss of absolutely unlimited life opportunity.

Depression has many forms. It may last a day or much longer. It can make you feel blue or absolutely overwhelm and paralyze you. There is, obviously, a huge difference between these two extremes.

Many of us may link depression with certain situations—a hurtful remark from a classmate, a romantic breakup, or failure to attain a goal. Psychiatrist Helen De Rosis, coauthor (with Victoria Y. Pellegrino) of *The Book of Hope: How Women Can Overcome Depression* contends that the so-called depression in these instances may differ dramatically from true depression.

"This so-called depression that many teens may have is a reaction to a specific, immediate situation," she says. "Often, these feelings don't last very long. You may feel very bad initially but, within a day or so, the mood will be gone. While you're in this mood, however, you may do a lot of talking and complaining. There may be a lot of activity, in other words. In true depression, you are immobile."

What are the characteristics of a true—or significant—depression?

"Significant depression is slower to develop," says Dr. De Rosis. "It may involve feelings of helplessness or inferiority. When you have a constant sense of falling short, you may have significant depression. This kind of depression may have, at its core, feelings we all have, but that are experienced here in more extreme forms. These feelings include anger, guilt, self-hate, helplessness, and hopelessness. When you attempt to keep these terrifying feelings of rage, self-hate, and anxiety from emerging (in other words, you keep them *de-pressed*), you become depressed. Depression is numbing. It is a move toward deadness."

Sometimes such depression is obvious. In other instances, it may be marked by things like addictive or compulsive behavior or vague physical symptoms.

How do you know if you or someone close to you may be suffering from depression? Consider the following questions. If you can answer "yes" to a majority of these questions, you may be a victim of depression.

- Do you feel tired all the time, no matter how much sleep you get?
- Do you feel that doing *anything* (even phoning a friend) is more trouble than it's worth?
- Do you say "no" to all suggestions of activities, even if you have nothing else to do?
- Do you find that you've lost interest in things that used to excite you? That you can't even get interested in, for example, a good meal or sexual fantasies?
- Do you fantasize a lot about being someone else?
- Do you find that you're not taking care of yourself much these days—from eating well to grooming—because you feel it's just not worth the effort?
- Do you dread getting up most mornings because you don't want to face the day?

- Do you feel that you're in a state of suspended animation, waiting for someone to make your life worthwhile?
- Have you lost a significant amount of weight—without trying?
- Do small annoyances make you fly off the handle?
- Is it difficult—or impossible—for you to make *any* kind of decision?
- Do you suffer from symptoms like headaches, insomnia, stomachaches, or constipation?
- Do you find yourself crying a lot—without really knowing why?
- Do you find yourself unable to express feelings like anger, even when you have a *right* to be angry?
- Do you feel a sense of hopelessness, that one day will be just like another, that there's no way you can make a difference?
- Have you thought recently of taking your own life?

In some instances, you can help yourself out of depression by forcing yourself to take some positive action.

A Change of Pace May Help. Dwelling on a problem or mood to which there seems to be no immediate solution is going to keep you on the downward emotional spiral. Try something different. Go for a walk. Listen to some of your favorite music. Dance. Jog. Force yourself to call a friend. Try to do things you would do if you weren't depressed, like *giving* to your friends as well as bending their ears!

Resist the Temptation to Anesthetize Your Feelings with Alcohol or Drugs. Depression is already an anesthetic. To take another will only deepen your problems. "Trying to solve problems by anesthetizing your feelings doesn't solve anything—just *postpones* the solutions," says Dr. De Rosis. "Dealing with feelings is an *opportunity*. Suffering can help you to grow."

Get Daily Exercise. Even if you have to force yourself, do some form of exercise—bicycling, running, or just walking.

Release Your Pent-Up Emotions in Ways That Feel Safe to You. "Cry, pound pillows, and complain to friends who can take it," says Dr. De Rosis. "This is a safe way to permit feelings of anger to surface. Anger is a very important part of depression and unless these angry feelings are released in some way, it is just about impossible to overcome depression."

Keep a "Feelings Diary." This is another suggestion from Dr. De Rosis' book. "Write what you say, do, and how you feel about all of this," says Dr. De Rosis. "Ask yourself what impossible expectations you were trying to meet when you began to feel depressed. If an answer doesn't occur to you right away, don't worry. You may think of it a few days later.''

Plan Each Day So That You Have Something to Anticipate.   You need something to look forward to every day. Your reward may be a soothing bath, a favorite food, time spent at a pleasurable hobby, or a walk to a favorite place—anything, in short, that pleases you and makes you anticipate, rather than dread, the new day.

If your depression persists despite these self-help measures and the loving support of family and friends, it's time to seek professional help.

You may wish to check with your regular physician just to make sure that there is no physical condition that may be contributing to your depression. It's important to realize that there is no stigma in asking for help. Sometimes you can't help yourself.

"If you're stuck with this ongoing feeling of hopelessness, you may have trouble getting out of it without special help," says Dr. De Rosis.

It is this ongoing hopelessness that can drive people to suicide—or suicide attempts. This is a very real danger for teens. It is estimated that suicide is the number-two or -three cause of death in this age group and that the rate of adolescent suicides has nearly tripled in the last 20 years.

Suicidal feelings are not particularly unusual, but they *are* danger signals, signs that you may need help in dealing with your feelings.

In many suicide attempts, young people are not saying that they want to die, but that they simply want life to be different. They don't want things to go on as they have been, yet feel powerless to change the order of things. A suicide attempt, or suicidal feelings, are a definite cry for help, help in regaining power over one's destiny.

Unfortunately, help comes too late—or not at all—to some.

The writer of the following letter is one of the luckier ones.

SUICIDAL FEELINGS

I have attempted to take my own life three different times and I am only 17. I was depressed over a boyfriend leaving me and the fact that my parents didn't seem to care how I felt. My first two attempts were with pills. It was terrible. They tasted awful. I was lucky in that I only got sick, and broke out in a stinging rash. I talked to my best friend about suicide once and said I thought I might shoot myself in the head. She was horrified and said she cared very much about me

and would like to help me. Things were fine for a while, but one day, I felt down and decided to cut my wrists. I went into the bathroom and cut one, just a little bit, and started crying. My mother heard me and came into the bathroom. I saw the horror and pain in her eyes as she came over to me and put her arms around me. I decided I didn't want to die for anyone then. I think I grew up right there with the razor in my hand. I have a long way to go even yet, but now I realize that people do care and, most important, I'm beginning to care a lot about myself. I won't do anything like that again. I wish millions of others were as lucky as I am!

Katie B.

People—family and friends—*do* care and are anxious to help. And if you happen to be related to, or a friend of, someone who is talking about suicide, take ALL he or she says seriously. Contrary to the old myth, people who talk about suicide sometimes *do* follow through! So if someone you know seems so inclined, do listen and try to help him/her explore alternatives *and* sources of possible professional help.

Such help is available at Suicide Prevention Centers, special crisis Hotlines, or at one of some 300 community mental health centers across the nation (as well as some of the more obvious sources of help—like a personal physician, college student health center, and so forth). See specific listings in the Appendix of this book.

Help is available—if you reach out for it. And, in reaching out, you may gain new insights into your life and the many options you do have—as the writer of the following letter did.

I have been a victim of depression for the last four years and have attempted suicide six times, the last time eight months ago. At that time, I took an overdose of speed. When I did this, I was suddenly terrified. I didn't want to die. Suddenly, death seemed more lonely and isolated than my life. I went right to a teacher for help before I collapsed. Since then, I have received special help and counseling and it has enabled me to help myself and to fight my depression. Now I am making plans for the future. I also realize time to be a great healer and life to be full of surprises. I would like to help other teen-agers to realize that they, too, can rediscover the surprises of life. There really is hope!

Terri

This feeling that you *can* make a difference in your life may also help combat a rather common teen complaint . . .

BOREDOM

I'm bored all the time now. I can't get turned on over anything. My town is superboring. Maybe life would be less dull if I could move somewhere else, but I can't do that until I'm 18 and that's three years away! Is there something I can do now so my life won't be so boring???

Curt Y.

When people talk about how they feel, I feel left out because I honestly don't know how I feel most of the time. It's like I feel blah . . . I really don't know how I feel except maybe bored.

Kevin W.

I think I have a common problem: Sometimes I get bored with life. There doesn't seem to be a reason for me to be here. If I have a goal in mind, I have something to work for instead of taking what comes day to day. I want to be useful and to help other people, but what can I, at 14, do now? I feel so helpless. I mean, I feel that nothing I do really makes a difference. Can you help me understand this? I've always wanted to be a writer and/or a psychologist, but what can I do about these goals now?

Jamie T.

Boredom, which may be closely allied with depression, can stem from a number of related causes.

Some of these may include nonparticipation in life due to lack of confidence or motivation, or fear and a sense of hopelessness because the goals you do have seem so far away. Time stands still while you wish for something—anything—to happen.

You can make things happen.

First, take a close look at your feelings of boredom. Try to discover when and why you started feeling this way. Boredom may well be a symptom of depression. What could be behind this? What feelings are you suppressing? What impossible or distant goals could you be piling on yourself? Perhaps you have become so future-oriented that your present couldn't possibly measure up to your dreams for the future. It may seem, then, just like empty, meaningless, and boring time that stands between you and your distant goal.

How can you beat boredom? Some of the depression-fighting tips we gave just before this may also work for boredom. In addition, you might want to try some, or all, of the following.

While Planning for the Future, Don't Forget to Live in the Present! Give yourself intermediate goals. Planning for a bright, fascinating future can help com-bat boredom in many ways. However, if you depend on this future as your only source of excitement, your present may seem even *more* boring by comparison. You may wonder, like Jamie, how you might make a difference in your future NOW.

Jamie, who wants to be a writer, a psychologist, or both, can do a lot at present to help herself in the future—and have a good time right now! She can study the people she knows, trying to understand how and why they feel and act as they do. She can experience closeness and committed friendship, learning to give as well as take. She can keep a daily journal, which will help her to develop the *habit* of writing even when she doesn't *feel* inspired *and* to sort out her feelings. She might write for school publications and, when she feels increasing confidence in her work, contribute to young reader pages in local newspapers and youth-oriented magazines. If she's feeling especially strong and confident, she might even try more competitive markets.

Another teen, who dreams of a faraway career in medicine, might try working as a volunteer at a local hospital to see how she likes it *and* to get a sense of helping others now.

Even if you don't have specific career goals (you just want to get as far away from your small hometown as possible and lead a happy, glamorous, and independent life), you can get a sense of purpose now by looking for ways to make a difference, such as volunteering to work with an organization, spending time with someone who is lonely, or taking a part-time job that may give you a little more economic freedom now. There are a number of things you can do that may help to give you a renewed sense of purpose—and joy in living right now!

If Everything Seems Boring, Try to Think of the Least Boring Activity You Know—And Do It. Action—any kind of action—can break the cycle of boredom and get you out of that rut.

Try to Learn One New Thing Every Day. It may be a word or something you read about in a magazine, newspaper, book, or an encyclopedia. Learning something new *every day* will help you to feel in touch with the world and *growing* again.

Be Open to New Experiences. This suggestion comes from Dr. Sol Gordon, a noted New York psychologist, writer, and educator who talks about boredom extensively in his delightful teen self-help (and fun) *Book You.*

Many times in adolescence, you may feel that to grow up is to leave youthful exuberance and curiosity behind, that some things are cool, other things are not, and it's definitely not cool to reveal that anything turns you on.

The reverse, of course, is true. It is curiosity, joy,

and diversity in your life that will help you to retain the best qualities of youth, even as you attain maturity.

"You can enjoy so many different kinds of experiences, many of them totally unrelated," says Dr. Gordon. "You can enjoy exchanging ideas with a stranger you meet on a plane. You can enjoy trying something you've never tried before—like writing a poem. You might go someplace you'd never ordinarily go voluntarily. Maybe you've never been to an art museum except when you were literally dragged there on a school field trip. So visit an art museum and spend some time there trying to figure out why some people visit this place voluntarily. There are so many opportunities in life, so many experiences that can be unexpectedly meaningful."

Make a List of Things You Love in Life. "I don't love anything," you may grumble at first. But think about it. What things have you loved in the past? What things could you—possibly—if you let yourself, still enjoy?

Dr. Gordon has found that bored people, once they get into making a list of what they love, may get excited all over again. He loves to muse over his own list. "I feel good when I think of chocolate cake, the Sunday *New York Times,* old Beatles records, T. S. Eliot, and Chicago when the wind doesn't blow," he says.

That's a pretty diverse list, isn't it? And it's a list that can grow constantly as you rediscover the excitement of being alive. Even the simplest things can be a turn-on!

One 14-year-old girl we know tried this exercise and discovered, as she compiled her "Love List," that she had a lot of love in her life. Also, to her initial surprise and continuing joy, she found *herself* on her own list!

I've made my list and I'd like to share what I love in life with you:
I love a cool, fresh breeze in early winter.
I love the tiny, sparkling stars at night.
I love camping, summer nights, and cookouts.
I love music, especially country, John Denver, Donny and Marie.
I love the "Baretta" show.
I love sharing a room with my sister.
I love school.
I love being loved.
I love myself and everything around me. . . .
Cathie

Cathie's letter represents a significant step in her journey toward finding herself.

For it is in finding and accepting your many feelings—from joyous to sad, from angry to ecstatic, from repulsion to love—that you grow to find, to accept and, finally, to love yourself.

CHAPTER FIVE

Healthy Body / Healthy Mind

I'm 18 and have a friend who drives me crazy talking about how you are what you eat! I'm pretty healthy, not overweight and still eat a good amount of junk food. Is there anything to all this health food stuff? I don't know a lot about nutrition. It seems so boring! But I wonder if my friend is right about what you eat having a lot to do with your health. I think it's dumb to be caught up in minute details about your body and what you eat. I'd rather be free!

Erin M.

I'm 17 and never had a date because I'm so overweight. I want to have a normal life, but I can't stick to any diet. I hate myself!

Hopeless

I'm into jogging, but have problems with my right knee. How can I keep from injuring it again?

John K.

Is it true that sunbathing is bad for your skin? I have good skin and want to keep it that way. Any tips for keeping a good, clear complexion?

Nancy A.

I hate doctors, but I hate dentists even worse. Do I have to have a checkup every year? How come? I brush my teeth pretty regularly.

Clancey C.

My dad just came down with diabetes and he also has heart trouble and he's only in his forties! Does this mean I'll get these things, too, when I'm his age? I'd like to stay healthy and live a long time because I enjoy life so much. What can I do to avoid getting health problems like my dad's?

Myles R.

Living a long, healthy, happy life is just about everyone's dream. It can become reality, but it means work, awareness, and more work! Having and maintaining a healthy body means being concerned with all aspects of your health—from nutrition to regular exercise, from taking good care of your skin, hair, and teeth to understanding how preventive measures on your part may keep you healthy for years to come.

There seems to be a correlation between health and happiness. It's hard to be happy if you're not feeling well or if you're unhappy with yourself, you may tend to neglect your body and thus become caught up in a spiral of bad feelings, both mental and physical. Your body plays a major part in how you do generally. If you feel well, you'll do better in all aspects of your life.

Your body is you, and it's vital that you build a strong, healthy body to go along with your active, healthy mind. You may get tired of the same old advice: eat well, take vitamins, exercise, get sufficient sleep, take care of your skin, exercise(!), watch your weight, visit your dentist once a year, exercise (enough already!).

We'll admit it may all sound superboring . . . *until* you begin to turn into a highly personal action plan, one that will help you to stay active—and attractive—all your life!

Contrary to Erin's fear of the health-conscious young person getting caught up in "minute health details," an awareness of your body's needs and possibilities will *free* you to become the best possible you!

ARE YOU WHAT YOU EAT?

Yes! What you eat has a huge impact not only on your physical health and appearance, but may also influence your emotions.

The Basic Food Groups

You've probably heard more times than you'd like about the basic food groups. We'll go over them once more—briefly—before exploring *why* some foods are essential to good health.

The four basic food groups are:

1. *Meat and Other Foods Rich in Protein.*   These include all types of meat (beef, pork, lamb, poultry), fish and seafood, eggs, cheese, and peanut butter.
2. *Fruits and Vegetables.*   This second category includes all fruits from apples to watermelon and green

68

and other low-calorie vegetables such as asparagus, broccoli, mushrooms, green beans, lettuce, cauliflower, and celery.

3. *Breads, Pasta, Cereal, and Other Vegetables*. This group, which furnishes you with needed carbohydrates, includes bread, pancakes, waffles, crackers, cereals, rice, beans, carrots, corn, peas, onions, and potatoes.

4. *Milk and Milk Products*. This includes all kinds of milk, from whole to nonfat and buttermilk. It also includes all types of cheese (including cottage cheese), yogurt, and ice cream.

Extras include foods like margarine, sugar, and nuts.

Although the basic food groups contain a wide variety of possibilities, many teens, and older people, too, fail to take advantage of this infinite variety.

Many medical experts worry most about teen-agers, however.

"According to the Department of Agriculture studies, the worst diets in America today are those of teen-agers," says Dr. Emanuel Cheraskin, chairman of the Department of Oral Medicine at the University of Alabama and coauthor of the best-selling book *Psychodietetics*.

Dr. Cheraskin, who is both a physician and a dentist, adds that "teen-age girls have the very worst diets of all. Too many teens of both sexes have diets heavy on junk foods, but girls often combine this with attempts to diet, often with fad diets, which means they may eliminate whole categories of food."

These extremes may be typified by two teen-agers we'll call Peter and Caroline.

Peter's usual breakfast is a sweet roll and coffee. He munches a chocolate bar during his 10 o'clock study hall and favors macaroni, cake, and soft drinks for lunch. After school, he snacks on ice cream, cookies, and more soda. Dinner varies. It may mean meat, potatoes, and a vegetable at home, but it often means a hamburger, fries, and chocolate shake at a local fast-food outlet. Before going to bed, Peter likes to have some crackers or cookies and hot chocolate.

Caroline, on the other hand, is *very* conscious of her weight. She always skips breakfast, has coffee for lunch, and may have a salad for dinner.

Both Peter and Caroline are starving themselves nutritionally in somewhat different ways. Caroline (who is not overweight) is not taking in nearly enough calories. Peter is taking in plenty of calories, but many of these calories are "empty"—with no accompanying nutrients.

What is a calorie?

A calorie is a measure of heat energy, the amount of energy in the form of heat that the body is able to produce from a food substance. A pound of weight contains 3,500 calories of energy. To gain a pound, you must take in and store that amount. To lose a pound, you must get rid of that amount. Carbohydrates, fats, and protein contain calories. Water, minerals, and vitamins do not. Girls between the ages of 12 and 18 need from 2,000 to 2,400 calories a day. Boys in the same age range require from 2,500 to 3,000 calories a day. These calorie requirements are to maintain your current weight. Obviously, if you need to lose weight, you must reduce the number of calories you take in each day. Excess calories, ones the body cannot manage to burn up, are stored as body fat.

But calories aren't all you require.

Some teens—like Peter—may take in plenty of calories, and because they are active, may be able to avoid becoming overweight. They will still be undernourished, however, because we need not only calories, but also vitamins and minerals. Some foods, like sugar-laden, sweets, furnish *only* calories without essential nutrients. Nutritionists call these "empty calorie" foods or junk foods.

To see why junk foods may, as a steady diet, be harmful, it's necessary to know what you're missing when you subsist on snack foods.

What you may be missing are the essential vitamins and minerals that are all supplied in a good, well-balanced diet.

Vitamins

Some of the essential vitamins include:

• *VITAMIN A*. Helps you to grow normally and to maintain healthy skin, teeth, gums, and eyes. Vitamin A also aids the repair of body tissue. It is found in milk, butter, margarine, carrots, liver, eggs, and dark green and yellow vegetables and fruits.

• *VITAMIN B_1 (Thiamine)*. Also promotes healthy eyes, skin, and body tissues. It is found in meat, fish, poultry, and in some cereals.

• *VITAMIN B_2 (Riboflavin)*. Is essential for smooth skin and clear vision. It is found in dairy products (including ice cream), enriched bread and cereal, eggs, poultry, fish, and meat.

• *VITAMIN B_6 (Pyridoxine)*. Helps to maintain the health of the skin, the red blood cells, and the nervous system. It is found in meat, liver, cereals, and vegetables.

• *VITAMIN B_{12} (Cyanocobalamin)*. Is important for a healthy nervous system and helps to protect you against certain types of anemia. Important sources of vitamin B_{12} are liver, meat, and milk.

• *VITAMIN C (Ascorbic Acid)*. Promotes healthy capillaries, gums, bones, and teeth. Delicious sources of vitamin C include citrus fruits, cantaloupes, berries, tomatoes, green peppers, and broccoli.

- *VITAMIN D.* Also helps you to make use of calcium and phosphorus in building strong bones and teeth. You can get this vitamin via fortified milk, liver and other organ meats, eggs, and fish (especially salmon).
- *VITAMIN E.* While the exact function of this vitamin has been open to debate, it is theorized that vitamin E prevents abnormal breakdown of fat in body tissues and helps the body to utilize other nutrients. Seeds, nuts, soybeans, wheat germ, and whole grain cereals are all sources of vitamin E.
- *NIACIN.* Converts food to energy and plays a part in forming certain hormones. Niacin is found in red meat, poultry, liver, milk, eggs, and peanut butter.
- *FOLIC ACID.* Helps cell formation, most notably in red blood cells, and may help prevent certain types of anemia. Folic acid is found in asparagus, broccoli, spinach, lima beans, and liver.
- *PANTOTHENIC ACID.* Helps you to metabolize carbohydrates and fats as well as other vital substances. Sources of this vitamin include eggs, broccoli, nuts, and liver.

Minerals

There are certain minerals that we need, too, to keep the body healthy and strength constant. Some of these include:

- *CALCIUM.* This not only helps you to have healthy teeth, bones, nerves, and muscles, but it also helps your blood to clot normally. Milk products (including yogurt and cheese), shellfish, and green, leafy vegetables all contain calcium.
- *PHOSPHORUS.* Helps get energy to your cells and is found in meats, cheese, and milk.
- *FLUORIDE.* Found in soybeans, lettuce, and onions as well as specially treated water, this mineral helps you to have strong teeth and bones.
- *POTASSIUM.* Is necessary for growth, a healthy nervous system, and a strong heart. It also helps to regulate the balance of water in your body. Potatoes, orange juice, leafy vegetables, bananas, dried fruits, and lean meats all contain potassium.
- *IODINE.* Found in seafood and iodized salt, iodine is an essential aid to your thyroid gland in regulating your energy and metabolism.
- *IRON.* This mineral is essential for young women who may lose iron via the menstrual flow and for pregnant women, but it is also necessary for all of us. It prevents some forms of anemia and increases one's resistance to disease. You can get iron from lean meat, eggs, dried fruits (especially raisins), whole grain breads and cereals, and liver.

Balanced Diet

A truly balanced diet does not eliminate any of the major food categories and contains a blend of vitamins and minerals, water, carbohydrates (vegetables, fruits, and grains) as an efficient source of energy, fats (like safflower oil) as a concentrated energy source, and proteins.

My mom is forever nagging me to eat a balanced diet. I like sweets and snack foods mostly, but she goes on about how I should eat things like eggs, milk, meat, and vegetables. Milk makes me gag, eggs are sickening, and I hate vegetables and don't like steaks or hamburger. What can I do?

Cecile K.

A balanced diet *is* important, but keep in mind that within the basic food groups, you have many choices. Milk products like yogurt and cottage cheese or even ice cream (in moderation) may be more to your taste than plain milk. Frozen yogurt seems to be a particularly popular—and nutritious—food choice among teens these days. You can also use milk in soups, casseroles, and puddings. Eggs can be ingredients of casseroles, soufflés, omelets, custards, and other dishes. If you hate vegetables, try new varieties—or the same variety in a different form. If, for example, you find canned green beans disgusting, try fresh or frozen green beans. The taste may be quite different. Steaming vegetables or cooking them in subtle seasonings may make a big difference, too. A little cinnamon sprinkled on yellow squash can make it a delicious side dish. A bit of cheese sauce can do wonders for vegetables like broccoli, asparagus, and cauliflower. If you're a hard-core vegetable hater, eating your vegetables in a soup or stew or in a Chinese dish like chow mein may make them infinitely more palatable. If you don't like red meat, that's OK. Cultivate a taste for chicken, fish, and seafood. There are many wonderful ways to prepare these—from salads to hot entrées.

The point is . . . you can eat a balanced diet and still make highly individual food choices!

I'm thinking of becoming a vegetarian. My best friend became one several weeks ago. My parents are having a fit, saying that I'll wither away and that there's no way I'll get enough nourishment. Is this true?

Kevin J.

It depends on the vegetarian diet you choose to follow.

A diet confined to brown rice (as in the Zen Macrobiotic diet) is severely deficient in necessary nutrients. According to the American Medical Association's Council on Foods and Nutrition, "The concepts proposed in Zen Macrobiotic constitute a major public health problem and are dangerous to its adherents."

However, a carefully balanced vegetarian diet, particularly a modified one, may be very healthy.

Betty Waldner, staff nutritionist for the Los Angeles County Health Department's Van Nuys Youth Clinic, sees a number of teens who are interested in becoming vegetarians.

"I advise common sense above all," she says. "I tend to discourage teens from choosing a strict vegetarian regimen because it's hard to follow and low in calcium and protein. However, if you add a balance of milk, eggs, and cheese, your diet may be quite adequate. Some teens also elect to include fish and seafood in their diets and this, too, may be good."

Before beginning a new way of eating, it is a good idea to make up a week-long menu plan and check it out with your physician, school nurse, or a nutritionist, to make sure that such a diet will be sufficiently balanced to meet your nutritional needs.

My buddy is into organic foods and vitamins. He says that these are much more nutritious. Is that true?
Paul S.

There is a lot of controversy about the whole subject of so-called health foods. At this time, there is no evidence that organic foods and vitamins are, indeed, more nutritious.

Vitamins are vitamins—and are identical in structure whether they are natural or synthetic. The only difference between the two may be in price rather than quality. Vitamins are best obtained by good eating habits. Certainly, vitamin pills are no substitute for a balanced and varied diet.

Organic foods, generally, are those fertilized by compost with no sprays or pesticides. There is no scientific proof at present that organic vegetables and fruits are better than those you'd find in your supermarket. In fact, the ones in the supermarket may be fresher and therefore more nutritious. Washing supermarket fruits and vegetables thoroughly should remove any pesticides.

The only harm organic foods might do is to deplete your food budget (they are more expensive) and, possibly, fool you into an unbalanced diet. Keep in mind that no one food is a ticket to good health. You need a balance of the four basic food groups for good nutrition.

As long as the essential balance is there and economic considerations aside, it probably doesn't matter much to your body whether you eat supermarket or health store fare.

Diet-Related Health Problems

I'm constipated a lot. What causes this? I exercise a lot and drink plenty of water, but I'm only fine when I take laxatives.

Worried

I have bad pains in my stomach at times. What could be causing these? I've had them for over a year. If it matters, I'm 17.

Bill T.

I have this really embarrassing gas problem! Could it be because I eat too much fruit? I only eat about an apple a day. This is a terrible problem for me— you'd better believe it! Help!

Mortified

If you are a victim of chronic constipation and your physician has not found any organic disease, your eating habits may be at fault. Regular meals, plenty of water, and a lot of fresh fruits, vegetables, and salads with oil-based dressings may help a great deal. A tablespoon of mineral oil a day may also help to keep you regular. *Do not* take laxatives unless your doctor so advises.

Pains in the stomach may come from a variety of causes. One may be gastritis or hyperacidity. This causes severe stomach pains that may be felt in the middle of the chest, too. When this happens, people often call it heartburn. Gastritis occurs when the stomach secretes excess acid and digestive enzymes that digest all the food in the stomach and then start in on the stomach wall! If this is allowed to continue, it may be the beginning of an ulcer. While the major factor here may be emotional upset, diet may also figure largely in the problem. Skipping meals, eating very acidic and/or unbalanced meals (for example, too many colas, fried and greasy food) may aggravate—if not cause—the condition. Alcohol, coffee, and cigarettes (even in moderate amounts) may cause excessive stomach acid secretions in some individuals. Eliminating these factors may help. In addition to three regular, well-balanced meals a day, it may be necessary to take antacids to neutralize excess stomach acid. Milk and milk products (including ice cream) are natural antacids. Nonprescription antacids in tablet or liquid form are also available. If pain continues, despite these measures, it is important to consult your physician.

A number of teens complain about flatus, or gas. Medical studies have shown that food may be a major factor here. The worst culprits seem to be apples, apple juice, apple cider, radishes, and cabbage. Avoiding some of these gas-producing foods as much as possible may help. Eating your food slowly—to avoiding gulping air along with your food—may also play a part in alleviating the problem. If you have an unusually stubborn case of flatus, you might want to try one of several nonprescription, over-the-counter drugs that contain simethicone. This helps by dissipating gas, breaking the surface tension of the gas bubbles in the intestines.

I wonder if too many soft drinks with sugar could rot your stomach. I say yes. My brother, who drinks a 64-ounce bottle of cola every day, says no. Who's right?

Holly L.

I've read some stuff about junk food and especially sugar that says this can affect your feelings as well as your physical health. Is this a bunch of BS or is it true? I like sweets a lot. Can this hurt me?

Jim P.

Soft drinks, in moderation, are not necessarily harmful, but there are several possibilities that concern us about Holly's brother (who is putting away a half gallon of cola a day!) and other teens who drink large quantities of these beverages.

First, these drinks (except for the diet variety) contain a fair amount of empty calories and may be replacing the more beneficial calories that might be acquired through a balanced diet.

Second, in some cases, the acidic, carbonated content of cola may be harmful to the stomach (which already secretes acid). When such fluids are taken in excess and to the exclusion of other fluids, such as milk, which neutralize the acidity of the stomach, problems (like gastritis) can occur.

Finally, most nondiet soft drinks are high in sugar content and the effect of so much sugar on one's teeth—and general health—must be considered.

Drinking large quantities of diet drinks is not a good idea either since the safety of the artificial sweetener saccharin is currently being investigated. Some preliminary findings have indicated that it may be a cancer-causing agent, but study results are not yet conclusive.

What impact *can* a heavy intake of sugar have on your health?

Theories and estimates vary, but the fact is that young people in general consume great quantities of sweets. A poll by *Progressive Grocer* revealed recently that those in the 10- to 14-year-old age group consume an average of 33 pounds of candy per person a year! Those in the 15- to 19-year-old age group scored a close second—with 30 pounds of candy per person annually.

Sugar, of course, is not only found in candy, but in all sweet snacks *and* in convenience foods. There is, for example, sugar in ketchup, hot dog relish, canned vegetables and soups, most cereals, frozen dinners, and bottled salad dressing.

Sugar consumption, of course, has been heavily implicated in tooth decay, but many medical experts believe that its effects may be much more far-reaching. Many believe that there may be a link between excessive sugar consumption and health problems like obesity, heart disease, hypoglycemia, and diabetes, to name a few.

The *main* problem with sugar may be that it adds large amounts of empty calories to our daily diets and may be replacing essential vitamins and minerals. Thus, we may become more prone to disease and to obesity (which may be a factor in developing diabetes in middle age).

Many physicians believe, too, that excessive consumption of sugar may also cause personality and behavioral problems.

"We hear from educators that eliminating junk foods results in less rambunctiousness, better grades, attention and obedience, and less absenteeism," says Dr. Emanuel Cheraskin, the physician/dentist we quoted a little earlier in this chapter.

Preliminary findings of studies conducted at Kaiser-Permanente Medical Centers in San Francisco, Ohio, Oklahoma, and Canada seem to suggest that high levels of sugar, combined with various chemical additives in junk foods, may trigger violence and/or possible mental problems, particularly in those who may have so-called hidden allergies to these ingredients.

Many physicians insist that a lot of sugar isn't good for *anyone*.

"During World War II, Denmark and Norway were deprived of sugar due to the German blockade and, as a nation, their health improved!" says Dr. Cheraskin. "The rates of cancer, heart disease, tooth decay, and so on were noticeably lower. I believe that the following message should be printed on all candy wrappers: 'This product can be dangerous to your mental health!' The sugar-laden American diet may be leading to a national epidemic of hypoglycemia, which may have among its symptoms irrational behavior, distorted judgment, and emotional instability."

We will be discussing hypoglycemia in detail in

Chapter Nine, but will simply point out here that hypoglycemia, or low blood sugar, may happen when the pancreas overproduces insulin in the wake of too much sugar and may be the result of poor eating habits—like the coffee, sweet roll, and cigarette breakfast of many Americans. This, with its combination of caffeine, sugar, and nicotine, triggers a flood of insulin into the system and dramatically lowers the blood sugar. Other symptoms of low blood sugar may include: dizziness, fainting, headaches, fatigue, muscle pains, insomnia, irritability, crying spells, inability to concentrate, forgetfulness, temper tantrums, and shortness of breath. Some physicians feel that an addiction to sugar may mimic hypoglycemia.

"I see only five or six cases of true organic hypoglycemia a year and I see nothing but metabolic cases!" says Dr. Rachmiel Levine, a renowned specialist in metabolic disorders and executive medical director of the City of Hope National Medical Center in Duarte, Calif. "What may seem to be hypoglycemia may be an addiction to sweets or to put it bluntly, cookie-itis. Some people will have a cookie and claim to feel better immediately, long before the cookie is even *digested,* let alone absorbed into the bloodstream!"

An addiction to sugar may lead to vitamin deficiencies that can have a considerable impact on your physical and mental health.

"Medical investigators have known for many years that severe nutritional deficiency can cause mental illness," says Dr. Cheraskin. "In some cases we've treated, diet corrections alone helped the patient. In other cases, diet correction plus other forms of therapy have helped long-term patients to recover. We have found that a lack of calcium may cause symptoms like nervousness, exaggerated fears, and sleep disturbances. Low levels of vitamin B_3 may cause you to be humorless and overly emotional. A lack of niacin may also affect your sense of humor. If nothing seems too funny these days, don't be so quick to blame the world situation. Plentiful servings of raw green vegetables, whole grain cereals, eggs, organ meats, and nuts might help you to laugh again!"

Many young people tend to be leery of reports that sugar may be so harmful. After all, few of us have ever keeled over after eating a candy bar or even a whole bunch of cupcakes!

When we talk about harm, we're talking about habitual and excessive sugar consumption. The effects of too much sugar—and too many empty calories—aren't always immediate. But in long-term, total health planning, it makes sense to limit sugar intake as much as possible. This may not mean a drastic change of diet, but simply a few wisely chosen substitutions in your daily diet.

I love fast-food hamburgers, fries, and shakes. I'm 15, active, and not overweight and I like to have these as dinner at least three times a week. I have a coach who is a nutrition nut who hates the whole idea of this. Now we're arguing because of a magazine article I found where a nutrition expert said that a meal like this isn't harmful for an active teen-ager. Naturally, the coach pulls an article by another big expert out of his files and this guy says that this meal is high in fat and could be harmful. Now we're back to where we started. Would YOU like to referee this???
                                              Ron H.

The meal that Ron describes, which is a favorite with many teens, is the center of a fair amount of controversy.

A number of nutrition experts believe that these fast-food meals, although high in calories, will not be particularly harmful when eaten in moderation by an active young person, especially if supplemented with fruit, vegetables, milk, and salad.

There are others, however, who voice considerable concern. These meals, they point out, are not only high in sugar, but also in fat content. High-fat diets—like many Americans who favor steaks, potatoes piled with butter, hamburgers, and so forth tend to eat—may be linked in later years with heart disease and certain cancers. Some believe that with high-fat diets, you don't always have to wait until middle age to see the consequences.

A recent survey by the American Health Foundation of nearly 22,000 12- to 15-year-olds revealed that more than 30 percent of the young people had abnormally high cholesterol levels. And autopsies of young soldiers killed in action in Vietnam and Korea often revealed the clogged arteries of old men in the superficially healthy young bodies.

It's never too soon, many nutrition experts believe, to establish good dietary habits. This is especially true in adolescence when many of your lifetime food habits and preferences are being formed. At age 30, you may not be able to eat great quantities of junk food and fast food without piling on weight. A drastic change of diet may be difficult at that age, after your weight gain is under way and your preferences set on high-fat, high-calorie food. Growing up with healthful food habits—salads, vegetables, seafood, chicken, and veal—will help you to maintain your weight and your health throughout adulthood.

I'm a 16-year-old girl and I'm afraid that I'm going to have a problem with my weight if I don't do something soon. Right now, I'm pretty OK—maybe three to five pounds over my ideal weight. I hate the whole idea of dieting. I enjoy eating and need the energy. I think I'm eating too many calories, but I really need my snacks. I don't like diet food, but I can tolerate diet sodas sometimes. What I'd like is a way to keep my weight down and even lose some weight gradually without going hungry. I'm attaching a list of my present typical day's diet. What changes could I make? Could you please help me?

Sally W.

Although we will be talking in much greater detail about weight control soon in this chapter, we thought that Sally's question here might help many teens who may not have weight problems now, or who may have very minor weight gains, maintain a healthy, trim body.

Controlling a minor weight problem does not call for drastic dietary change, simply for wise substitutions. If you have more than a few pounds to lose, of course, you may wish to read the upcoming section on weight control *and* consult your physician before beginning *any* diet.

There are a lot of teens like Sally, though, who are anxious to stop minor weight gains before they become major problems. Looking at Sally's typical day's menu, we agree with her that her calorie intake during a typical day is too much. In our revised version of her daily menu plan, we have cut the calories in half via simple food substitutions, while staying close to Sally's food preferences.

This diet revision, as you can see, does not spell "deprivation." Snacks and desserts are a part of this sensible eating plan that will enable Sally to halt weight gain and even shed a few pounds in time. This action plan to maintain her ideal weight has worked well for Sally. A similar substitution plan may help you to stay trim, too.

"MY PROBLEM IS . . . MY WEIGHT!"

This is a common lament among teens—both boys and girls, and both those who are (or feel that they are) overweight or underweight. There are many differences, of course, among these weight-conscious adolescents.

There is the guy who is teased because he is skinny and the guy who carries around 20 extra pounds of what his mom still insists is baby fat.

There is the girl who weighs over 200 pounds and who has just about given up the dream of ever being slender and the girl who can't seem to gain weight, no matter what she eats!

Then there is the already slender girl who diets constantly because her friends do or because she'd like to wear an even smaller dress size.

What you would like to weigh and the best weight for your height and build may differ. You can check a weight chart to see the average weights for your age, height, and build.

Help! I'm too skinny and all the other kids tease me. I'm 14 and just starting to get breasts, but mostly my figure still looks like a dumb kid's! I want to look like everyone else. Would eating more candy help me to gain weight? My aunt says I ought to count my blessings that I'm thin, but I don't see it that way. I'm too thin!

Tina S.

A lot of people might agree with Tina's aunt, but if being thin is a problem for *you*, you've probably had it with such comments, right?

If you are thinner than you'd like to be, you might want to try the following suggestions:

Consider Your Age, State of Physical Development, and Body Type. Some young people in early adolescence who are just beginning to develop may be temporarily expending a lot of calories in growth. As your growth rate slows down a bit, you may tend to fill out. It may take time, too, to develop a mature figure, whether you're male or female. There are a number of young teens who still have a child's figure. Time will help. Also, there are people who have more angular bodies than others. You may be one of these.

Keep a Diary of Everything *You Eat for at Least a Week.* Note your eating habits. Do you eat three well-balanced meals a day or do you snack a little here and there and tend to skip meals a lot? Do you have trouble eating when you're nervous or upset? Are you extremely active? Are you a nibbler who tastes lots of food, but who never finishes anything? Linda, for example, told us that she had "pot roast with potatoes and vegetables, milk and chocolate cake" for dinner the night before. When asked how much she actually ate, her countdown was "three small bites of roast, one bite of potato, one carrot, half a glass of milk, and two tiny bites of cake." In your food diary, *do* note how much (or how little) you actually eat!

Take Steps to Change Behavior That Keeps You Skinny. Eliminate snacks before mealtimes if this tends to spoil your appetite, and eat larger meals. Never skip a meal! Try to stop nibbling and start eating, even if it takes you longer than anyone else. (Some teens are very conscious of not wanting to be the last to finish a meal. Enlist the aid of your family. They may be very glad to help you by not making a big deal about it if you do eat slowly.) Even if you're feeling upset, try to eat regular meals. Your body needs essential nutrients, no matter what you're feel-

Typical Day's Menu

Original Breakfast

1 orange	65 calories
1 pecan roll	240 calories
1 fried egg	110 calories
1 glass milk	160 calories
TOTAL	575 calories

Revised Breakfast

1 orange	65 calories
1 plain English muffin	145 calories
1 poached egg	75 calories
1 glass nonfat milk	90 calories
	375 calories

Original lunch

Tuna fish sandwich (oil-packed tuna, 2 tbsp. mayo, 2 slices of bread)	510 calories
1 glass milk with 1 scoop ice cream	325 calories
½ cup corn	85 calories
1 slice pineapple (canned, syrup)	90 calories
TOTAL	1,010 calories

Revised Lunch

Tuna fish sandwich (water-packed tuna, 2 tbsp. low-cal mayo, 2 slices of bread)	280 calories
1 glass nonfat milk	90 calories
½ cup broccoli	20 calories
1 slice pineapple (canned, in its own juice)	65 calories
	455 calories

Original Afternoon Snack

1 slice apple pie	350 calories
1 slice Cheddar cheese	115 calories
12 oz. cola	145 calories
TOTAL	610 calories

Revised Afternoon Snack

1 medium apple	70 calories
1 slice Cheddar cheese	115 calories
12 oz. diet cola	2 calories
	187 calories

Original Dinner

Salad with 2 tbsp. French dressing	145 calories
1 chicken breast, fried	420 calories
½ cup mashed potatoes with gravy	120 calories
½ cup mixed vegetables	85 calories
½ cup lima beans	90 calories
1 glass milk	160 calories
1 piece of chocolate cake, with frosting	235 calories
TOTAL	1,255 calories

Revised Dinner

Salad with 2 tbsp. low-cal French dressing	33 calories
1 chicken breast, broiled	205 calories
½ cup mashed potatoes with margarine	90 calories
½ cup spinach	20 calories
½ cup lima beans	90 calories
1 glass nonfat milk	90 calories
1 piece of Angel Food cake, with no frosting	135 calories
TOTAL	663 calories

Original Evening Snack

4 1-inch chocolate chip cookies	200 calories

Revised Evening Snack

1 tbsp. peanut butter on four saltines	145 calories

TOTAL CALORIES FOR DAY: 3,650

TOTAL CALORIES FOR DAY: 1,825

---

ing. And a well-nourished body may give you extra strength to cope with a crisis!

Supplement Your Daily Diet in Little (But Nutritious) Ways! A sudden frenzy of candy eating or a cupcake binge may do more harm than good. Besides making you ill (and even less inclined than ever to eat), these foods will only give you empty calories.

It's better to pamper your body with more nutritious foods—that also happen to be delicious! Add snacks like granola, bread and peanut butter, and milk products to your diet. Fruits and vegetables are important, too.

If You're Only a Little *Underweight, You Might* Consider *Counting Your Blessings!* A slender body that is, nevertheless, well-nourished can be a healthy, attractive one. As time goes by and your calorie needs decrease, you may tend to put on weight anyway. You may want to start a little low and thus reach (and then maintain) the average weight for your height after your growing years are over.

If You're Active—Don't Stop!   Regular exercise is a health *must* for everybody. If you're set on gaining weight, simply increase your caloric intake, but *do* keep exercising.

There are thin teens who fit into quite a different category: those suffering from a disorder called *anorexia nervosa.*

We will be discussing this in detail in Chapter Eight, but a brief explanation here may be in order. Teens afflicted with anorexia nervosa diet and exercise compulsively and may even starve themselves to death. These teens, however, usually have a distorted body image, and do not see themselves as underweight (even at 50 or 60 pounds!). They imagine that they are either heavy or just right and are very resistant to efforts to help them gain weight. Because this is a psychological as well as physical disorder, which happens to manifest itself in drastic weight loss, we will be discussing this in detail in ''Mind Over Body,'' Chapter Eight.

I'm 17 and never had a date because I'm so overweight. I want to have a normal life, but I can't stick to any diet. I hate myself so much! Help!
                                        Hopeless

I'd like to lose about 10 to 15 pounds. What is the best way to do this? One friend told me about a banana diet and another about a high protein diet and I've read about the liquid protein diet and wonder if it's safe. Which one is best?
                                        Beverly P.

I'm a yo-yo dieter. I go up and down, up and down. I've tried every diet there is and I do lose weight, but I put it right back on again. How can I get weight off and keep it off?
                                        Ellen J.

I've always been overweight and my parents say it's just something to do with my glands and maybe I'll outgrow it. I'm 16 and still waiting. Both my parents are heavy. Could fat be hereditary?
                                        Janet

I feel like someone from a different planet! I've been about 30 pounds overweight for the last four years.

Whenever I'm nervous or upset, I eat (with my friends it's just the opposite). Also, I notice that I never really feel full and finish everything and can eat more, while my sister can have a plate half filled with her favorite food, feel full, and be unable to eat another bite! I used to feel different because I was heavy. Now I wonder if I might be heavy because I'm different . . .
                                        Claudia Y.

Did you see yourself in any of these letters?

If you're weight-conscious, you could probably identify with at least one of them. A number of physicians treating adolescents report that overweight has become a number-one concern among teens.

For some seriously overweight adolescents, this is a very real problem. For some others, this concern may be exaggerated. Some, while maintaining a very normal, healthy weight, feel fat after looking through fashion magazines at the often underweight and sometimes downright emaciated models. This, however, is an unrealistic measure of health and beauty. Some of these models must follow unhealthy regimens (like one meal a day!) to maintain below-normal weight. The emaciated look may sell clothes, but it is *not* conducive to good health. And nothing is more beautiful than a healthy body.

A more accurate measure of your weight would be to check a weight chart and also check with your physician, school nurse, or local clinic to determine the *healthiest* weight for YOUR body.

Weight isn't the only determination of whether or not you are too fat. Although people tend to use the terms *overweight* and *obese* almost interchangeably (though, admittedly, obese may be more synonymous with *gross*), there is a difference between them. And you can be obese without being gross at all!

Overweight means that you weigh more than other people of your sex, height, and body build.

Obese means that you carry too much fat on your body.

An athlete may weigh more than others his or her age and height, but may not be obese. He or she carries extra weight in muscle mass, not fat.

A teen-age television addict, on the other hand, may fall within the average weight category and yet, due to his or her long hours immobilized in front of the tube and virtual lack of physical exercise, he or she may have too much body fat.

You can test yourself to see if you are carrying around excess fat via the simple pinch test. Pinch a fold of skin on one side of your waist or on your upper arm. If this fold of skin measures more than one inch, you have excess fat.

Another test for fat (if you're a real glutton for guilt

and need more proof!) is the infamous ruler test. Take off your clothes, lie down on the floor, and place a ruler on your body, with one end at your rib cage and the other at your pelvic bones. Ideally (if you're not too fat), the ruler will rest on these bones. If the situation is less than ideal and you do have excess fat, the ruler will seesaw—even bobble—back and forth.

Once you discover that you have excess fat (if you weren't already painfully aware of it), what can you do about it? One of the first steps you can take is to learn the truth behind some common myths about fat and dieting.

Fat Is Hereditary.

UNTRUE! Whole families can be fat, but this is usually a case of shared (fattening) food preferences and eating habits (like using food to deal with tension, depression, boredom, or anger). These "inherited" habits can be broken.

Sometimes, hereditary factors make it especially important for you to go against family tradition and keep your weight down. This may be especially true if the older people in your family are heavy and tend to develop diabetes in middle age.

"There is a strong relationship between obesity and diabetes," says Dr. Rachmiel Levine. "Particularly if you have a family history of diabetes, your chances of developing the disease are greatly increased if you are overweight."

If You're a Fat Teen-ager, Chances Are It's Baby Fat.

UNTRUE! Fat is fat, So-called baby fat, or fat developed during childhood, may be the most stubborn fat of all.

"Some of the most difficult obesity cases are those who have been fat as babies and small children," says Dr. Levine. "When you are obese in these early years, you experience an increase in fat cells in your body and these fat cells never really go away. It's harder to lose weight, and once you've lost it, it may be easier for you to regain it."

Even if you have had a lifelong battle with fat, however, you can lose it and, with careful diet maintenance, keep it off!

It's important that you start to shed that fat *now,* though. Don't wait to outgrow it. Hard work—not time—is the only way you'll get it off and keep it off. If that sounds like a grim possibility, consider this: It may be easier for you to lose weight now than it will be in five or ten years. And why spend any more time feeling fat and unattractive? Now is the very best time to begin to win the weight war!

"It's Your Glands . . ."

Exhaustive medical studies have shown that only a *very* small percentage of obese people can point to glandular or metabolic problems as the cause of obesity. However, obesity—as the result of chronic overeating—may affect your metabolism.

"The hypothalamus gland, located in the brain, is your own internal scale," says Dr. Levine. "It weighs you internally and usually maintains your weight. You may go for years at the same weight. Then something happens. The balance is tipped and you gain."

This tip of your weight balance may happen with a drastic change of activity or eating patterns, Dr. Levine adds.

Lisa, for example, was an aspiring ballerina until a year ago. She spent about six hours a day at lessons and practice. Then a serious injury to her Achilles tendon shattered her dreams of a classical dance career and kept her relatively immobile for a time. She gained weight rapidly.

Alex found the same to be true when he stopped playing football. His activity went down while his calorie consumption remained high, so his weight soared.

Marilyn, a bride at 19 and a mother at 20, found that her weight started creeping up after her first baby was born. Feeling trapped, exhausted, and bored at times by the constant responsibility of the baby, she began to nibble and soon found that not only was her weight increasing, but also the sense of feeling full after eating was gone.

It may well be that chronic overeating may interfere with the "Stop! Enough!" message from the hypothalamus, the message that makes you say "I'm full." It has been found that many obese people can eat large quantities of food without getting the message that they are full.

You Should Eat When You Feel the Need to Eat.

UNTRUE! Some people's *feelings* of need exceed their actual needs.

Researchers have found that so-called hunger cues in obese people may differ a great deal from true hunger.

In his award-winning studies of obese rats and humans at Columbia University, Dr. Stanley Schacter discovered that people of normal weight feel hunger only when their stomachs contract. Obese people, however, may feel prompted to eat at the sight of food, at the ready availability of food, out of boredom, or in the face of rejection. The worse they feel, the more they eat.

It's important to learn to distinguish between true hunger and psychological hunger. As you hurry to the kitchen, stop and ask yourself "How am I feeling?" You may be truly hungry. But then again, you may be feeling bored, restless, angry, depressed, or any number of feelings that may trigger your "hunger cues." It's important to begin to know how you're feeling and to learn to distinguish between hunger and your emotions.

There Are Diet Aids That Melt Off Fat Effortlessly.

UNTRUE! If a skinniness pill existed, its inventor would be the richest person on earth!

Unfortunately, there are no shortcuts, wonder drugs, or miracle substances that melt away fat.

Diet and exercise are the only weight-control measures that *really* work.

The Faster You Lose Weight, The Better.

UNTRUE!   There are diets that enable you to lose weight quickly, but these have three major disadvantages:

1. They're difficult, and often unhealthy, to sustain over a long period of time. Therefore, you tend to go back to your old eating habits and preferences after the diet is over.

2. They do nothing to change your behavior about food. What you're doing is a temporary sacrifice to achieve an ultimate goal—a slender body. You're not learning a new way to deal with your eating habits for a lifetime.

3. As soon as you go off such quick-weight-loss diets and eat normally, the weight tends to come right back on.

Via a quick, crash diet, you may only join the ranks of yo-yo dieters (who are forever losing-gaining-losing-gaining), but also endanger your health.

A slow, but steady weight loss is better for you, both physically and psychologically. The commitment that it takes to stay with a long-range diet will also help you to *keep* the weight off once you lose it.

What You Need Is a Diet with a Gimmick.

UNTRUE!   What you need is a diet you can live with. There are countless gimmicks around. Some—like an unsupervised liquid protein diet—may endanger your health and even your life. Others—like the ubiquitous grapefruit diet, banana diet, and other one-item "miracle" diets—may bore you into cheating before you have time to endanger your health. Still others may represent more of a threat to your pocketbook than to your health.

Remember that *any* diet that promises you can eat as much as you want and not exercise is a rip-off! Still other diet gimmicks—like having your jaws wired shut—attempt to get rid of the symptoms of your weight problem (overeating) instead of really curing the problem. Unless you actually work to find out why you overeat and try to change your behavior, you will start gaining back the weight you lost as soon as those wires are clipped.

For most of us, weight control is *not* a miracle nor a short-term project. It requires a lifelong effort and revision of eating habits and behavior. The initial step in this battle against excess weight is to find out *why* you behave as you do.

In her letter earlier in this section, Claudia Y. asked if overweight people behave in different ways from people of normal weight. The answer is "Yes!" in many cases.

If you think that you may have a problem with your eating habits and behavior, ask yourself the following questions.

1. *Do you eat when you're upset, angry, nervous, or bored? When you want to reward yourself? Do you have special foods to fit specific feelings?*

Dr. Harvey Einhorn, a specialist in nutrition and metabolic disorders, contends that the foods you choose to eat may reveal a great deal about your emotional history. Eggs, milk, and butter, he claims, are security foods. Reward foods are ice cream, cake, cookies, and chocolate. Many overweight people use these security and reward foods to comfort them in times of stress and crisis, and to celebrate as well after a difficulty has passed.

2. *Are you a breakfast skipper?*

Studies show that one of the worst habits that obese teen-agers have is that of skipping breakfast. You may start the day with the best intentions, but eventually hunger and a feeling of deprivation may get the best of you. You'll tend to load up on food—and calories—late in the day. A good breakfast is essential for everybody, but especially for dieters.

3. *Do you eat faster than most people you know?*

In his studies at Columbia University, Dr. Stanley Schacter discovered that fat people eat 39 percent faster than those of normal weight. Fat people eat faster and they eat more. If you shovel your food in, you may be finished with a meal before your brain gets the message that your stomach is full. That's why you may be able to reach for a second helping you don't really need—or to raid the refrigerator right after a huge meal.

If you eat slowly, really tasting your food, you will feel full—and eat less. You can learn to eat slowly by setting your eating utensils down between each bite, by swallowing one bite before you take another, and by talking to your family during a meal.

4. Do you spend time preparing your food or do you tend to grab the first edible thing you happen to see?

Dr. Schacter also discovered that the obese are less likely to work for their food than those of normal weight. They are much more likely to grab convenient snack foods, usually high in calories and offering little nutritional value.

5. Do you dream about having dates and an active social life, but think that, in reality, this might be scary?

Fat can be a protective shield against pressures to date or against expressing your sexuality with another person. There are undeniable pressures involved in dating, particularly with regard to sexual choices. Some teens, often unconsciously, may try to avoid such pressures altogether by making themselves unattractive to others. This may be especially true for someone who has experienced some sort of sexual trauma at an early age. Dr. William Shipman of Michael Reese Hospital in Chicago did a study of obese women falling into this category and found that they were "affected for the rest of their lives . . . seeking solace in something safe like food rather than in something as dangerous as human contact, friendship, sex, and love."

6. Are you a stress eater?

Do you find yourself gobbling cupcakes after an argument with a friend? While you're trying to write a tough term paper? While waiting for someone special to call you?

If so, you're far from alone. Dr. Neil Solomon of Johns Hopkins Medical School in Baltimore has found that 75 percent of the obese people that he has studied respond to stress by eating. He adds that very often the stress eater feels underlying hostility toward some person or some situation, but would rather eat than voice such hostilities.

If you happen to be a stress eater, stop and think for a moment. How could you deal with stress in a more constructive way? It is a lot less fattening to pound a pillow, write an irate passage in your diary, exercise, or say how you feel.

7. Do you tend to eat when you're bored and have nothing else to do?

A lot of obese people fall into this trap. You have nothing to do, so you eat and gain weight. And the more weight you gain, the less inclined you are to do things, particularly if it involves exercise. So you stay sedentary and even more bored—and continue to eat. It can be a vicious cycle! Organizing your time around activities and well-spaced meals and snacks can help break this cycle of misery.

8. Are you rebelling against someone?

Before you dismiss this as an incredibly dumb question, think about it for a minute. Is it *very* important to your mother (or to someone else who is very close to you) that you be popular and have lots of dates? Does your mother want you to be prom queen just as she was (or wasn't!)? Is she always going on about beauty and fitness? Is she extremely weight-conscious? If so, you may be rebelling against your mother with fat.

Dr. Johanna T. Dwyer studied a group of obese women at Harvard University and discovered that many of them had mothers who had pushed them to succeed at everything and who talked about thinness as some kind of moral virtue—and being fat as the worst possible fate.

So how does a teen fight back against such pressure?

Some teens may choose to fight back by becoming fat and making their mothers' vision of the worst possible fate reality.

I want to lose weight really bad and I'll do anything to lose it! Please give me a diet that works. I need to lose about 40 pounds and I'm even thinking of going on that diet with the shots.

Kay S.

I want to fast to lose weight but my parents are against it. Lots of people do it. I can't see why I can't. I'm 17 and want to lose about 20 pounds fast.

Chris H.

I'm kind of upset. I just got back from an appointment with my doctor who talked to me for a long time about my weight. He said I'm much too heavy. I'm 15, 5 feet 4, and weigh 163 pounds. He suggested that I go to Weight Watchers, but I don't know. I'm not exactly a joiner type of person and like my privacy. I hear they weigh you in public and make fun of you if you don't lose a lot. Also, it is pretty expensive, isn't it? Do people lose this way? Or is it just another rip-off operation?

Charlotte K.

What many people seek in a diet is nothing short of a miracle: a diet that works fast and that requires little or no effort or deprivation as the pounds simply melt away. In search of such miracles, many people endanger their bank accounts—and their health.

Kay's letter, for example, mentions her willingness to try anything, notably "the diet with the shots." Kay is referring to injections of HCG (human chorionic gonadotrophin), combined with a 500-calorie-a-day diet used by a number of weight clinics across the nation.

These hormone shots, prepared from the urine of pregnant women, have been found in some studies to be virtually worthless in themselves. The *Journal of the American Medical Association* reported not long ago that a control group of patients getting saltwater shots fared just as well as those getting the hormone injections. This was seconded by an Air Force study that revealed no significant difference between obese patients receiving HCG injections and those receiving injections of a placebo. However, some people do lose weight on this regimen. Who *wouldn't* on a 500-calorie-a-day diet?

Not only is this treatment usually quite expensive, it may also be dangerous for teen-agers. Five hundred calories a day is *far* too low for teens, who should never go below 1,000–1,200 calories a day (and who shouldn't go even that low without medical approval and supervision).

What about fasting?

Fasting is not a healthy way for *most* teen-agers to lose weight. When you fast, you lose fat, but you also lose muscle tissue. This loss of muscle tissue is something you can ill afford when your body is still growing and developing. Fasting may also affect your bones and stunt your growth as well as putting a strain on your kidneys and liver, causing possible hair loss and, for women, menstrual irregularities.

There has been much interest in fasting, however, in the wake of the liquid protein diet fad, a modified fast that is, at this writing, causing a great deal of concern in the medical community due to reports of deaths among dieters using this method. The Food and Drug Administration has issued a warning against the public's using this diet plan without medical supervision, and there has been discussion of a possible ban.

This diet, which is much like a regular fast except that the dieter takes protein and vitamin-mineral supplements to help prevent the loss of much-needed body tissue, was originally developed for extremely obese people who would use the plan under strict medical supervision.

In recent months, however, bottles of liquid protein and diet kits have mushroomed on drug and department store shelves. Many people—a number of them only moderately overweight—have been following this diet regimen without any medical supervision.

Most physicians seem reluctant to put teens on such a diet unless they are *massively* obese and such obesity is contributing to other health problems, such as high blood pressure. If you fit into the massively obese category, you should check with your physician, who may supervise your diet or who may refer you to another doctor with more experience with the modified fasting program.

Actually, whether you have 15, 50, or 100 pounds to lose, you should check with your physician before beginning any diet. Besides checking your present health and possible health needs, your physician may be able to recommend a diet plan that may work for you.

Many physicians—like Charlotte's—recommend the Weight Watchers® program. Weight Watchers combines a sensible, well-balanced eating program with behavior modification, recommended physical exercise, and group support. There are some Weight Watchers branches that even have special teen groups. Even when only a general, all-ages group exists, teens seem well-represented.

A number of young people may be leery of the whole idea of organized dieting.

Charlotte, for example, wonders how much a diet group would cost—both financially and psychologically. She wonders whether the Weight Watchers diet works.

The eating program does work—the way a diet should. That is, it provides you with a balanced eating plan you can live with, one that allows you to eat normal food in controlled quantities. It enables you to lose weight at a steady pace and then, with the aid of a Maintenance Plan, to keep it off.

At this time, Weight Watchers cost $4.00 a week. You weigh in once a week, but can attend as many lectures that week as you like. The weekly fee includes weigh-in, lecture, and special materials—like "Eating Management Techniques"; a series of behavior modification pamphlets by Dr. Richard B. Stuart (a noted psychologist) with titles like "Breaking the Chain," "How to Use Rest, Relaxation, and Resistance to Manage Eating Binges," "How to Manage the Blues, Tension, Anger, and Boredom," and "How to Get Help from Loved Ones and Friends"; recipe sheets, and, in some chapters, small cookbooks, with delicious, diet-wise menus.

When you join Weight Watchers, you are given a Program Handbook that includes all versions of the program, which has variations for men, women, and youth. Weight Watchers don't count calories per se. (But calories in a typical WW daily menu plan might equal about 1,200.) Weight Watchers *do* weigh portions and follow a carefully outlined, balanced eating plan with a lot of room for individual food preferences.

What about possible ridicule and violation of privacy? At Weight Watchers you are weighed in private and nobody but you, your lecturer, and the weigh-in clerk *ever* know your weight! If you lose weight in a particular week, you are congratulated in a nice, low-key way. If you gain, you are *never* humiliated. The lecturers at Weight Watchers are *not* professional skinnies who can't understand how you feel. They've all fought and won their own weight wars. It's a requirement for the job. So they never do things like add to the pain you're already feeling for having gained by humiliating you in public. You may talk about an eating problem in private with your lecturer or you may share experiences and feelings with the others in your class, but only if you choose to do so. There is a lot of group spirit in many classes, but privacy is always respected.

There are a number of other diet groups, including the Diet Workshop and Overeaters Anonymous (which has more of an emphasis on group support than on diet per se). All of these groups are nationwide and you may find local chapters in your telephone directory.

Planning a Personal Diet

Maybe you're not a joiner.

You can diet effectively on your own, in many cases, but, if you plan to lose more than a few pounds, *do* let your physician in on your plans and let him or her help you to map out a sensible and healthy diet.

We are not including specific diet menus here for two reasons: One, you (with your physician) may best be able to plan a diet that will meet your own, individual requirements, and two, the most successful, long-range diet will adhere closely to your own food preferences—within reason, of course. (For an idea of how this might work, look back to our substitution plan for Sally's diet on page 75.)

There are some important points to remember in planning your own, individualized diet, however.

Your diet should include at least 1,000 or, better still, 1,200 calories a day, should not eliminate *any* of the major food groups (including carbohydrates), and should include a schedule of regular exercise.

Remember that you need the following foods every day:

• Two or more servings of protein, which is found in eggs, meat, cheese, beans, or dried peas.
• Three servings of vegetables and fruits.
• One serving of a citrus fruit.
• Half-cup servings of rice, cereal, or pasta *or* three slices of bread.
• Two or three servings (8 ounces each) of skim milk.

There are some inexpensive books that may help you a lot.

If you choose to count calories carefully, send for a pocket-sized calorie counter from the U.S. Department of Agriculture. You can get *Calories and Weight*

by sending $1.00 to: Superintendent of Documents, U.S. Government Printing Office, Washington, D.C. 20402.

You may also find calorie charts and excellent diet tips just for teen-agers in *'Teen's Diet and Exercise Fitness Manual,* available for $1.95 from: Petersen Publishing Company, Magazine/Circulation, 6725 Sunset Boulevard, Los Angeles, Calif. 90028.

Rating the Diets, which is published by *Consumer Guide* and which is available on newsstands for $1.95, offers an excellent discussion and critique of the best-known diets (and diet groups), which are rated according to safety and effectiveness.

As you plan your diet—and live with it—you may find some of the following suggestions helpful.

• Watch your portions! A 4-ounce lamb chop is 400 calories and a 3-ounce rib roast is 375 calories. As a rule, most of us are accustomed to eating much larger portions than we need. Buy a small food scale and use it to weigh everything you eat.
• Learn to take your time when eating so that you can really taste and enjoy your food. If you do this, you won't feel deprived, even though you are probably eating less.
• If your portions look tiny on your plate, switch to a salad plate. Your meal will look more bountiful—and you may feel more satisfied.
• Eat small meals more frequently. Three major meals with a fruit or vegetable snack saved for prime hunger times—like midmorning, midafternoon, or evening—may keep you from getting extremely hungry—and cheating!
• Eat a good breakfast!
• Plan to get out of the house after a meal if you have trouble breaking the chain of your eating (if you feel like snacking right after a meal). Take a walk. Jog. Ride your bike. Go see friends.
• If you're going to a party or on a date, fill up on liquids like skim milk and/or diet sodas or some fruit juice. Researchers have found that drinking liquids can keep hunger under control.
• Learn to ask "Why?" when you're reaching for a forbidden food. Ask yourself if that triple-scoop ice-cream cone will really solve anything!
• Keep an "Alternative Activities List" of things you can do instead of eating when you're tense or angry or bored. Exercise. Call a friend. Take a walk. Take a bath. Daydream. Chew sugarless gum. Write a long passage in your diary. Write a letter to someone.
• Keep a chart of what you eat, when you eat, and how you're feeling at these times. This may help you to find out what your own overeating triggers are. Keeping a food chart may keep you on the straight

and narrow, too. Somehow you feel *silly* writing down "half a chocolate cake and three pieces of fudge."

• When tempted, reach for a pen instead of food. This bit of advice comes from Dr. Martin M. Schiff, a specialist in weight control and the author of several books on the psychological and physical aspects of weight control. "Write what you're feeling at this very moment," Dr. Schiff suggests. "Do this *instead* of eating. This will help you to identify your danger times. You have to know what your eating habits, hurtful feelings, and rationalizations are before you can change them. Writing at moments of temptation may help you to understand and help yourself. Remember that *you* are totally responsible for your life. Take each day at a time. Tell yourself that *today* you will write unhappy feelings and joyous thoughts, too. Promise yourself that *today* you will write when tempted to eat improperly."

• Don't let a friend lead you into temptation. If he or she is really a friend, he or she will understand and not push you to take "just one bite . . ." when you say no to a forbidden food. That first bite can be a real diet-breaker.

• If you do fall off your diet, get right back on! Don't wait until tomorrow. Reward yourself by eating sensibly for the rest of today, too.

• If you feel like a freak (it seems that everyone else can eat as much as they want and never gain weight), take heart. There are many young people who are weight-conscious. Find a friend who is watching his or her weight, and diet together. You can even do this by mail with a faraway friend, encouraging each other with letters, diet recipes, and so on. *'TEEN Magazine* occasionally offers a Diet Pen Pal Exchange; thousands of teens have made new friends, and shed excess pounds, with the help of this very special service.

• If it seems like you've been on this diet forever, it can get depressing. Maybe you've lost 20 pounds, but you have another 20 to go. Maybe you've reached a plateau and just aren't losing much this week. It happens. To keep your spirits up, find an object that weighs as much as you've lost. Ten, 15, or 20 pounds is a lot! Try to pick up a 20-pound object and you'll see. Think that that much excess weight is now off your body. That's pretty terrific! You're doing just fine.

• If you're getting bored with so-called diet foods, give yourself more variety. We can't think of anyone who salivates at the sight of cottage cheese and carrot sticks for lunch every day for a week. Try a variety of menus and recipes. Don't fall into a diet rut. Even the traditional diet foods like cottage cheese and tuna can be fixed in a variety of ways. Experiment and you'll find yourself enjoying your meals more.

• Enlist the aid of your family and friends in your personal weight war. It may help if they can encourage and praise you for sticking to a diet as well as losing weight.

• Take things day by day. Don't think "Oh, my . . . I have 25 pounds to lose!" Say instead: "Today, I will eat in a healthy way. I will be good to *me*."

• When you're tempted to stray from the diet . . . remember! Call on your memory to furnish you with new motivation. Remember bad things (like being ridiculed or being shunned) that happened to you because of your weight. Remember, too, that it is your choice whether you will continue to be overweight or whether you will be slim. Give the diet—and yourself—a chance!

EXERCISE: THE HEALTHY, ACTIVE YOU

Exercise is a must for everyone, whether you're overweight, underweight, or normal weight.

I'm 15 and am on a diet to lose weight. What kind of exercise would be best to trim my body and make me physically fit?

Suzi N.

I'm a boy who is 14 and pretty much of a runt, to tell the truth! I'm short and skinny. How can I build my muscles up and keep up with the others?

Frank T.

Spot exercises may help Suzi to fight flab and tone her muscles in specific places.

A supervised regimen of weight lifting—in gym class or at his local "Y," Youth Club, or Boy's Club—may help Frank to build up his muscles and physique.

To be *physically fit,* however, Suzi and Frank need a regular program of exercise that involves the entire body. This kind of exercise is called aerobic exercise and includes swimming, cycling, jumping rope, walking, some forms of dancing (ballet is especially good), and running or jogging.

Aerobic exercise not only gets your muscles in shape, but also gives a much needed workout to your heart, lungs, and blood vessels, getting increased oxygen to all parts of your body. And the more oxygen you have in your body, the less fat you will have.

Such exercise, too, not only burns calories, but also helps your body to keep essential protein and minerals—like calcium. It also aids digestion and helps to give you more energy and stamina. In short, it's a great way to safeguard your health.

What are the best forms of aerobic exercise?

It depends. To reap the benefits of such exercises, you must do them at least three times a week. Ask yourself which exercise or exercises you would like best and would do on a regular basis. In building physical fitness, consistency is very important!

Many experts believe that running or jogging regularly may be the best exercise of all. Medical research has found that there are numerous long-range (as well as short-range) benefits to running. Most important, perhaps, is the fact that runners tend to live longer and suffer fewer heart attacks in later life.

However, if you absolutely hate running and question your ability to stick with it, you'd be better off choosing something you like better.

It might be swimming. A number of physical fitness experts believe that swimming is the ideal sport, one that gives every muscle of your body a workout. Such swimming, of course, does not mean splashing around for half an hour or struggling across the pool once and then resting for ten minutes afterward. To gain maximum benefits, you must swim for a minimum of 20 minutes nonstop. Of course, if you're a beginner, this may not be possible, but you can gradually build up your stamina.

Bicycling is another excellent way to exercise. It can be fun and it also helps to firm leg muscles.

Dancing is also an excellent—and fun—way to exercise. Ballet is, perhaps, the most beneficial (for *both* men and women!), but tap and jazz are also helpful.

I'd like to start jogging. I hear it's a really good form of exercise. But when my older brother tried it, he hurt his knees. This kind of discourages me. I tried to read some books on running, but they're so discouraging because they all talk about running for an hour or for several miles, which I know for a fact I couldn't do right now. Any tips for a beginning jogger?
Joe W.

Yes. Start sensibly!

We know lots of people (and you probably do, too) who start running regimens with a burst of speed—like modern-day Paul Reveres—only to limp off the track minutes later: stiff, sore, winded, and muttering *"Arrgghhh!* Never again!"

Jogging can be fun . . . IF you approach it in a sensible way.

A good warm-up before you start to jog is essential. Do exercises, particularly those involving stretching, for five to ten minutes before you start to jog.

After your initial warm-up, take it slow and easy on the track, or wherever you're jogging. (If you're a beginner and aren't using a track, the soft grass in a local park may be a better surface for you than hard concrete sidewalks.)

You might want to start by walking and gradually increase your speed until you're jogging or running. Then you might alternate between walking and run-

ning. Run for one minute. Walk for one minute. Repeat this over a ten-minute period.

After running your last minute, walk a while longer to "warm down." This will reduce the chances that you'll feel tired and sore.

Other important points to remember:

• Don't run on your toes (or you may experience leg cramps). Run flat-footed or, preferably, in heel-toe style.

• Get a good pair of training shoes. They may be expensive initially, but they'll last a long time and, most important, will help to protect you against injuries by cushioning your heel.

• Don't overdo! Check your heartbeat (by taking your pulse, counting the heartbeats over a 10-second period) just after exercising. If you're female, this shouldn't exceed a count of 30. If you're male, it shouldn't be more than 28 beats during that 10-second period. To get your Working Heart Rate, multiply your 10-second rate by 6. In women under 30, the WHR should not exceed 180; in men, 168.

• Do not exercise intensely (this does *not* include your warm-up and warm-down periods) for more than ten minutes a day during the first month.

• Schedule jogging sessions on *alternate* days three or four days a week if you can. This will lessen the chance of muscle or joint problems. Later, as your body gets used to the new exercise, you may want to exercise every day.

• Don't eat a full meal just before jogging. Wait at least two hours after a meal before you exercise strenuously.

• If it's extremely hot or humid, you may want to try an alternate form of exercise, like swimming.

The advice "Don't overdo at first!" applies to ALL strenuous forms of exercise. It's far better to start jogging and stay with it than to be so sore after your first session that you don't try exercising again for a week or, worse still, to sustain an injury that will keep you inactive even longer.

The Runners Handbook by Bob Glover and John Sheppard is an excellent book with a lot of helpful information for beginning and experience runners; we highly recommend it.

I'm 15 and into weight lifting. I've been working out for about a year now. I've been doing this every day recently and my brother says that's not a good idea. Is this true?

Stan R.

I'm a junior in high school and interested in weight

lifting. I'd like to make it my main exercise, but my coach says I ought to be running or something, too. How come?

John S.

I can't believe it. I asked my gym teacher about exercises for the muscles under my bust and she suggested lifting small weights! I don't want to get big weight-lifter muscles! Is she crazy?

Beth B.

Weight lifting is, like isometric or spot exercises, a static exercise. That is, it is stressful in short sessions and is excellent if you want to build up certain muscles.

However, it doesn't give you the steady workout that running or swimming does, for example, and it doesn't speed circulation. So, ideally, you should combine weight lifting with one of the aerobic forms of exercise for maximum fitness.

However, as with other stressful exercises, you should use your head when weight lifting. Build your strength gradually and don't work out more than three times a week. Weight lifting every day at this point may cause undue stress on your body without making you any stronger in the long run.

More and more women these days are weight lifting, and contrary to common fears, this exercise does *not* build huge, knotted muscles in women. Male hormones, especially testosterone, plus strenuous exercises do build such muscles in men. However, women, lacking this hormone, simply grow in strength, but not in size of muscles the way men do.

I like to bowl. Is this a good exercise for overall fitness?

Julie K.

Bowling is fun and can be an excellent part of an exercise program. However, bowling (like golf) is not an aerobic exercise involving the entire body; the heart, lungs, and blood vessels in particular. For this reason, you should also try to fit some form of aerobic exercise—running, swimming, or bicycling, for example—into your schedule to supplement the fun exercise of bowling.

I recently saw the play A Chorus Line *and I'd love to start studying ballet and maybe even be a professional dancer. My mother doesn't like the idea very much because she says it will give me bulgy leg muscles, but my dad says it's OK. Do you know whether plain ballet or toe dancing is better to do? Also, I'm*

13. Is this too old to start training? One of my friends, who has studied ballet since she was six, says it is.

Mara D.

My basketball coach told me that if I want to learn to jump higher, it might be good to take some ballet lessons. I never heard of that before. I can't see how some sissy dance can make me better at sports. What do you say?

Peter A.

Ballet dancers may be among the greatest athletes in the world, and some of the world's greatest athletes have studied ballet. In fact, ballet is considered a vital part of basic training among outstanding European male athletes.

To learn more about ballet and ballet training, we visited Joyce and Houston Johnson, directors of the Ballet Petit Studio in La Canada, Calif. Ballet Petit has an outstanding reputation nationwide for training professional dancers. In fact, of all the ballet schools in the nation, it has consistently had the largest number of students winning Ford Foundation grants, scholarships, and apprenticeships with the major ballet companies.

What can ballet do for an active teen athlete who sees it as a "sissy" dance?

"It's helpful to know that ballet began as a masculine art form, was developed by men, and is the best body developer there is since it builds the body geometrically," says Joyce Johnson. "Good ballet training produces a graceful, strong, and healthy body. Special attention is given to attaining muscle tone without overdevelopment and, as I said, it develops the body geometrically; that is, all movement is performed equally on *both* sides of the body."

The Johnsons, who have a special class for boys (some of them aspiring athletes), say that ballet can help you in many ways—in terms of strength, endurance, and elevation, enabling you to jump higher if you happen to be a budding basketball star or pass receiver! It can be of great benefit whatever your sport or your aspirations.

What if, like Mara, you haven't had previous training but are interested in ballet—maybe even as a career?

Most professional dancers seem to have started as young children. Among the teens studying in the professional development program at Ballet Petit, most have been dancing for years.

"To do it right, to make a young professional, takes about nine years of good training," says Houston Johnson. "It takes a minimum *maybe* of six years of intensive training. We like to take students through adolescence to get them stretched and turned out right. Sufficient stretch and turnout are vitally important.''

You don't have to wait until adulthood to see the benefits—a lovely body and beautifully shaped leg muscles—that ballet can give you.

It takes careful training to build beautiful bodies, however. The Johnsons are extremely concerned about the detrimental effects of careless training, which *may* cause big muscles or back or foot problems. These often come when teachers allow students to do toe—also called *pointe*—work at too young an age or after insufficient training and strengthening.

"We don't allow any student on pointe until she is at *least* nine-and-one-half years old and only then after several years of training," says Houston Johnson. "The bones of the feet aren't completely developed until late childhood and you could wind up with foot problems if you try too much too soon. Also, if your back doesn't have enough strength, you can end up with back problems if you try pointe work prematurely."

Good turnout, which emphasizes tucking in your buttocks and turning your feet and legs out, will fully utilize the muscles in your inner thighs as well as those on the outer section of your leg. Using all these muscles together will prevent overexercising the outside "quad" muscles and ending up with lumpy leg muscles, Johnson says.

Although some teens may have larger leg muscles to begin with, all can be helped with good dance training. This is also generally true of those with weak knees and other physical problems.

"If someone has a supple back or a knee problem or pre-Osgood Schlatter disease [See Chapter Nine], we watch that student carefully," says Houston Johnson. "We may not let them do grand pliés or certain jumps until they can get sufficient muscle buildup to avoid injury to that vulnerable area." But, if you have a special problem, discontinuing exercise might cause even more problems. It's usually better to continue dancing—or exercising—with caution and build your muscles up gradually.

Diet is also important for the would-be dancer. Joyce Johnson also has a college degree in nutrition and insists that her students follow healthy diets. Those who are in the intensive professional preparation program are weighed weekly and are suspended from classes for two days if they are overweight. Carbonated beverages and sugar are banned. Raw vegetables are considered the ideal snacks for the growing young dancers.

"It's really beautiful to work with these young people," says Houston Johnson. "Some of them will go on to become professional dancers. Many won't. But it's a joy to teach all of them love of dance and exercise and healthy eating and living habits!"

I'm 15. I want to build myself up to make the football team. Should I take vitamins? What can I do besides eat a lot of stuff that's fattening to gain more weight?

Ryan H.

Don't take loads of extra vitamins. This can be harmful. Instead, follow a good diet with 12 servings daily from the four basic food groups. If you need a supplement to gain weight, consult your physician and use such brands as Sustacal (Mead-Johnson) or Ensure (Ross), which will help you to add weight without adding high cholesterol.

I need to maintain my wrestling weight of 140, but after a long lazy summer, I'm up to 155. Should I try a fast?

Bruce C.

No, never! As we mentioned earlier, a 1,200-calorie-a-day diet, approved by your own physician, and mixed with exercise, should work well for you. NEVER go below 1,000 calories! Deaths have been reported among teen wrestlers on starvation diets to maintain wrestling weight. Use your head—for a healthy life *and* a thriving wrestling career!

I want to take karate lessons, but I wonder if it's dangerous. Is it good exercise?

Gary

There is a risk of injury in all the martial arts (as well as in most strenuous exercise), but karate can also be good exercise if you're careful in choosing a good school. A good school has well-trained instructors and takes precautions to help avoid student injuries.

I'm a girl, 15, and I'm interested in surfing. I've done a lot of body surfing, but I want to be a real surfer—with a board. My parents say I'll end up paralyzed or something and they don't want me to. They say to just keep on body surfing. Is surfing really dangerous or not?

Kim J.

Guess what? A study by physicians in Hawaii (which was reported by Dr. Robert H. Allen in the *Journal of the American Medical Association*) reveals that surfing with a board is much safer than body surfing and that surfing overall ranks as a fairly safe sport.

Head and spine injuries are most likely if you body surf. If you board-surf, the most common problem could be getting hit with the surfboard. It's important, however, to use safety precautions to help keep the odds on your side, the Hawaiian doctors contend.

Among their suggestions:

• If you're a body surfer—Avoid crowded beaches, especially those where board surfers are present and *do not* attempt to body surf unless the waves are breaking in deep water. Arch your body with your head back while riding a wave. This will help you to avoid hitting your head in the sand. When leaving a wave, roll to one side. Don't somersault!

• If you surf with a board—Avoid crowded beaches, but *do* surf with a companion and try to stay with your board. (Runaway boards are a major hazard.) If you wipe-out in deep water, try to fall *behind* the board, diving deep and staying under for a while. When you do come up, protect your head with your arms. If you have a wipe-out in shallow water, try to fall flat, feet or buttocks first.

SPORTS INJURIES—AND HOW TO AVOID THEM

I'm active in school sports, but have had a few injuries—a sprained knee and some strained muscles. What is the difference between a sprain and a strain and what is the best thing to do when you're injured like this? Also, what should you do about a blister?
Patrick M.

A *strain* is a muscle injury. It may cause mild aching or stiffness after you exercise strenuously for the first time or after a long period of inactivity, or it may be more severe—with pain and swelling. Although a strain usually means "muscle strain," it may also include a strain of your tendons, which are the ends of your muscles that attach to the bones.

A *sprain* is an injury of the ligaments (the connections between one bone and another, stabilizing your joints). These ligaments are, by necessity, not too elastic and a sprain happens when the joint is forced to bend in an unnatural way, as when you "turn your knee," for example. Pain, swelling, and more pain on movement may indicate a sprain. (It may also be a symptom of a broken bone, so in case of doubt, a trip to your physician might be in order.)

What causes the swelling in injuries like strains and sprains? The swelling is caused by bleeding of the affected muscle into the tissue surrounding the muscle.

It's important to stop this internal bleeding before the body reacts with an automatic healing response and starts growing connective tissue—called adhesions—around the joint, muscles, and ligaments. These adhesions can be painful and can restrict your movement even further. So it's best not to let your body develop them. This is done by clearing the injured area of fluid and blood as soon as possible.

How do you do this?

With the I-C-E formula: ice, compression, and elevation!

As soon as possible after the injury, put an *ice pack* on the affected area to constrict blood vessels and stop further internal bleeding. *Compression*—possibly with an Ace bandage—again helps to constrict the blood vessels and retard bleeding into the tissues, and *elevation* of the injured area may help to reduce swelling.

Some people like to alternate hot and cold treatments, using ice compresses until the area feels numb and then applying wet heat (like hot towels) and then cold again. This can be an especially effective treatment during the first 24 hours if combined with compression and elevation. *After* the first 24 hours, wet heat treatments—hot wet towels and, if available, a Jacuzzi or hot whirlpool—are best. Some well-equipped college athletic departments may also have Ultrasound, a form of electrotherapy, available to help injured tissues and muscles.

What about blisters?

Open them with a sterilized needle, apply antiseptic cream, and cover with a bandage. To prevent blisters on your feet, make sure that your shoes fit well and that they are tied tight enough to prevent rubbing.

I love sports, but have a problem with muscle cramps—especially in the lower part of my legs. What's the cause of this? What should I do when it happens?

Penny W.

Cramps may be caused by a lack of potassium, which can come with water loss due to perspiration during strenuous exercise. When a cramp hits, moist heat, pressure at the center of the cramped muscle, and brief, slow stretches of the affected area may help.

I'm on the basketball team at school and have noticed recently that I have sharp pain in my knees when I'm climbing stairs or jumping during a game and it's sort of a dull ache otherwise. My doctor says he can't find anything wrong, but I hurt! I'd hate to stop playing basketball!

Carole

What Carole is describing may be *patellar tendini-*

tis, an inflammation of the patellar tendon, and her pain may be caused by stretching of the scar tissue due to torn fibers that haven't healed properly. As long as this doesn't keep you from playing a particular game or sport, such activities aren't likely to make the condition any worse. It may eventually go away by itself. If it doesn't and, certainly, if it gets worse you should consult a doctor about special treatment.

I'm an avid tennis player now that I've been taking lessons for two months. My friends and I play a lot. Two of these friends had to quit playing tennis for a while recently because they had "tennis elbow." I'd sure hate to get this. Is there any way I can avoid it?

Jenny S.

The best prevention for tennis elbow is playing the game well! The power for your swings should come from the shoulder—with your forearm used for control only. A lighter tennis racket, bouncy (rather than dead) tennis balls, a two-handed backhand, and a band worn just below your elbow (which may keep the muscles of your forearm from squeezing bone ends) may also help to prevent tennis elbow.

If you do get this condition, stop playing and apply the principle of I-C-E—ice packs, compression with an Ace bandage, and elevation. If the problem persists, see your doctor.

I've been jogging for a couple of weeks now and have started to have throbbing pains in the lower part of my leg. My mom says it's probably shin splints. What's that?

Jerry H.

I like running a lot, but my right knee has been bothering me lately. What can I do about it?

Melissa N.

I'm 17 and my knees have started hurting. This makes it hard for me to ride my bike, which I've been doing a lot. Why could they be hurting?

Katie W.

Joints, particularly the knees, are subjected to stress in many sports. So are the muscles. It's important to know how common injuries occur so that you'll know how to prevent them.

Throbbing pains—like Jerry's—in the lower part of the leg may, indeed, be shin splints, which are considered to be tears in the tissue covering the shin bone when the two bones of the lower leg separate slightly. This can happen when you run on hard surfaces.

To *avoid* shin splints (and to build up muscles in

that area) jog on the beach, the grass at a local park, or on a soft track instead of a hard sidewalk.

Proper running technique—flat-footed or heel-toe—is important, too. If you run on your toes, you might feel pain at the back of your legs caused by straining the Achilles' tendon.

Proper shoes—with cushioned soles—and arch exercises may also help prevent foot and knee problems. It is also important to warm-up and cool-down before and after running.

Knee injuries can be avoided, in many cases, by sufficient warm-up and proper running (or cycling) technique. Although cycling is one of the safest of all sports, generally, some people put stress on their knees by trying to ride in too high a gear. If you're straining to push the pedals, go to a lower gear.

My best friend just broke her leg skiing. I was thinking of taking it up, but now I don't know. How come people get hurt so much when skiing?

Pat G.

The people most likely to have skiing accidents are those who are young (under 25), who ski when they're tired or in poor weather conditions or with inadequate equipment—or recklessly. Statistically speaking, those at greatest risk are young women who are just learning to ski. The rate of injury for women decreases quite considerably with competence, however, so lessons and practice may be your best defense against injury. It is also important to be careful. Watch for other skiers. (Many accidents happen during collisions or near-collisions between two skiers!) Also, when you start to feel fatigued, stop for a rest.

A physically fit body may be your best defense against skiing injuries. You can build endurance, flexibility and strength by running, walking up and down stairs, swimming, bicycling and jumping rope. Preparing your body in advance for the physical demands of skiing is an excellent preventive measure.

Are there any common kinds of injury you can get from swimming? It seems like a pretty safe sport to me.

Brian B.

Swimming is fairly safe, but those who swim a lot should watch out for two common problems.

The first, a middle ear infection, may occur if you go swimming with a head cold. Water pressure, added to the problems the cold presents, could cause the Eustachian tube (the passage between the mouth and ear) to close, and an ear infection lasting as long as six weeks may result. Staying out of the water for a few days to get over your cold is far preferable than being dry-docked for six weeks—with a painful ear infection yet.

Swimmers Ear is another problem that serious swimmers may have. This condition, which can cause tenderness, itching, drainage, and pain, comes from repeated exposure of the ear to water. Such constant exposure causes the skin in the ear to change from acid to alkaline and, in the long run, infection may set in. Keeping your ears clean and dry and using, with your physician's direction and consent, alcohol-based eardrops may help to prevent this from happening to you.

I'm interested in gymnastics, but have knee twist problems sometimes. My dad wants me to give up gymnastics. Do I have to?

Colleen

I love all sports and hope to be active all my life. How can I best avoid injuries?

Susan H.

Sports accidents and injuries can be avoided with adequate precautions. Ninety percent of sports injuries are abrasions, so proper clothing and appropriate padding for specific sports are in order. If, for example, you enjoy skateboarding, don't do it with bare feet and legs. Helmet, elbow pads, good shoes, and knee pads—at least—will help to avoid abrasions that are so common in this sport.

Other safety tips for skateboarders: avoid heavy traffic areas and learn proper falling techniques (rolling and somersault) to minimize the possibility of serious injuries.

What if you are a sports lover who seems to have a penchant for getting hurt? A tendency toward injuries may not be a dictum to stop activity, but simply a warning to be careful!

Sufficient warm-up is vital. In fact, physicians have found that a major reason for sports injuries is the fact that some athletes do not warm up long enough prior to starting the strenuous activity. Warming up—especially with stretching exercises—is essential to get the muscles ready for the upcoming workout.

It's also important to remember to build up to strenuous activity if you're a beginner. Too much, too soon can also cause injuries. You should also develop a sense of when you've had enough. Most sports injuries seem to happen when people are tired and reflexes, coordination, and judgment slack off. An injury, however, should not discourage you from being active. Rather, it should encourage you to become more physically fit—and thus less prone to injuries.

Coaches, dance teachers, and athletes all complain that too many people are likely to become quitters if they get hurt. There's usually no reason to be a quitter. You can strengthen muscles so that the injury is less likely to happen again, or in the event of a more serious injury, even switch to a different sport.

Sixteen-year-old Sue Soffe of Woodland Hills, Calif., is a prime example of a sports-loving teen who refuses to quit. Two years ago, Sue was an aspiring Olympic gymnast with a major problem: repeated serious injuries to her leg muscles and tendons suffered during vaulting and tumbling exercises. Finally her doctor said: "That's *it!* You're going to have to give up gymnastics!" Sue was heartbroken. Then a very special coach came to her rescue.

Alla Svirsky, an outstanding Soviet gymnastics coach who had immigrated to this country only a few months before, began to teach Sue Modern Rhythm Gymnastics (MRG) with her doctor's approval.

MRG, which is a mixture of gymnastics and dance utilizing props like ribbons, balls, and hoops in free exercise routines, is wildly popular in Europe and a major part of the training of outstanding Russian gymnasts. There is a good chance that MRG will be included as an event in the 1980 Olympics in Moscow—and that Sue Soffe will be among the contenders for an Olympic medal. Only three months after beginning MRG training, Sue placed among the top five in the national MRG championship. In the years since, she has consistently won the national title.

Even a serious motorcycle accident last year, when she suffered a leg injury so extensive that doctors feared they would have to amputate the leg, failed to keep Sue down. With incredible determination, she was back in training within a few months. To see her perform today, you would never guess the extent of her injuries.

"Regular gymnastics is more challenging physically," Sue says. "But you need more *endurance* for MRG—and I have plenty of that!"

It is endurance, above all, that you need to build a strong, healthy body. The better shape you're in, the less likely you will be to suffer serious injuries—and the more likely you'll be to stay healthy, active, and attractive ALL your life!

THE HEALTHY, ATTRACTIVE YOU

A well-nourished, active body is likely to be an attractive one, but there are some special problems that may concern young people especially.

I'm 14 and have pimples galore and it's just making me sick! What can I do about it?

Monica

I'd love to have long, healthy hair like the models I see. How can I do this? My hair is so dull now.
                                    Jeanine P.

I'm a teen-ager (15) and sweat like you wouldn't believe. It's awful! How can I dry out?
                                    Tom B.

I have stretch marks on my breasts. Will they ever go away?
                                    Debbie K.

I've got an embarrassing problem: warts. Five of them on my right hand. Short of a magic spell (ha, ha!), how can I make them disappear?
                                    Dick T.

I'd like to get contacts. How can I convince my parents that it's OK for someone my age (16)?
                                    Paula Y.

My dentist says that if I don't start taking care of my gums, I'll lose all of my teeth before I'm 25. I only have a few cavities. What do gums have to do with losing my teeth?
                                    Bill C.

Head-to-toe attractiveness starts out with a good diet and exercise program.

Eating *protein,* for example, can help your skin to stay smooth and your hair to grow strong and shiny.

Vitamin A (acquired via diet, not extra supplements) is great for healthy skin and the B vitamins help you to have healthy hair.

Cleanliness, too, is important. A daily bath or shower—plus extra face cleansings if you, like most young people, happen to have oily skin—helps to clear away dirt, oil, and dead cells, preventing the accumulation of bacteria on your skin that can cause body odor.

However, there *are* some well-nourished, active, and clean adolescents who have special problems and concerns about their health and attractiveness.

"My Problem Is . . . My Skin"

Skin, not surprisingly, is a number-one concern among teens and acne is the most common skin problem that young people seem to have.

A recent report from the National Center for Health Statistics revealed that 86.4 percent of all 17-year-olds suffer in varying degrees from acne. Only 27.7 percent of American adolescents between the ages of 12 and 17 have clear skin, free from significant lesions or scars, the report added.

So if you've been feeling ugly, ashamed, out of it, and alone because you suffer from some degree of acne, you have a lot of company—as the following letters may reveal!

I have awful zits and can't figure out why. I've always kept my skin superclean and I don't eat greasy food or chocolate. I watch my diet very carefully. My dad had a bad complexion when he was a kid. Could this be an inherited thing?
                                    Deb A.

I am so ugly I can hardly stand myself! I had good skin until I started my periods two years ago. Since then, it's been terrible! The other kids at school make fun of me and even my own family thinks I'm ugly. How can I help myself before it's too late?
                                    Sandy F.

My skin is pretty clear, but I get occasional pimples around the time of my period. Why does this happen then? And what causes these pimples in the first place?
                                    Shannon H.

Heredity, which determines your skin type along with other important characteristics, may have a lot to do with whether or not you have acne.

The condition of adolescence, however, seems to be a major factor. At this time, there are many changes going on in your body: growth spurts, physical maturation, and a surge of—and possible imbalance of—hormones. These hormones—progesterone and testosterone—become part of your lifelong body chemistry. So acne can flare up at any time later in life, too. But it seems most common in adolescence. Acne may be a problem for you for a short time—like a year or so—or for a number of years.

How do your hormones trigger acne?

As hormone levels increase, the oil, or sebaceous, glands (which are quite numerous on your face, shoulders, chest, and back) become more active, producing a fatty substance called *sebum.*

This sebum travels from the gland to the pore (opening of the skin) and produces the oily skin so common in teens.

If this passageway becomes blocked with sebum, the first step of acne—blackheads—may develop. Blackheads are black, *not* from dirt, but from oxidation of sebum and skin pigments in the pore.

If these blackheads are not removed, the sebum continues to fill the duct of the gland, pressure will build, and bacteria may invade the area. The resulting infection may cause red papules and pustules (filled with pus), which teens call "zits" or "pimples." In more serious cases of acne, these may progress to cysts and subsequent scarring.

Can washing your face and other affected areas help to prevent this progression?

It may certainly help. Removing oil from the skin surface and keeping the pores open through cleansing with ordinary or antibacterial soap two or three times daily is the first step.

Frequent shampoos—to keep oily, greasy hair from adding oil to the affected areas—may also be helpful.

If you're troubled by acne on your back, a shower once or twice daily with antibacterial and abrasive soap, using a backbrush to scrub the back thoroughly, may help, too.

If you have blackheads, a pulverized soap may help to remove the blackheads and open the pores, but *do* be careful! These soaps are abrasive to the skin, so don't use them more than once or twice a day. Wash your face in hot water and rinse with cold water to help close the pores again. You may even wish to swab your skin with an alcohol-soaked pad after washing to help remove the last trace of oil and dirt. Used in moderation, alcohol is a good astringent. If your skin starts to feel dry, however, you may be using too much, depleting your skin's natural oils.

Washing isn't always enough, however, since sebum and blackheads start below the skin surface. Blackheads may be removed with a device called a *comedo extractor*. When used correctly, this device can be very effective in removing blackheads (also called comedones). When applied over the blackhead, this device exerts uniform pressure, causing the blackhead to be expelled and thus removing the blockage of the oil duct. This extractor works well and does not leave scarring, which might happen if you pick at a blackhead with your fingertips.

Although the area around the blackhead may be a little red (from the pressure) right after removal, this will fade quickly.

Your physician may use this comedo extractor to remove blackheads for you or you can learn to do it yourself. You can buy a comedo extractor at a surgical supply store (easy to find in most large cities) or, in some instances, at a drugstore or pharmacy.

We'd like to emphasize that a comedo extractor is useful for *blackheads only!*

When the blackhead becomes infected and turns into the classic red bump we usually call a pimple, the comedo extractor will do more harm than good. At this stage, exerting pressure could damage the skin and cause scarring. So don't use this device for pimples *and* don't pick at or squeeze your pimples in any way!

In mild cases of acne, some over-the-counter acne lotions and creams may aid drying of the skin.

If you're female and wear makeup, be very careful about the makeup you use. Oil-based makeup will only clog your pores more. However, a nonoily and/or medicated makeup that may even have astringent qualities may be helpful.

My mom says that I shouldn't eat chocolate because it will cause pimples. Is this true?

Steve S.

This is a common—and controversial—question. Many studies have been done in an effort to determine whether or not chocolate, nuts, salted foods (like potato chips), and greasy, fried foods—among other alleged culinary culprits—really do cause excess oil in the skin, resulting in acne.

At this time, there is no conclusive evidence showing that certain foods cause acne. In one study, in fact, acne patients ate large amounts of chocolate without experiencing any noticeable skin changes.

However, there may be some who find that certain foods do seem to aggravate their acne. If chocolate (or soft drinks or shellfish or nuts or salted snacks or ?) seems to make matters worse for you, try to avoid such foods as much as possible.

I find that my face breaks out just before my period. Why does this happen?

Janet J.

I always seem to have a pimple attack just when I want to look my best: like just before senior portraits were taken, the day before the prom, and the morning of my sister's wedding (I was maid of honor). Is it my imagination or do pimples have a sort of sixth sense about when they're most unwanted?

Ann C.

I usually have a pretty mild case of acne, but it really got bad when I went on a Hawaiian vacation with my family a few weeks ago. I didn't eat a lot of junk food and got a lot of sunlight, which I always thought was good for your skin. Could it have been the hot weather? It's pretty hot where I live, too, in San Bernardino, Calif., but I don't have problems like that at home!

Tim L.

There are several conditions that may aggravate acne.

Fluctuating hormone levels, present just before a woman's menstrual period, cause increased oil production, and the chance of an acne flare-up.

Stress, which may be present before an important

event, may also be a predisposing factor. While there is no absolute scientific proof that this is so, such ill-timed pimple attacks are seen by many doctors and suffered by many teens.

While sunlight combined with dry heat (such as Tim might find at home in Southern California) may help dry out oily skin, hot humid weather—like that in Hawaii and Florida or in most of the nation during the summer—may aggravate acne.

Also, Tim may find that his acne was aggravated by salt water. If you're a beach-lover, but find that you seem to break out more after a dip in the sea, try washing your face with clear water as soon as possible after you finish swimming.

In most cases, a moderate amount of sunshine (enough to cause reddening of the skin, but not enough to bring about a second degree burn) can help your skin. If it's winter and the sun rarely shines, a *carefully used* sun lamp may be a good substitute but once again, getting just enough exposure to ultraviolet to cause slight reddening of the skin.

I've tried everything—washing, lotions, a good diet—and nothing seems to help. I'm thinking about going to a doctor about my skin, but my parents are skeptical. They say that if I'd just stop fiddling with my face and wait a few years, my acne will go away. But it's been here for almost three years already and shows no signs of going away. Is there any way a doctor could help me?

Terri

One of the most harmful myths around concerning acne (especially severe acne) is the old saying "Leave it alone! You'll outgrow it!"

If nothing is done to treat acne, particularly if it is more than a mild case, the pimples will progress to cysts and scars may be the ultimate result.

The worst damage, though, may be inside. As you know, the self-image of a teen plagued and scarred by acne may suffer a great deal. You may feel ugly and out of it, scorned by your peers. You may feel very much alone.

Such damage to the skin—and to the psyche—can be tragic. But it doesn't have to happen. If your acne doesn't respond to self-treatment, a physician can help you. You might seek help from your personal physician or from a *dermatologist,* a doctor who is a skin specialist.

What can he or she do for you?

One method of controlling acne is the combination of good hygiene and oral antibiotics like tetracycline. Tetracycline, which must be prescribed by a physician, can be quite effective in controlling acne. It works in two ways: First, it has been shown to inhibit

the formation of the fatty acids which, in turn, form sebum, and thus it cuts down the amount of oil secreted by the skin; second, as an antibiotic, tetracycline has an effect on the superficial infection that causes papules and pustules. Although tetracycline may be effective, it isn't a trouble-free miracle cure.

The drug must be taken only under your physician's careful supervision and there are side effects. Although these are the exception rather than the rule and are usually mild, some people experience nausea (particularly if they are consuming a lot of dairy products while taking the drug) and a number of others may develop a condition known as photosensitivity, which means that the skin becomes very sensitive to sunlight. You may go out on the beach with your friends for a quick game of volleyball and come home with a severe sunburn! Patients taking tetracycline, then, must be especially cautious about overexposure to the sun. Women taking tetracycline may also have a higher incidence of vaginal yeast infections.

Tetracycline therapy for acne, however, has been judged safe by a task force of the American Academy of Dermatology. It works well for some, not so well for others.

An antibiotic in *lotion* form, which is applied directly to the skin, is now in the experimental stage and shows promising results.

One of the most promising new treatments for acne, however, seems to be vitamin A acid (also called Retin A), which may be used alone or, for best results, in combination with benzoyl hydroxide. This treatment, too, is available only through your physician.

How does Retin A work? Following your doctor's instructions, you apply it to your face for several weeks (or longer, in some cases). At first, you may wonder how in the world this will ever help you! It will seem oily when you put it on and then it begins its work—by inflaming your skin. In the first week or so of treatment, your skin may actually look worse.

"Oh, *terrific* . . ." you may be saying. Actually, it can be rather terrific in the long run. In succeeding weeks, your outer layer of skin—with the active, inflammatory stages of acne—will peel, leaving a soft, pink layer of skin. This new skin is usually clear and blemish-free, very similar to the skin's appearance after you have peeled from a sunburn. Your skin may be clear of active blemishes, but old acne scars will remain. (For removal of these scars, see Chapter Six for information about a form of plastic surgery called *dermabrasion.*)

Unfortunately, this treatment with Retin A can be used only on the face. In other areas (such as the back) the skin does not have the tremendous regenerative (regrowth) aspects that facial skin has. Also, some people with very sensitive skin may not be able to tolerate this treatment at all. In such cases, another form of treatment—such as antibiotics—might be used.

My best friend told me that birth control pills can help clear up acne. Is this true? Would a doctor give me the Pill just to clear up my skin?

Jean H.

Hormones, as we have seen, *do* exert a strong influence on acne.

The hormone estrogen, which birth control pills have always contained, seems to suppress oil gland secretions and, in the process, may help to control acne. In the past, some doctors have prescribed birth control pills to help battle acne.

Now, however, the estrogen level of birth control pills is much lower than before. In the opinion of a number of experts, these pills today contain too little estrogen to be consistently helpful or to justify the side effects and risks that may be involved in taking birth control pills. (For more on birth control pills, see Chapter Twelve.)

In some very severe cases of acne in women, however, a physician *might* consider using a high-estrogen birth control pill to help alleviate the condition. However, this is an option that must be seriously weighed and considered first.

I'm a 15-year-old girl who has bad eczema. I've had this for a long time. How can I get rid of it?

Desperate

Eczema is a chronic skin allergy and, like many allergies, there is no sure cure. There are ways to control it. Treatment with steroid creams to control the inflammation and itching may help a lot, but this is available by prescription only, so check with your physician.

I can't wash my face because I'm allergic to soap. Whenever any soap gets on it, my face breaks out, gets red, and burns. How can I wash my face?

Grimy(!)

Try a hypoallergenic soap such as Neutrogena® or Lowilla. These soaps are made especially for people who have very sensitive skin. If the problem persists, however, do see a physician.

I'm black, 14 years old, and try to keep my complexion clear. Our school nurse warned us black kids against using cleansing grains or harsh soaps on our skin, but she didn't say why. Why??

Wondering

Black teens are well-advised to avoid abrasive products because black skin has a tendency to react to even slight injury or irritation by getting lighter or darker in patches. (This is called *hypo*pigment and *hyper*pigment.) Black skin, incidentally, is more likely to get raised scars, called keloids, when injured. So if you're black, be especially gentle with your skin.

I practically live on the beach in the summer and love to get deep tans. I've read some stuff, though, about too much tanning making you wrinkle like a prune before you're even old and that you might even get skin cancer. I hate to think about giving up my tans. Is any of this stuff true?

Mary B.

Long-term sunworshipers may be prone to premature aging of the skin and skin malignancies, but there are ways you can bask in the sunshine and still protect yourself.

First, it's vital to know how the sun and your skin interact.

Melanin, a brownish pigment that determines skin color, acts as a shield to protect the skin from damaging ultraviolet rays from the sun. People with black or brown skin or even olive-skinned brunettes have more melanin and therefore more (but not total!) protection from these ultraviolet rays. Light-skinned people have a much smaller quantity of melanin and so are much more likely to suffer from overexposure to the sun.

Action of the sun's ultraviolet rays on your skin's surface makes you burn—or tan. When these rays are unfiltered (fair skin with no sunscreen products added for protection), they can cause blood vessels under the surface of the skin to swell, causing redness and, in some severe cases, blisters on the skin.

In tanning, ultraviolet rays cause melanin in the skin to darken and stimulate the body to produce *more* melanin, which will darken the skin. While darkening of the present melanin may be evident the same day, production of the new melanin may take several weeks. A tan, then, is something you build gradually. Staying out in the sun for long periods of time will only damage your skin, not speed up the tanning process.

A gradually acquired tan, with its increase of melanin, may protect your skin. In the meantime, sunscreen products and common sense may keep you from suffering painful burns.

If you, like many young people, practically live outdoors in the summer, here are some commonsense tips that may help minimize skin damage from the sun:

• Try to avoid direct sunbathing during the danger times of 10 A.M. to 2 P.M. when the sun's rays are most powerful and direct.

• If you're swimming, remember that water is no protection. It admits the sun's rays, too. In fact, wet skin is more receptive to ultraviolet rays than dry skin, so apply a sunscreen before swimming *and* after you get out of the pool or the surf.

• Your nose, ears, lips, knees, and shoulders are more exposed and will burn faster than other parts of your body, so give these extra protection.

• Don't use a sheer, gauzy cover-up when you're at the beach. Ultraviolet rays penetrate these fabrics easily.

• You can burn as easily on a cloudy day as on a sunny one, so use a sunscreen even when haze hovers over the beach.

• DON'T use a sun reflector unless you want to risk a serious burn!

• Black skin *can* burn, though not as easily as lighter skin. So, even if you're black, use a product with some sunscreen properties for added protection.

• If you do get sunburned, cool, wet compresses, soothing lotions, and aspirin may bring some relief.

• If you get a severe sunburn, see your physician. Drugs can be prescribed to reduce swelling and the associated pain.

While we'll be talking more about suntan preparations—along with cosmetics—in the next chapter, we do want to emphasize here that a sunscreen can filter out damaging sunrays and still permit a gradual, protective tan. Look for a sunscreen with the ingredient PABA—para-aminobenzoic acid. The better sunscreens will have this.

What are some of the long-term consequences of constant sunning without adequate precautions?

Most of these don't show up for years after a sun-loving adolescence, but they can and *do* happen.

Damage to the elastic fibers of the skin by overexposure to the sun can cause wrinkles. These fibers, which keep the skin soft and elastic, cannot function well if damaged and this may lead to wrinkled, saggy, leathery skin at a fairly early age. You may find yourself at 35 or 40 looking like you're 50 or 60.

Skin malignancies (cancer) have been linked with ultraviolet radiation and there are an estimated 300,000 new cases in this country every year. Fortunately, however, most types of skin cancer are quite treatable and curable. However, by using common sense and

a bit of foresight, you can avoid these problems and enjoy the sunshine, too.

I'd like to get a sun lamp with a timer for safety. Could it still hurt my skin? I really would like to have a year-around tan.

Sunny

Sun lamps are not as effective as the sun in giving you a good tan, but they can give you a nasty burn if you're not careful. If you use a sun lamp, one with a timer may be the safest bet. Also, it is best if a friend or family member is close by to make sure that you don't fall asleep under the lamp. (The worst burns seem to happen this way!) And before using the lamp, *do* read the instructions thoroughly.

Help! I'm 14 and desperate! I have stretch marks on my hips and breasts. Is there any way to get rid of them? Will they go away?

Sue S.

Stretch marks, which are medically termed *striae*, are breakdowns in the elastic fibers of the skin and may be caused by any one of a number of factors. Most commonly, they are seen in instances where the skin has been stretched excessively—as in rapid growth and development, overweight, or pregnancy. Also, certain medical conditions and taking synthetic steroid medications such as Prednisone (which may be used in the treatment of certain chronic illnesses like asthma) may cause striae.

These stretch marks cannot be removed, generally, nor do they usually go away entirely. In many cases, however, they will fade and become much less obvious in time.

I have several moles on my neck and chest. Are they dangerous in any way? Should I have them removed?

Don R.

Moles, medically termed *nevi*, are very common in all age groups.

Basically, a mole is an area of the skin where there is a heavy concentration of the skin pigment melanin. Generally, moles are harmless, though, in some instances and locations, they may be cosmetically unappealing.

If you have a mole that begins to enlarge or change in color, however, this is a reason for concern. This could be a symptom of a rare, but serious condition called malignant melanoma, a cancer that can kill young people as well as older ones—and can do so rather quickly without prompt treatment. So if you do notice any changes in a mole, do see your doctor.

If you elect to have your moles removed for cosmetic reasons or otherwise, this can be done by a dermatologist or a plastic surgeon.

I've got an embarrassing problem: warts! Five of them on my right hand. Short of a magic spell (ha, ha!) how can I make them disappear?

Dick T.

What causes warts? Are they contagious? My boyfriend has a wart on his hand and I'm almost afraid to hold hands with him.

Shelley

Warts are caused by a virus and come in many varieties.

Some, like venereal warts, which occur around the genitalia (and which will be discussed in further detail in Chapter Eleven) are quite contagious. Others, such as those occurring on the arms, legs, hands, and feet, are usually not contagious.

There is a great deal of speculation about how one gets these warts. We do know that warts are caused by a virus—not by frogs as the old myth goes—but, beyond that, we have very little conclusive evidence about what exactly causes this virus to happen in some people.

Some warts on the hand can be treated at home with topical application of an over-the-counter preparation like Compound W. This type of treatment usually requires persistence and repeated applications, however, so don't get discouraged if your warts don't disappear on the first try.

If your warts seem immune to nonprescription preparations, your physician may be able to help in several ways. He or she may remove the warts via electrocautery (burning off the warts with electrical heat), topical applications of certain prescription medications, liquid nitrogen (which turns warts white, "freezing" them and causing them to die and eventually to fall off), or even via a systematic approach, using vaccines to remove and prevent the recurrence of the warts.

There is another kind of wart that is something else altogether: the plantar wart. This type of wart, usually found on the sole of the foot, is not raised like most other warts, but burrows deep into the skin. This wart, which may be very painful, is also caused by a virus, which may be picked up by a minor break in the skin at places like gym shower rooms.

Plantar warts should *not* be treated with home remedies. If the wart is not particularly painful and does not appear to be multiplying, some physicians prefer to leave it alone. These warts will often disappear in a month or so when the body begins to reject the wart. However, if the wart is painful and/or starts to multiply, the physician may remove it, usually by electrocautery or by treatment with an acid solution.

"My Problem Is . . . My Feet"

Help! I keep getting athlete's foot and I hate it! I'm not even an athlete, although I do wear tennis shoes a lot. Could this be adding to my problem?

Melanie S.

Contrary to some popular opinions, athlete's foot does not seem to be highly contagious nor is it likely to be picked up in gym showers. It seems to be connected with athletes only by the shoes they may wear.

The fact is, athlete's foot is most likely to happen when the feet are hot and moist, often in the warm months of summer, but this problem can strike in any season under the right conditions. Constant use of rubber-soled, nonventilated shoes (like some tennis shoes) can provide an ideal condition—warm, moist feet—for the growth of fungi and bacteria.

Athlete's foot causes the skin to be itchy and scaly with cracks between the toes and on the sole of the foot. If the toenails are also infected, they become discolored and brittle.

Going barefoot as much as possible in the summer or wearing sandals may help to prevent this problem in the warm-weather months.

In the winter when you usually must wear closed shoes, take extra care to wash your feet at least once a day and use talc or baby powder to help keep your feet dry. Also, wear absorbent cotton socks (instead of nylon or wool) and change them at least twice a day. Alternating shoes—wearing one pair while the other dries out—may help, too.

There are a number of over-the-counter products designed to kill the bacteria and fungi and to help dry the skin; these are available in powder, spray, lotion, or ointment form. Which you use is a matter of personal choice, but do combine such treatment with the precautions we listed above.

I love to wear sandals in the summer or go barefoot, but at the beginning of every summer, my feet are so ugly from wearing shoes all winter. I have blisters and corns sometimes. I know how to care for them and they go away, but how can I make my feet look good all year round?

Diane T.

Many young people are having foot problems these days and the culprit could be the shoes you're wearing. A recent study revealed that, by college age, 88 percent of Americans' feet need medical help.

Well-fitting shoes, combined with clean and powdered feet, can keep a lot of blisters and corns from happening.

Bathe and powder your feet every day and when shoe-shopping, do it in the afternoon when your feet tend to be bigger.

Beware of certain types of shoes. Platform shoes can cause bone-breaking or ankle-spraining injuries. Flats may also cause foot problems and tight-fitting boots may restrict blood circulation in your legs. Your best bet: comfortable, well-fitting shoes with a slight heel.

"My Problem Is . . . Perspiration"

What is wrong with me? My hands always get all wet and clammy when I'm around guys. I'm afraid to go out with a guy on account of my hands. I've heard that it's just my nerves. Whatever it is, I hate it. Help!
The Clam

For the past two years, I've been perspiring under my arms—a lot! I've tried to hide my perspiration by wearing light-colored tops, but forget it! I take a bath every day and use a deodorant and an antiperspirant, but nothing seems to help. I'm perspiring so much that I have yellow stains on my new clothes. Other kids tease me and I'm worried that this will happen all my life. I'd appreciate any suggestions you might have.

A Real Sweathog

In adolescence, when the body is growing and changing in so many ways, the sweat glands are also developing fully and, at times, they may seem to be working overtime.

Wet, clammy hands seem to be the special curse of adolescence—and something we've all experienced. With the body changes come circulation changes as well, as your body grows from child to adult. This, plus the stress that you may feel in certain situations, makes it possible for your hands to be cold *and* sweaty. How can stress and/or an emotional crisis do this?

In times of emotional crisis, the adrenal gland secretes the hormone *epinephrine,* which causes constriction of the blood vessels, especially those in the hands. Blood supply to the hands decreases and the area becomes cold—and moist.

Learning to deal with stress and overcome some of your social fears (see Chapter Four) may help. Time will, too. Many people find that after adolescence their hands become considerably less clammy, even in times of stress.

Perspiration under the arms, which is a normal bodily function that may be aggravated by stress and adolescent body changes, is another complaint that many young people have.

Younger adolescents especially may be very conscious of this because it is a new occurrence. Children, whose sweat glands under the arms aren't so developed yet, don't generally perspire in that area, so when it begins to happen in puberty, it can be a shock.

Sometimes, the more you worry about it, the worse it gets. One high school student told us that he was so worried about perspiring that his shirt was soaking wet before he even left for school. Another student, convinced that she was the only girl in her whole high school who perspired noticeably, insisted on wearing a sweater all the time to hide the evidence. Both of these students found that when they were able to deal more effectively with all the stresses in their life and worried less about perspiration, their perspiration problems became less acute.

It's important to realize that perspiration is not, invariably, a problem. It is a normal bodily function, one of the ways that the body cools off and is able to maintain a constant temperature. Without such built-in temperature controls, our body temperature in hot weather or during strenuous exercise might reach dangerously high levels—enough to cause convulsions and serious complications.

There are ways, however, that you can deal with excess underarm perspiration.

Regular showers or baths and absorbent (for example, cotton), well-ventilated clothes may help. So will one of the several excellent antiperspirant/deodorants on the market today. Those with *aluminum chlorohydrate* as the major, active ingredient are most effective. There are some brands, too, like Gillette's Right Guard "Double Protection" that have ingredients to help keep you dry and your clothes stain-free.

If it seems that no product ever seems to work for you, read the instructions on the label very carefully. Some product labels will advise you that, for maximum effectiveness, you should use the product at bedtime rather than first thing in the morning. Others may suggest, too, that you do not apply an antiperspirant right after emerging from a steaming shower. Your perspiration from the hot shower may simply wash the antiperspirant away. Dry yourself thoroughly and let your body cool down a bit. Then apply the antiperspirant.

If you find that you have a closet full of clothes marred with perspiration stains, don't despair. There are several excellent stain removers that can be sprayed on the stains before you put the clothes in the washer. One or two treatments and washings usually will give you stain-free clothes again.

Probably the worst thing about problem perspiration is that it can make you feel like a freak. You may be totally convinced that you're the only person in your whole school who sweats noticeably.

The fact, is, everybody perspires. It is more of a problem for some people, but you can make things easier on yourself by good grooming, learning to deal with stresses, and by avoiding things that only add to your problem—like wearing a sweater or jacket all the time or keeping your upper arms stiff and tight against your body to hide any signs of perspiration.

Time helps, too. We've seen a number of young adults, plagued with perspiration problems as teenagers, dry out remarkably when they hit their twenties. This may simply be an adjustment of the body to adult functioning or more expertise at dealing with stress or, perhaps, a combination of the two.

"My Problem Is . . . Leg Veins"

I'm 16 and have a part-time job at a hamburger stand. My job requires me to stand for hours at a time and I've noticed that the veins in my legs are becoming more noticeable. Could I be getting varicose veins?? What can I do about this?

Concerned

It is unlikely that an adolescent would have varicose veins, although many teens are concerned about this. (We've had a lot of letters much like the one above.)

Varicose veins are usually seen in older people when the veins lose their support from the skin and connective tissues and when the wall of the vein itself loses strength. The vein then enlarges due to blood pooling in it and can be very painful.

Teens may experience something quite different. If you're especially active in sports or have a job that requires you to stand for long periods of time, the veins in your legs can become more prominent due to the increased demands of the venous system of the legs to return blood to the heart. These are not varicose veins, however, because there are not degenerative changes that are characteristic of aging.

Support hose can give added support to the legs, enabling the veins to return blood more quickly to the heart. This will tend to decrease the number of prominent veins in your legs and will probably make you feel a little less tired, too, after a day on your feet. Many support hose are made by popular pantyhose manufacturers and tend to be almost indistinguishable from regular hose. Some long socks for men may also have support characteristics, if you're a guy and have this problem.

"My Problem Is . . . My Nails and Hair"

My nails are flaky and chip easily. Would drinking gelatin help? I want to have pretty nails like everyone else.

Betty

If your nails are brittle or chip a lot, analyze your habits. Do you have nervous mannerisms, like drumming your nails on a hard surface (like a desk), flicking them, or picking or biting them? All of these can retard nail growth and cause things like chips, spots, and pits in the nail. So can a fungal infection or poor circulation. If there seems to be a skin infection involved, you may want to visit your doctor for treatment. If there is no infection involved, you might try taking iron supplement pills for a long-term effect and, for the moment, soak your nails in a combination of water and gelatin for temporary hardening—or use one of the nail hardener-lacquers available at your local drug- or department store.

I've been using artificial fingernails over my own nails, but I've noticed lately that my own nails are getting separated from the skin and really look gross. What's wrong?

Jill J.

You may have *onycholysis,* a condition usually caused by a fungal or bacterial infection or by an allergic reaction to the glue used on artificial fingernails. Stop using the artificial nails (and the glue) immediately and see your doctor. Usually, removing the cause of the infection will cure the problem and the nails will grow back.

I have oily hair and like to wash it every day. My mother objects because she thinks I'll lose all my hair. I have acne, too, so I feel it's especially important to keep my hair clean. Am I right?

Chrissy

It is a good idea to wash oily hair every day if desired, not only to keep from aggravating any acne that may be present on the face or back, but also to stimulate the scalp. This stimulation, in combination with a mild shampoo, may actually enhance hair growth by stimulating the hair follicles and the scalp's natural oils.

Recently when I shampoo my hair, I lose more hair than usual. Is something horrible wrong with me?

Worried

It is normal to lose some amount of hair every day. Hair follicles have distinct cycles, involving active growth of hair followed by shrinkage of the follicle and then rest. After producing hair for several years, a follicle may shed its hair and rest for a few months. This is occurring on a constant basis with countless hair follicles on your head.

There are some factors that can trigger some of the hair follicles to take an unscheduled rest and shed hair. Some of these factors include: bodily upsets like stringent dieting (as with anorexia nervosa) or severe illness; certain anticancer drugs; infection of the scalp (which can be caused by allergies to a hair product like shampoo, conditioner, or a hair-coloring agent); and hormonal changes brought about by birth control pills or pregnancy.

If you have a problem with profusely shedding hair, do see your physician.

My hair is dull and looks faded. How can I make it look shiny?

Carla A.

There may be a number of reasons for dull-looking hair.

A buildup of dirt or hair products (like conditioner or hair spray) on the hair can make it look dull. So can a residue of shampoo if you don't rinse your hair thoroughly after washing it. Frequent shampoos—possibly with a protein shampoo product—may help to make your hair shine.

As we have discussed, your diet is extremely important to your looks. Dull hair may be an indication that you lack vitamin B_{12} and could use some more lean meats, fish, eggs, milk, and liver to start feeling— and looking—your best.

"My Problem Is . . . My Eyes"

Your eyes, too, can be a reflection of your general health. A specially trained physician may be able to see symptoms of diabetes, liver disease, or high blood pressure—to name a few disorders—while examining your eyes.

Your vision may also have a huge impact on how you do in school. If you suffer from headaches after reading or find it hard to keep your place while studying, you should get your eyes checked.

Whether or not you experience any troublesome symptoms, periodic eye examinations are advisable.

Our school nurse said that we should get our eyes checked and talked about different kinds of eye doctors once. Now I'm confused. Which one do you go to for what?

Nancy K.

An *ophthalmologist* is an M.D.—a physician— whose specialty is diagnosing and treating diseases and defects of the eye. He or she performs surgery when necessary.

An *optometrist* is not a physician, but has a Doctor of Optometry degree (O.D.) and is highly trained and licensed by the state to diagnose eye problems and diseases. He or she may prescribe glasses, contacts, or other optical aids.

An *optician* is the technician who grinds lenses, fits them into frames, and then adjusts these frames to each individual.

If you go to an ophthalmologist, he or she may refer you to an optometrist or an optician for glasses or, if you desire, contact lenses.

I wear glasses now, but would really like contacts. My girl friend says that the new soft contacts are great. Are they really good? Are they better to have than hard contacts?

Tom J.

Soft contact lenses, which were introduced in 1971, do have some advantages over hard lenses. They are more comfortable and can be worn for longer periods of time. They don't have the penchant for popping out at inopportune moments that the harder lenses have. However, they do not give adequate vision correction to all forms of vision defects. They also tend to be expensive and somewhat less durable than hard lenses.

Soft lenses may be great for your girl friend, but they may not be right for you. Individual needs vary widely and no particular type of lens is right for everyone. Check with your doctor to see if soft contact lenses may be right for you.

My best friend and I both wear contacts. She wets hers by putting them in her mouth. She says it's perfectly OK to do. But I heard it's not good. Who's right?

Amy L.

Amy is right. Placing your lens in your mouth may spread infection. Other practices to be avoided are: rubbing your eyes with contacts in, wearing them too long, or sleeping with your contact lens in place. If you are careless, your eyes could suffer serious irritations.

I have normal, good eyesight, but my eyes get bloodshot and water sometimes. Why does this happen?

Alex G.

Bloodshot, tearing eyes can be the result of several possibilities: allergies, eye strain, and pollution being the most likely. Washing the eyes with water may help. If a person has a chronic problem involving allergies, an eye preparation like Visine may help. However, if the problem is severe or chronic, see a physician.

Is it true that you're not supposed to wash just under your eyes? Someone told me that and I just can't believe it. Why should that be true?

Bev W.

It's *half* true. The truth is . . . the skin around the eye is very delicate, should not be scrubbed, and needs to be moisturized regularly. However, you can clean the area and remove eye makeup with a cleansing cream or a special makeup remover that is made just for the delicate eye area.

For some time, the white parts of my eyes have had a slight yellowish color. Could this be serious?

Worried

A condition like this—called *icterus*—may or may not be serious, but it's certainly worth checking with your physician. Icterus may be a sign of a liver disease, like infectious hepatitis. Then, too, it may mean nothing. There are some entirely healthy people who may have slightly icteric eyes. However, only your physician can tell whether this condition is normal for you or a symptom of a serious health problem.

"My Problem Is . . . My Mouth and Teeth"

Help! I have bad breath and nothing, even mouthwash, does any good! What's the matter with me anyway?

Embarrassed

What causes bad breath?

Persistent bad breath can be a symptom of indigestion or one of a number of diseases. However, it is often caused by decaying teeth and/or a gum infection.

Many people, young and old alike, worry about bad breath and the social problems this may cause, and try to mask the symptom rather than to cure the underlying causes by seeking dental help.

The fact is . . . your teeth and gums are an intrinsic part of your total health. Too many young people seem to be ignoring this fact. Among the statistics compiled by the American Dental Association, one in particular stands out: Fifty percent of young people 15 and under have *never* been to a dentist.

Many adolescents may share the sentiments of one young teen who, feeling a bit under the weather, checked in with her school nurse. After asking the girl when she had her last medical examination, the nurse asked her how long it had been since she had visited her dentist.

"My dentist? What do my teeth have to do with anything?" the teen snapped. "I can't remember the last time I went to a dentist!"

Your dental health is an important part of your total health.

"Your dental health is just a sign of what's going on with the rest of your body," says Dr. Cherilyn Sheets, a dentist in Inglewood, Calif. "If you are having a lot of cavities or bleeding gums, it's a sign that you are doing something that isn't good for your body. Your mouth is the barometer of your body's health."

"In a way, we're lucky that teeth show decay relatively quickly," adds Dr. Helyn Luechauer, a Los Angeles-based dentist. "It may take a long time for the heart or muscle cells to show decay. A tooth, on the other hand, can show some decay in six months. Teeth can serve as early warning signals that what you're doing—especially what you may be eating—is not good for your body. And dental problems are widespread among young people. The ages of 13 to 16 are particularly cavity-prone years."

Teens in this age group may be especially prone to cavities because these are busy years: You're always going places, often eating on the run. You may not be taking time to clean your teeth properly. Also, you may be eating a lot of junk food or convenience food that may be laced with sugar.

How can sugar consumption and a fair amount of neglect add up to dental problems? Neglect plus sugar can equal a buildup of plaque on the teeth.

What *is* plaque? It is a film of harmful oral bacteria that forms on the teeth. Combined with sugar, certain bacteria in the plaque form acids that attack tooth enamel, leading to decay and, even worse, to gum disease. Although you can remove some of this plaque by brushing and flossing your teeth twice daily, regular visits to a dentist for a more thorough cleaning are essential to remove plaque from the hard-to-reach areas on your teeth.

Too often, people put off going to a dentist until an emergency—like a toothache—hits. But good preventive care can keep such painful emergencies from happening.

Although tooth decay is extremely common in young people (it is estimated that, by the age of 17, the average young American has nine decayed, filled, or missing teeth), it is the possibility of gum disease that causes the most concern, perhaps, among dentists. Gum disease, called *periodontal* disease, is what usually makes people lose their teeth later on in life.

A third of all Americans have no natural teeth left at all by age 60.

Sixty may seem a long way away, but the damage can start now.

I have had a problem with my gums bleeding when I brush my teeth for a couple of months now. Is this serious or not? If it matters, I'm 14.
Allen J.

During a visit to my dentist, I found out I had gum disease. My parents think that sounds strange, since they say that usually happens to older people. Can somebody who is 15 have gum disease?
Lisa R.

Periodontal disease—or advanced gum disease—is seen most often in adults, but teen-agers can show signs of the early stage called *gingivitis*.

What is this and why does it happen?

Irritating poisons and enzymes, produced by the bacteria that grow in plaque, invade the area below the gum line and can cause your gums to become inflamed and to bleed slightly during brushing. This "pink toothbrush" symptom is the most common sign of gingivitis. Other symptoms are gums that are swollen and inflamed.

What happens in more advanced gum disease?

The plaque on the teeth, extending below the gum line, starts to harden, building up into a substance called *calculus*. This causes even more irritation of the gums and eventually the gums begin to separate from the teeth. Bacteria begin to fill the spaces in between and attack the gums *and* the bone structure that supports the teeth, causing the teeth to loosen and, possibly, to be lost.

Removing plaque by regular brushing and flossing of your teeth plus regular visits to your dentist are the most effective preventive measures against gum disease. Most dentists recommend brushing at least twice a day (and rinsing your mouth after eating in between).

"If you can, it's best to brush immediately after eating, especially if you have been eating sweets," says Dr. Sheets. "Carry a toothbrush in your jeans pocket and brush after lunch at school. My father, who is also a dentist, made me do this when I was in high school. I liked sweets as much as any teen, but because I brushed immediately after eating—even at school—I have yet to develop a cavity! Flossing between your teeth is important, too. Lots of teens think that they don't have time to do this, but it's so easy. Do it while you watch TV!"

Is fluoride toothpaste better for my teeth? What kind of toothbrush should I have? And is it really nec-essary to use dental floss? (It gives me the creeps!)
Gail

It's true that some fluoride toothpastes do seem to reduce the possibility of tooth decay. Those recommended by the American Dental Association will have a notation about this on the label, so check labels! And choose a nonabrasive toothpaste for best results.

A soft-bristled toothbrush is also important. Check carefully for signs of wear. A toothbrush full of loose and bent bristles isn't going to do you much good. Plan to replace yours about every three months.

In brushing your teeth, it's important to be thorough, covering the teeth and gum line up with a gentle, circular motion, and to follow up the brushing with dental floss, to reach the cavity-prone areas between the teeth—where your toothbrush can't reach.

In addition, your dentist may recommend using "disclosing tablets," which are pills that you can put in your mouth to color any remaining plaque red (with a harmless food coloring). This will help you to see—and clean more thoroughly—areas you may have missed.

Perhaps the most important preventive measure of all, however, is a good, healthy diet.

"Your best health defense is a good diet," says Dr. Sheets. "It is basic to good dental *and* total health . . ."

"These two—dental health and total health—can't be separated," adds Dr. Luechauer. "Some dental problems can affect your whole body. For example, a tooth abscess can affect the kidneys and liver. Even when you have sore or bleeding gums, this creates a stress load on your body. It's like having a constant infection."

Both dentists insist that even slight changes in eating habits may be very beneficial.

"Don't risk failure by trying to revise your eating habits drastically all at once," says Dr. Sheets. "Eat protein-rich snacks. Learn to like salads and raw vegetables. Carry strips of bell peppers, carrots, and celery sticks with you to school. If you happen to have a party, try serving raw vegetables with a yogurt or guacamole dip. Your friends may think you're quite a gourmet!"

Dr. Luechauer believes strongly in the value of vegetables in a good diet. "Balance your diet with five vegetables for every piece of fruit you eat," she says. "You'll begin to glow after a while. When you eat protein and vegetables, it makes a big difference in the way you feel *and* look. Your complexion will glow. Your skin will be smooth and your hair will shine."

"To be healthy from a dental standpoint and overall, you need all of this: a good diet, a regular exercise program, and good hygiene. When you work to give yourself the best, you'll see wonderful results," says

Dr. Sheets. "Your mouth will be healthy and your whole body will benefit. This is what you deserve. See all this work now as a journey toward the best health you can possibly have."

I'm real depressed. My dentist said I ought to have braces. I don't have horrible buck teeth. My teeth are just a little crooked. I can live with that. What I can't live with is the thought of having those awful braces. A friend of mine has had hers for three years! I don't want to spend three years of my life like that. My parents tell me I'm being really dumb about this, but I feel that straighter teeth wouldn't be worth all the hassle. What do you think?

Chrissy L.

While many young people associate braces with eventual cosmetic benefits and present social detriments, the actual function of braces is much more crucial than simply helping you to look better.

"The main function of braces is to help the teeth to work in proper coordination with the skull," say Dr. Sheets. "If your teeth are not properly aligned, you may have jaw pain and headaches in the years to come and you may even wind up losing your teeth! Crooked teeth are a real disease factor. They decay faster because they're harder to keep clean. Periodontal disease is more likely to occur. Due to poor occlusion, your teeth may become loose. These problems tend to occur later in life. I have a number of patients in their thirties, forties, and fifties who are just now getting braces to avoid losing their teeth. Psychologically, it seems to me that it would be easier to have braces during the teens—when so many others have them, too."

The time that you will have to wear braces depends a great deal on your stage of growth, your dental condition and your co-operation.

"If your teeth are straightened about the time of your growth spurt and while you're young and your bones are softer, this can be to your advantage," says Dr. Sheets. "Also, your co-operation is important. If you wear the necessary headgear regularly and follow instructions carefully, this might shorten the time you must wear braces."

While most dentists have their own detailed instructions for patients, there are some that are practically universal.

"Avoid sweets because these not only promote tooth decay, but also irritate your gums more," says Dr. Sheets. "Stay on a good diet, floss your teeth and use a Water Pik for hard-to-reach places."

Despite any temporary disadvantages they may have, braces have two major advantages.

"First, there is the cosmetic change—lovely, straight teeth—and this lasts a lifetime," says Dr. Sheets. "A lifetime of lovely teeth makes two or three years with braces seem minimal in the long run. Second and most important is the functional change—the proper positioning of teeth—made possible by braces. In this way, braces can help you to live a happy, healthy dental life."

CREATING A HEALTHY FUTURE

My boyfriend and I just got engaged and we plan to marry next June. We're both 20 and looking forward to a lot of happy years together. Last night we talked about growing old together and how we hope we CAN do this! How can we make sure we live a long, long time?

Patti G.

My father just came down with diabetes. He also has high blood pressure and heart trouble and he's only in his late forties! Does this mean I'll get these things, too, when I'm his age? I'd like to stay healthy and live a long time because I enjoy life so much. What can I do to avoid having health problems like my dad's?

Myles R.

We would all like to live long, healthy lives.

Whether or not YOU live a long life relatively free of debilitating illness may depend very much on you and what you do now to safeguard your health!

In recent years, the concept of *preventive medicine* has become popular among health-care professionals. The purpose of this concept is to try to prevent, as much as possible, common killers like heart disease, cancer, strokes, high blood pressure, and diabetes.

Although the possibility of developing such disorders may seem remote to you right now, the fact is . . . what you do or don't do in your teen years may have a great impact on your health in later life. And the beginnings of some of these common killers may even be seen among teen-agers!

A recent survey, sponsored by the American Health Foundation and *Current Science* magazine, examined the health, habits, and food preferences of almost 22,000 young teen-agers in 46 states and came to the conclusion that many of those in their early teens are already in trouble.

Analyzing the results of the survey, which was one of the most extensive on health ever done, Dr. Christine Williams of the American Health Foundation observed that:

• As many as 30 percent of the 11- to 14-year-olds surveyed already have high cholesterol levels. High cholesterol level, which can stem from a diet high in animal fats and cholesterol, is related to atherosclerosis, or hardening of the arteries, and may in later life lead to heart disease and strokes.

• Close to half (41 percent) of those surveyed said that their food was always salted during cooking at home and more than one fourth admitted that their favorite snacks were salty ones.

Overuse of salt, Dr. Williams observes, can lead to such problems as hypertension (high blood pressure), a widespread health problem among Americans and one that may lead to life-threatening crises like heart attacks, strokes, and kidney failure as well as serious vision problems.

"The high salt intake of American teens is the most disturbing result of the *Current Science* survey," says Dr. Williams.

• A number of teens have habits that may be health-threatening. Nearly 10 percent of the younger teens surveyed smoke cigarettes and it is estimated that up to 40 percent of them (more girls than boys) will be smokers by high school graduation.

It is estimated that cigarette smoking will cause about 75 percent of the nation's 89,000 lung cancer deaths this year. Smoking may also be a factor in cancer of the lips, mouth, and esophagus, and in emphysema.

High numbers of teens—the 11- to 13-year-olds included—drink some form of alcohol regularly and some of these drink heavily. Alcohol abuse can have a number of tragic consequences: shattered lives and increased accidents now and fatal liver damage and possible cancer later on.

• American teen-agers—especially girls—do not get sufficient exercise. Only 58 percent of the girls surveyed were getting *any* form of strenuous exercise!

Lack of exercise can lead to obesity, which carries with it a greater risk of developing diabetes, high blood pressure, strokes, atherosclerosis, and heart attacks later on. Even if you *don't* become obese via a sedentary existence, you are at a greater risk of having a heart attack or stroke if you continue to avoid regular exercise.

The American Health Foundation, which conducts "Know Your Body" programs for young people to identify and correct health risks early in life, did another survey of some 4,000 adolescents up to the age of 14 in the New York City area.

The findings of this smaller survey were no less alarming. Two out of five young people who were examined had one or more of these heart-risk factors: high cholesterol (17 percent), obesity (15 percent), regular smoking habit (10 percent). A smaller percentage had other disorders like high blood pressure.

Such health screenings, says a spokesman for the foundation, are to identify and change habits that may shorten lives, early enough in life so that any damage might be reversible.

You can cut your risks of developing major health problems—and increase your chances of living a healthy life—by following these precautions:

• Eat a Balanced Diet and Watch Your Fat and Salt Intake.
• Have Your Cholesterol Level Checked by Your Physican.
• Get Down to—And Maintain—Your Ideal Weight.
• Don't Smoke and Avoid the Overuse of Alcohol.
• Get Regular Exercise.
• Learn to Deal with Stress.

These are simply the basic health maintenance musts.

It's important that you work to maintain your good health while you're young and healthy and while whatever damage there may be is reversible and/or not extensive.

It is impossible to predict how long you will live or to say "If you do this and this, you will never have a major health problem."

It is possible for you to be healthy—and happy—for many years to come. But whether or not you will be is very much up to *you*.

CHAPTER SIX

"I Need Help to Be Beautiful!"

I'm feeling guilty. I'm lucky in a lot of ways. I'm healthy and have a good figure and a nice family that's pretty well-off. There's just one problem: my nose. It's really ugly—big with a hump. It ruins my whole face. Otherwise, I'd be pretty. My family says I ought to be grateful that I have my health and people who love me. That's true. But my nose is a problem for me. I'd like so much to get it fixed so I can be pretty, too. Would a plastic surgeon do a nose job for someone who is 17 if I got my parents' consent?

Brenda R.

I want to get my ears pierced. But I'm afraid, first, that it will hurt and, second, that I'll get an infection like my girl friend did. Is ear piercing pretty safe? Should I do it?

Sheri J.

I'm ugly. Really, I'm just ugly overall. My family isn't rich, so plastic surgery is OUT! Besides, it's everything, not just one thing that's wrong. I'm tired of feeling ugly. It seems like if you're not pretty, no one wants to know you. . . .

Sad and Lonely

Although a healthy, well-nourished, and exercised body is a great start toward a more attractive you, it may not always be enough. What you may want most of all, perhaps, whether you're male or female, is to be attractive and be accepted by others.

You may have a feature that you feel keeps you from looking your best: a large nose, a receding chin, ears that stick out, or skin pitted with acne scars.

You may be plagued with excess body or facial hair.

You may wonder about the safety of ear piercing or the safety and effectiveness of cosmetics and beauty aids—like bust developers.

You may be willing to settle for something less than stunning beauty. You may just want to look, essentially, like everyone else, minus an embarrassing flaw or two.

People see so-called flaws in a variety of ways. Many contend that flaws add to your character, your individuality. Many people aren't bothered at all by a prominent nose, for example. There may be others,

on the other hand, with much less obvious physical irregularities who feel that their lives are being ruined because of these.

"Size of a deformity may have very little to do with how you feel about it," says Dr. Richard B. Aronsohn, a well-known Beverly Hills, Calif., cosmetic plastic surgeon and author of the book *The Miracle of Cosmetic Surgery* and the upcoming book *Aesthetic Surgery: A Way to a Younger and More Attractive You*. "Some people may get hysterical about a slight bump on the nose. Others with huge, horrendous noses may not be bothered at all. I see this quite often. A patient will come in with a horrible nose, but be worried about something else, like a mole! So I never try to second-guess a patient. I always *ask* what he or she would like to see changed!"

Many who do seek plastic surgery or help from cosmetics or special beauty aids may feel a bit guilty.

"I'm really self-conscious about my ears and the other kids laugh at me," says one teen. "But I know if I mentioned plastic surgery, my family would say, 'With all the sick and dying people in this world, you're worried about your *ears*? They work, don't they? So count your blessings!'"

Others, plagued by self-consciousness and shame, find that, for them, a physical defect, however slight, is a major problem.

"If you're dying inside over a defect, that can be very destructive," says Dr. Aronsohn.

Special help is available. Plastic surgery is the answer for some. Special cosmetics may be fine for others.

It's important for all of us to realize, however, the limitations of these beauty aids. These may help you to look better, but how you feel about yourself and how you choose to live your life go far beyond these procedures.

Plastic surgery to reduce the size and shape of your nose, for example, may do just that. It is not guaranteed to turn your life around, make you the most popular person in school, or drastically alter who you really are. It may help you to feel better about your appearance, but it will not guarantee instant self-esteem or a sense of immediate self-worth.

Special beauty help, combined with your growing

sense of the worthwhile person you have always been, may add a great deal to the good feelings you already have.

Plastic surgery and cosmetics cannot give you bona fide miracles, however. This is important to know, for it is in search of such miracles that many people encounter disappointments, rip-offs, and even tragedy. A commonsense approach, understanding just what these special aids can—and can't—do for you, may keep YOU from becoming a victim!

PLASTIC SURGERY

I saw an ad in the paper today about plastic surgery to increase your bustline and to make your nose better. I'd like to have this done if I can save enough money from my summer job. Is an ad like this a good way to find a good doctor?

Diana P.

I heard from some kid at school that you can't just get a nose job because you want it. She said that this doctor she knows about turned down a friend of hers who wanted her nose changed. Why would a doctor do this?

Trish A.

Plastic cosmetic surgery can be a great help to someone whose life has been adversely affected by a defect.

It can also be a tragedy when practiced by an incompetent, inexperienced surgeon or when a patient is not given adequate screening to determine if he or she will be able to have cosmetic surgery without undue physical or psychological side effects.

These two concerns may often go together. The inexperienced surgeon, whose technique may be faulty, may *also* accept patients who have physical or emotional problems that may preclude the possibility of successful cosmetic plastic surgery—patients that a more knowledgeable surgeon will advise *not* to have such surgery.

How can such incompetence happen?

Any profession has its share of incompetent people, of course, but in the area of cosmetic plastic surgery, there is an added complication. The problem is that *any* licensed physician may do surgery, including plastic surgery, even if he or she has not had any specialty training.

Major surgery, of course, is usually done in a hospital and hospitals generally don't grant surgical privileges to physicians without specialized surgical training beyond medical school. Therefore, it would be highly unlikely to find a physician without specialized training doing open heart surgery.

Plastic surgery, however, may, in some instances, be done in an office or clinic setting. So a physician is not necessarily dependent upon hospital affiliations and may simply set up his own operating room in his office or clinic. (This is not to say, of course, that all plastic surgeons who do office or clinic surgery are incompetent. Many are well-qualified and may also have hospital affiliations.)

If you're like most people, you probably want the best surgeon you can find. So how do you find a qualified, well-trained, and licensed plastic surgeon?

1. Instead of looking for ads in the paper or in the yellow pages of your telephone directory, ask your family doctor for a recommendation or check with your county medical society.

2. Check the physician's credentials, making sure that he or she is a *board-certified plastic surgeon.* Most competent, experienced physicians who have specialties are board-certified in that specific specialty. Make sure that the plastic surgeon you choose is board-certified in *plastic surgery.* You can check this out in the *Directory of Medical Specialists,* which lists all board-certified specialists in the United States. You may find this in your public library. Membership in the American College of Surgeons is an additional indication of competence.

3. Choose a doctor who is affiliated with an accredited hospital. Even if the procedure that you're contemplating may not involve a hospital stay, it's important that your doctor has a hospital affiliation— both as a measure of competence and in case of an emergency.

A competent, experienced plastic surgeon selects his or her patients with care. As we said earlier, some people are not good candidates for cosmetic plastic surgery.

For some this may involve physical reasons: a tendency toward excessive bleeding or clotting difficulties, anemia, or diabetes. Those who suffer from asthma or other respiratory disorders may be advised not to have surgery that may involve general anesthesia. For others, psychological factors may make the plastic surgeon hesitate or refuse to operate at all.

"I have to screen patients very carefully," says Dr. Aronsohn. "I may spend more time talking with them than operating on them and I do turn down a lot of prospective patients. In a way, I have to be a sort of surgical psychiatrist. You see, in some people, neurosis may be situational, stemming from an ugly feature. Correct that and the neurosis is gone. Other people are basically neurotic. They are never happy with themselves, no matter what surgery is done. They keep coming back for more and more surgery. They practically become your relatives. Some, too, may use a defect as a convenient crutch, a cop-out. If you remove this, the person may have a crisis. For example, I recently talked with a boy who came in to have his nose done. He had, basically, no physical problem, but he did have deep psychological problems. He just used his nose as a rationalization for all the problems in his life. If I went ahead and changed the nose without this boy coming to terms with himself, I might do more harm than good. I might suggest that a person like this get psychiatric help. Also, quite frankly, I am very careful about the perfectionist type who may be very alarmed about the slightest flaw. The truth is that each patient and each surgical procedure is very individual. I can't predict who will heal well and who won't. I wish I could, but I can't. . . .''

Dr. Aronsohn and other experienced plastic surgeons are also careful to discuss expectations with patients before surgery.

''I will always ask a patient what he or she expects from cosmetic surgery,'' says Dr. Aronsohn. ''It's important to have a meeting of the minds. I draw a charcoal sketch of how I envision his or her new nose or whatever and then I ask, 'What do you want?' and we discuss it. People often have an idea of how they'd like to look that may or may not be possible. If you would come to me wanting to look like a certain movie star, you may want something I can't give you. You may be wanting not so much that person's features, but his or her life-style and that I really can't give you. That's why it's so important that we talk about expectations and realities before surgery.''

Pain and necessary recovery time is another reality that Dr. Aronsohn carefully discusses with patients.

''People talk about cosmetic surgery being miraculous,'' says Dr. Aronsohn. ''They may feel that you can have this surgery without pain or scars or convalescence. That just isn't true. There is discomfort involved. And any time you cut the skin, there will be some amount of scarring. Also, it takes time to recover from cosmetic surgery, as with any surgery. You may look temporarily worse before you look better. Most doctors will take a sick patient and make him or her well. I take a well patient and make him or her sick—temporarily—in an effort to improve a defect. Yet some patients get very upset when they realize that cosmetic surgery does not mean a miracle or a complete rebirth.''

Even if cosmetic plastic surgery is not a miracle, it can help to improve your appearance, sometimes dramatically. There are a number of different procedures. The ones that teens have asked us most about are rhinoplasty (nose), mammaplasty (breast), otoplasty (ears), and dermabrasion (skin).

The Nose (Rhinoplasty)

My nose is big and ugly and ruins my whole face. If it weren't for my nose, I'd be pretty.
Brenda R.

It seems that people notice a nose primarily when it is ugly, and an unattractive nose can nearly spoil the look of an otherwise handsome or pretty face.

A surgical procedure called *rhinoplasty* can correct cosmetic defects of the nose as well as physical defects that may cause breathing difficulties.

''The nose is one of the few features that can be changed dramatically with no outward evidence of surgery such as scars or suture marks,'' says Dr. Aronsohn. ''When you combine a nose operation with a chin augmentation (as in the case of a person who has a large nose and a receding chin—an often-seen combination) you can really change the face dramatically.''

Rhinoplasty is performed on a number of teen-age girls and boys. However, it is best performed when nasal bone growth is complete.

''This would be about 16 or 17 for girls and slightly later for boys,'' says Dr. Aronsohn. ''The late teens are, generally, a good time to have rhinoplasty.''

What happens during a typical operation of this type?

Each case is highly individual, of course, but the following account from 18-year-old Cheryl may be fairly typical.

''My nose was too big and had an ugly hump in it,'' she writes. ''After consulting with my surgeon, we set a date that would come during my summer vacation before college. The night before the surgery, I checked into the hospital for necessary tests and then early the next morning, I was given a sedative. I didn't have an anesthetic that put me out, just a local. But my doctor did tell me that if I was really scared, I could have what he called a basal general anesthetic, which wouldn't put me out, but give me a kind of amnesia about what went on. But even though I was scared, I wanted to know what was happening!''

''I got shots in the inside and outside of my nose,'' Cheryl continues. ''These didn't really hurt, but it sounds awful, doesn't it? It didn't bother me at the time. The surgery was done entirely within my nose. I didn't feel pain, just a kind of pressure and I felt a tapping on my nose at the hump. My doctor explained that to remove the hump he had to break the nasal bones first. As he finished the operation, my doctor put stitches—he called them sutures—inside my nose, so I have no outside scars at all! Then he packed my nose with gauze and put a splint on it. He explained that this would help to protect and to shape it. Afterward, nurses put ice on my eyes and nose to keep my swelling and bruises down. I did get some of both anyway. Guess it's inevitable!"

Did Cheryl experience any other discomfort after her surgery?

"Well . . . yes . . . some," she admits. "I hear that some people have more pain than others. Mostly, I was bothered by having my nose filled with gauze and having to breathe through my mouth all the time. My throat felt really dry."

How long does it take to recuperate from rhinoplasty?

"I was in the hospital for four days, but I have a girl friend who had the same thing done and she was only hospitalized for two days," says Cheryl. "And a friend of hers who had the same thing done in a clinic had the operation in the morning and went home late that afternoon. So it varies a lot, depending, I guess, on your own case and what your doctor thinks best. On my last day in the hospital, my doctor took the gauze out of my nose and removed the splint and I saw my nose for the first time. My face and nose were swollen and my eyes were black, but my nose still looked great. I looked pretty OK within a week and by the end of three weeks, the black-and-blue marks were gone. So was the swelling. I healed pretty fast, I think . . . and I can't tell you how glad I am that I had this done!"

Although swelling and bruising (which are normal reactions to the surgery) may subside after three weeks, it may take up to six months for the affected tissues to heal completely.

"How quickly and well a patient heals may depend a lot on the patient and how well he or she follows directions," says Dr. Aronsohn. "It's important, for example, to avoid a bump on the nose during the healing period, yet some kids will be out there surfing or skateboarding or, even worse, necking, which may actively engage the nose. I also advise patients to avoid the sun for a while, since this can cause swelling of the nose."

Physical healing is not the only postoperative concern. There are psychological factors to be considered as well. No two patients will react in quite the same way to his or her new attractiveness and attention from the opposite sex. One person may feel frightened or threatened by this, whereas another may relish the attention to such an extreme that other aspects of his or her life may be neglected. These examples tend to represent extremes, however.

It seems that the average teen who has rhinoplasty will find that while this operation can make him or her more attractive—sometimes dramatically so—it can't change all the negative aspects of life, bringing instant popularity, confidence, and nonstop happiness. There will always be moments of pain and of loneliness. Life won't be perfect, but it *can* be better.

Her new nose helped 17-year-old Marcia to grow in confidence and the realization that beauty isn't everything.

"Now, instead of worrying about how awful my nose is, I can say 'Oh, looks don't matter!' and then concentrate on other things," she says. "But I had to be *attractive* before I could do that."

How much does rhinoplasty cost?

Rates vary widely according to doctor, locale, and the difficulty of the individual operation, but you might expect to pay between $1,500 and $2,000 for rhinoplasty, with an additional $750 average fee for a chin augmentation if you choose to have it. This latter procedure is often done in conjunction with nasal surgery and involves putting a solid silicone implant through a small incision either inside the mouth or underneath the chin.

Most cosmetic surgery is not covered by medical insurance, but if your rhinoplasty involves correction of a breathing difficulty, insurance may cover part of the cost.

The Breasts (Mammaplasty)

I'm 15 and miserable. My breasts are really tiny. I'm almost as flat as a child. I heard that you can get your breasts enlarged by plastic surgery and I'd like to know how this is done and how much it costs.

Mary Lou S.

I'd like to have silicone shots to make my breasts bigger, but my doctor says they're illegal here. Is there a state where I could have this done? I don't want to have an operation to increase my bust size because I don't want any scars. I'm 21 and working, so I think I should be able to decide what I want to do with my body, don't you?

Janna P.

Cosmetic surgery on the breasts seems to cover two extremes: women who have tiny breasts and those who have breasts so massive that posture defects, breathing difficulties, and backaches have become a way of life.

Help is available for women in either situation, although *breast augmentation* (increasing the size of the breasts) is, perhaps, more common. This surgery can help women who are flat-chested or those who have breasts that differ a great deal in size.

Such surgery is generally not performed before the patient is 20 to make sure that normal breast development is complete. We would, therefore, advise Mary Lou, who is "15 and miserable," to wait a few years before seeking surgery. Breast growth may not be complete at her age and any type of breast surgery might be ill-advised.

We would advise Janna to listen to her doctor. Silicone injections, which were used for breast augmentation some years ago, are now illegal for a good reason: They can cause severe inflammation, infection, and severe scarring of breast tissues.

Silicone *implants* are now generally used to increase breast size. This is the safest and most successful breast augmentation method at this time.

How does it work?

A small (one- to three-inch) incision is made just below the breast and a contoured silicone envelope (filled with silicone gel) is folded and inserted through the incision. This implant, which comes in eight sizes, is placed in a surgically created pocket beneath the breast tissue, overlying the chest muscle. These tissues are allowed to penetrate the Dacron mesh backing on the implant, which further assures its adherence.

In the majority of cases, breast augmentation is done under general anesthesia with a three- to five-day hospital stay (or a six- to eight-hour stay at an outpatient clinic) and a basic recuperation time of several weeks. Bandages and sutures are removed about a week after surgery and an elastic support bra must be worn at all times for the next two to six weeks.

Although there is a small scar from the incision, it is usually well-hidden by the fold of the breast.

How much does a breast augmentation cost?

Again, the price varies widely, but you might expect to pay between $1,000 and 2,000.

My breasts are too big and all the guys at school tease me. I'm 15 and a 32D. I can't stand it. Can I get surgery to make my bust smaller?

Claudia L.

I can't tell you how bad I feel because of my breasts. I'm too embarrassed to tell you my bra size, but I'm so big that my bra straps (already wide and padded) are cutting into my shoulders. I have scars to prove it! I have backaches all the time. What can be done to help me? Would a doctor do surgery on my breasts?

Lori A.

Because breast-reduction surgery is neither simple nor without undesirable side effects (like noticeable scars), some surgeons do not perform this at all and many others do so only in instances of extreme necessity.

For example, a surgeon might not operate on Claudia, but might consider Lori, who is having detrimental physical symptoms related to her breast size. Women who fall into this category are often advised to consider such surgery carefully.

What does breast-reduction surgery involve?

The operation is fairly lengthy (three to five hours) and is done under general anesthesia in a hospital. Skin and excess breast tissue are removed via a circular incision around the nipple and areola, and an inverted T-shaped incision in the lower part of the breast. Usually, the nipple is not removed and relocated higher on the breast, so a young woman who has had this surgery may nurse any babies she may have.

However, if the breast is extremely massive, the nipple and areola may be repositioned higher up on the breast. When a young woman is involved, a surgeon may transplant the nipple on a flap with glandular tissue attached, in an attempt to preserve her breast-feeding function.

After surgery, the patient will usually remain in the hospital for several days. Bandages and sutures are removed after one or two weeks with a three-week general recovery period. The patient will usually be instructed to wear a well-fitting bra for one to two months. As we mentioned earlier, the inverted T-shaped scar on the breast will always be present, although it may fade somewhat with time. It is on the underside of the breast, however, and so cannot be seen if the woman is wearing a bra or bathing suit.

The cost of such surgery varies a great deal, but it may be as much as $3,000.

The Ears (Otoplasty)

People are constantly teasing me and always have on account of my ears. My ears are large and stick out. As long as I can remember my classmates have called me "Dumbo." I'm beginning to believe the name! I've heard about special surgery that can make your ears look normal and I'd like to know more about it. I'm 15 and have had just about enough of this teasing!

Richard P.

Ears can be reduced and recontoured in a surgical procedure known as *otoplasty,* or external ear surgery.

If the ear is of normal size, but simply protrudes, the surgeon may position it closer to the head by removing some of the stiff cartilage that is holding the ear away from the head. If the ear is also too large, the surgeon may reduce its size, making incisions in the outer part of the ear. A turban-type dressing covering the ears will be worn for two or three days following surgery. After that, the patient will wear an elastic circular headband while sleeping, to prevent the ear from curling under the head. This precaution is used for about two weeks.

In all cases, the incisions of ear surgery are inconspicuous, often made behind the ear in natural skin folds so that any scars that may result are hidden. Don't be alarmed if your ears have a distinct purple hue for a short time after surgery. This exotic coloring is just a temporary side effect of surgery and will disappear within a month, during which time you should avoid sunbathing and most sports.

This operation may be done in a hospital (with an overnight stay) or in an outpatient clinic (with about a six-hour stay) and is generally done with a local anesthetic.

Surgical fees vary widely for otoplasty, depending a great deal on the individual problem. Your physician can give you a more accurate estimate of the costs involved, based on your specific needs.

The Skin (Dermabrasion)

I'm 19, a college sophomore, and embarrassed about the acne scars that really ruin the skin on my face. Is there anything I can do to get rid of these scars?

Connie R.

Two years ago, I did something really dumb. I got a tattoo on my arm with a heart and the name DeDe (my steady at the time). Well, now I'm going with a girl named Karen and my DeDe tattoo really bugs her. I'm pretty sick of it myself. Is there some way I could get it removed?

Paul S.

Acne scars, pockmarks, and other facial scars as well as some tattoos may be removed (or reduced) by a procedure called *dermabrasion*.

Dermabrasion—a surgical planing of the skin—can bring a 30 to 60 percent improvement to an acne-scarred face the first time it is done. If there is severe scarring, two or three abrasions may be necessary.

This procedure is usually done on the face. Since the skin of the chest, neck, back, and legs tends to heal slowly, a physician will be most cautious about trying dermabrasion in these areas. In addition, dark-skinned people, who may be subject to changes in skin pigmentation after skin planing, may be risky candidates for dermabrasion.

Dermabrasion may be done in the doctor's office with a local anesthetic if a small area of skin is involved. If the whole face is to be planed, the patient will be hospitalized and given a general anesthetic.

What happens in the course of a dermabrasion?

The surgeon removes the outer layer of skin with a surgical planer, a high-speed rotary wheel with a wire brush, stone, or diamond fraise cover. Near the lips and eyes, antiseptic sandpaper is used.

A person who has had a dermabrasion in the doctor's office will usually go home within an hour afterward if there is no unusual bleeding. A person who has had a whole-face dermabrasion will usually remain in the hospital for another day. Generally, there are no bandages applied and, at first, the results may seem unsightly.

Initially, the skin is moist, oozing a yellowish serum that will harden into a crust after a day or so. The face swells and throbs under the crust for the next two days with swelling decreasing after the third day. After the first week, the crust will begin to crack and peel off. This peeling may go on for about two weeks.

"The new skin will look smooth and pink and is usually superior to the final result, since swelling tends to mask small remaining scars," says Dr. Aronsohn.

Once the crust has peeled, you will look like you've had a bit too much sun for about two months—and it's essential to avoid overexposure to the sun during this time.

"The skin will be tender and easily irritated for several months," says Dr. Aronsohn. "So it is essential to shield the new skin from sunburn or windburn until the skin has regained its natural color."

Salabrasion, which is similar to dermabrasion, may be used to remove a tattoo. However, in this procedure, a softer, felt-covered wheel is used. This may take a bit longer, but less scarring is likely to result.

How much do dermabrasion and salabrasion cost?

It is not really possible to give a fair range for all aspects of these various procedures, since prices may vary a great deal. A surgeon would have to see your skin to determine what your costs would be. However, for a full-face dermabrasion, you might expect to pay as much as $1,500.

Surgical revisions may also reduce scars.

"However, I tell patients that any operation that begins with an incision ends with a scar," says Dr. Aronsohn. "I'm very careful when I talk with people who want scar revisions. So many of them expect *no* scar for this surgery. This can't be done."

Fat Removal Surgery

I have lots of fat on my hips and thighs and can't seem to lose weight. I heard that you can get your fat cut out. I'd like to do it, so I could wear jeans and a bikini like everyone else. Could you give me some information about this?

Janet L.

Since obesity is such a concern among teens, Janet's question is only one of many we have received about surgical fat removal.

There is such an operation, but it is expensive, involves major surgery, hospitalization, extended recuperation time, *and* extensive scarring.

"A patient might look fine in jeans after the operation, but a bikini? Never! Not with those scars!" says Dr. Aronsohn. "It's a continual source of amazement to me that so many people ask about this, that so many would rather have fat cut out—even if it leaves serious scars—than go on a sensible diet and exercise schedule. The latter plus a real commitment to being thin is the best way to reduce. This commitment is so important. Changing the feelings behind obesity will help you to lose weight and, most important, to maintain that loss. That's why I think that Weight Watchers®, with its group concept and maintenance plan, is such a good idea."

Alternatives

I have a big nose, but there's no way my folks can afford plastic surgery for me. Is there anything else I can do to make it look less obvious?

Kim H.

My ears stick out a little and I'd like to have them fixed surgically, but this will have to wait until after I have a full-time job and can save some money. What can I do in the meantime?

Leslie L.

I have a problem that's really getting to me. My parents think I ought to have a nose job and want to give this to me as a twenty-first-birthday present next spring. I don't want one. I like my nose as it is. It isn't cute, but it has character and it's mine. I feel hurt that my parents can't see what it means to me to be unique and real. I like myself "as is." Am I wrong not to want surgery that could make me look more conventionally attractive?

Rachael R.

Plastic surgery isn't for everyone.

For some, the cost may be prohibitive, although some plastic surgeons and medical groups may give special consideration to needy individuals.

For a number of teens, however, special cosmetic tricks will have to do.

You might have your hair styled in such a way that it will camouflage protruding ears.

You could also de-emphasize a prominent nose with makeup and a new hairstyle.

"You might try shading your nose with a light tan foundation and accenting your eyes and mouth to draw attention away from the nose," says Dr. Aronsohn. "Also, stark, pulled-back hairstyles are not for you! These only advertise the size of your nose."

Some young people—like Rachael—may have a feature that *others* see as defective, but they may be quite content with it themselves. Irregular and/or unusual features can be fascinating and are definitely not a problem for many people. It all depends on how you feel.

You may find that you're basically comfortable with yourself and your body just as it is.

COSMETICS

Cosmetics play a big part in many of our lives.

Last year, Americans spent about $8 billion on cosmetics: soaps, shampoos, deodorants, perfumes, aftershave lotions, makeup, and moisturizers—among other items.

All too often, these products disappoint us, failing to live up to the promises of the ads. They may even cause more problems for us, triggering allergic reaction, irritations or, in some cases, infections.

They may also put a strain on our pocketbooks as the price of bottled beauty soars. As costs—and consumer expectations—rise, it's vital to choose cosmetics with care.

I try all kinds of cosmetics, but it never looks as good on me as it does on the models, I feel cheated. I try to buy good stuff but can't afford really expensive makeup. Would it be worth it to save up my money and get the most expensive? Is the quality that much better?

Janine G.

I notice that ingredients are now listed on cosmetics. Why? Most of it doesn't mean that much to me and most things seem to have pretty much the same ingredients.

Georgia B.

Along with cosmetics, this giant industry sells dreams.

"Hope springs eternal," says Dr. Aronsohn. "And the cosmetics industry sells hopes and dreams at a high profit!"

In an attempt to protect your health and your cash, the Federal Drug Administration now requires cosmetic companies to list the ingredients on product labels in descending order, with the major ingredient at the top of the list. If you read labels carefully, you may find that there is little, if any, difference between a cheaper brand and an expensive cosmetics line. In the latter case, you may be paying for a famous name and, perhaps, for more elaborate packaging.

The new labels can be health protectors, too, since if you do have an adverse reaction to a product, you and your doctor may be able to determine, possibly, which substances may be involved and which ones you might avoid in the future.

What are some of the ingredients you are likely to find on a cosmetics label?

Solvents—primarily water and alcohol—are liquids in which solid substances are dissolved. Purified water may make up a large percentage of some cosmetics, and generally, this is one of the cheapest and safest cosmetic ingredients. In fact, it may be better for your skin if you use a cosmetic with a high water content rather than one with a high oil content. This may be particularly true of makeup bases. In some cases, the cheaper brands, which tend to contain more water, may actually be better for you. Alcohol is a frequent ingredient in astringents, perfumes, and in aftershave lotions.

Emollients—like mineral oil, lanolin, and glycerin—make the skin feel smooth, either by preventing loss of moisture from the skin surface or by getting moisture from the air. These are found particularly in moisturizers and hand and body lotions.

Emulsifiers—like sodium lauryl sulfate—are a component of lotions and keep water and oil ingredients from separating, and *stabilizers*—like sodium citrate—work with the emulsifiers.

Preservatives—like the parabens—keep harmful bacteria from growing in cosmetics.

A number of teens claim to like the natural look in cosmetics and express a desire to shun products with artificial preservatives. Most cosmetics, however—even those claiming to be "natural"—contain preservatives. There is an important reason for this. Growth of bacteria in cosmetics, particularly in eye makeup, may endanger your health.

I'm not sure, but I think I may be allergic to makeup. I started using a new lipstick and got a blister on my lips. Could this be an allergy?
Paula W.

It could be an allergy or it could simply be a skin reaction, an irritation caused by a particular product. *Contact dermatitis,* as this is called, is usually confined to the site of contact and irritations, rather than allergies, account for most common adverse reactions to cosmetics. Such a reaction does not mean that you have to give up cosmetics. You may find that you can use another product that may contain a different concentration of the irritating ingredient with no adverse reaction at all.

Identifying the source of irritation isn't always easy. Cosmetics may not be at fault, in some instances. You may, for example, have an adverse reaction to the metal in earrings or hairpins. There are some common ingredients, however, that are more likely than others to cause irritation.

A recent study by the Federal Drug Administration found that the highest rate of adverse reactions were found in deodorants and antiperspirants, hair sprays, hair colorings, bubble bath, mascara, moisturizers, eye creams, and chemical hair removers.

So if you suffer from an irritation and use one or several of these products, you might examine the possibility that this may be a likely source of your problem.

You may keep a troublesome irritation from happening on a large scale by trying a preliminary patch test, recommended particularly in the instructions for hair-coloring products, permanents, and chemical hair removers.

If you're plagued with allergies, do a patch test on any product you're thinking of using, preferably before you buy it. Many stores have demonstrator samples available for such testing.

Are hypoallergenic cosmetics better than regular ones for any type of skin? Are they guaranteed not to cause problems? Just how good are they?
Pamela J.

"Hypoallergenic" on the label of a particular cosmetic means that it is less likely to cause adverse reactions.

The Food and Drug Administration now requires all cosmetics manufacturers using the term *hypoallergenic* to run numerous tests proving that these products really are less likely to cause allergic or irritating reactions than are competing products.

If you have a history of allergies or irritations, it's

a good idea to pick a hypoallergenic product. These days, there are a number of choices available in all price ranges.

However, it's important to note that while hypoallergenic products may be less likely to irritate your skin, they will not clear up or cure existing skin problems like acne.

I've heard that mascara may be dangerous. How come? Also, my girl friend says you should never share eye makeup with anyone else. Is she right or is she just being selfish?

Sue Y.

It's true that mascara and other eye makeup has been under close scrutiny by the Food and Drug Administration lately. The problem is that possible contamination of the cosmetic through normal use may trigger physical symptoms—some serious—in the user.

While most eye makeup is pure at the time of purchase, skin bacteria can reach the makeup in a number of ways, for example, when you put your finger in an eye shadow container or touch a mascara wand to your eyelid. This bacteria may grow in the cosmetic and may be dangerous to the eye, causing red eyes, sties, inflamed lids, or, at worst, an eye infection that, if unchecked, may lead to blindness. This kind of infection may happen, for example, if your hand would happen to slip while you were applying mascara and the cornea of your eye were to be scratched by the contaminated mascara wand.

A number of reports of corneal infections and ulcerations due to the use of contaminated cosmetics have reached the FDA, which is now strongly recommending that all manufacturers use special preservatives, particularly in eye makeup, to prevent the growth of such microorganisms.

There are several steps that you, too, can take to safeguard your eyes.

- Don't lend or borrow eye makeup.
- Be sure that the makeup you use contains a preservative. (Check the label!)
- Don't keep mascara too long. Preservatives may begin to lose their effectiveness after three or four months. Replace your mascara after that time, even if you have plenty still left.
- When you buy new mascara, *always* discard the old brush.
- Wash your hands before using cosmetics.
- Keep makeup containers tightly closed when not in use.
- If a product needs water, use water, *not* saliva! Never lick an eyeliner brush or spit in any makeup.

- Don't leave cosmetics or a purse containing cosmetics in the sun. Intense heat may make the preservatives less effective.

Another safety tip that may apply to all cosmetic products is this: read directions carefully and use the product exactly as instructed!

If the manufacturer suggests a patch test, do it.

Don't use a hair-coloring product on your eyelashes.

Don't put cosmetics on already irritated skin.

The more common sense you use and the more you know about what cosmetics can and can't do for you, the less likely you will be to be disappointed or ripped off!

SUNTAN PREPARATIONS

I'm a sun-lover, but want to protect my skin from harm while getting a tan. What kind of product should I use?

John M.

I'm wondering about "instant tan" products. Will a tan from this protect my skin when I do go out in the sun?

Laura J.

I like the tan look, but hate going out in the sun a lot. Also, I hear that's bad for you. What can I do? I don't like looking pale!

Tammie F.

As we discussed in Chapter Five, sun-lovers *do* risk prematurely aged skin among other problems, but there are ways to have a tan and protect your skin, somewhat, too.

If you like the tanned look, but choose to avoid long sessions in the sun, a temporary bronzer that will wash off with ordinary soap and water may be preferable to an instant tan product.

The instant tan products, which supposedly tan you without exposure to the sun, have chemicals in them that make your skin look brown, but this is not a true tan. It is not a buildup of melanin (see Chapter Five) and therefore offers you no protection when you do go out in the sun. Also, when an instant tan product begins to wear off, it can give you a stunningly *un*beautiful mottled look!

So if you are an inside person who likes the outdoors *look,* try a bronzer that you apply fresh each time you opt for a tanned look!

If you're a sun-lover or a sports-lover whose pursuits keep you out in the sun, here are some tips to add to the ones we already gave you in Chapter Five.

- Use a sunscreen—especially at first. Even if your skin is dark, you need such protection. Some sunscreens block all light and prevent tanning. These would contain zinc oxide or titanium oxide. Others allow some light to pass through for a slow, even tan. These products tend to contain chemical blockers like para-aminobenzoic acid.
- If your skin is fair, always use maximum protectors. If your skin is medium to dark, start with maximum protectors, and as you tan, move on to products giving you medium protection.
- Use special protectors for sensitive areas like nose, eyelids, and lips.
- Applying a moisturizer after sun exposure will also help to keep your skin soft. It doesn't have to be an expensive product. Baby lotion will do.

EAR PIERCING

I want to get my ears pierced, but don't want to get an infection like this one girl I know did. Is it safe to get my ears pierced at a department store or should I go to a doctor?

Sally N.

I just got my ears pierced (at a store) and so far everything is fine. I want it to stay fine. What can I do to make sure my ear holes don't close up and that I don't get an infection?

Linda B.

Ear piercing is a popular fashion trend among teens. Done properly, under antiseptic conditions, it can be quite safe.

However, if you have a tendency to bleed heavily, have allergies to metals, are unusually susceptible to infections, or tend to form keloid scars, you may want to approach ear piercing with caution. Consult your physician first. In cases like this, it is especially important to have ear piercing done by a physician.

Some people try to go the do-it-yourself route and pierce their own ears—or have a friend do it. We don't advise this. Most of those we have seen with adverse side effects—like infections—have been do-it-yourselfers.

Infections like this may cause swelling around the ear puncture and, if unchecked, may lead to more serious health problems as well as scarring of the earlobes.

The best way to avoid such complications is to have your ears pierced by a physician. The doctor will use a sterile stainless-steel needle or an instrument much like a stapler, which will insert a spring-loaded earring into your earlobe. Although the procedure is generally painless, the physician may use a topical local anesthetic on the earlobe to numb it.

Many department and jewelry stores have special technicians trained to pierce ears. Here, the ear is often pierced with the sterilized post of the earring itself. As long as your ear is sterilized with alcohol before and after the piercing and as long as the earring has been sterilized and has never been used by another person, such ear piercing is generally safe.

After piercing, surgical steel or 14-carat gold studs are immediately inserted into the earlobe holes and must be worn continuously for about six weeks until the ears heal.

Wearing post earrings for about six months before trying wires may also help your ears to continue to heal and may ensure that the holes in your earlobes will remain instead of shrinking down into mere slits.

Other after-care hints:

- As your ears heal, dab the lobes regularly with alcohol or mild soap to keep bacteria away.
- Always dip your earrings in alcohol before inserting them.
- Be patient! Allow your ears to heal before removing or changing your earrings, or you may find that your earlobe holes will close up, making it painful (or impossible) to put the earrings back in.

EXCESS HAIR

Help! I'm a 15-year-old girl who is HAIRY! I have hair on my chin and a few hairs around the nipples of my breasts. The hair on my chin really looks awful. What can I do about it? My mom says it runs in the family. Help!

Maria G.

I have a lot of hair on my back. It looks weird. I'd like to have it removed. Obviously, I can't shave it myself. Should I try something like electrolysis or waxing? I heard there are good ways to get rid of hair like this. I'm a 21-year-old male college student.

Mark M.

I have excess hair on my upper lip and chin and break out from using chemical hair removers. I've seen ads for do-it-yourself electrolysis devices. Would this be safe to try?

Eileen S.

Excess hair growth, particularly on the face, can be an embarrassing problem.

For many, the cause may be genetic. If your ethnic origin is from the Mediterranean area (Italian, Spanish, Semitic, Greek, and so forth), you may have a greater-than-average tendency to have more body and facial hair than, say, someone of Scandinavian or Oriental origin.

For a minority of young people, excess hair may signal a hormone imbalance or gland problem. If you are well into adolescence—in your late teens—and suddenly develop excess hair, you might want to consult your physician. For most, however, the cause is genetic rather than glandular.

What can you do about excess hair?

Many women, of course, choose to shave leg and armpit hair (which is perfectly normal—and superfluous only because of our fashion and grooming trends) or remove it with chemical hair removers called *depilatories*.

Depilatories dissolve hair on the skin surface, but do not remove hair permanently. They may also be somewhat irritating to the skin, so try them with caution (on a small area) first. If you have facial hair, use a depilatory designed for use on the face or a general one that is safe for facial use.

When a few hairs are involved on the chin or breasts, some women prefer to pluck the hair. This may be a bit painful and does not, again, remove the hair permanently.

Another effective, albeit temporary, treatment is the hot wax method for removing hair. This can be done at home (following instructions from a hot wax hair remover kit *exactly*), but, especially when a large area is involved, it is best done by a professional in a beauty salon or a special waxing salon. (These do not exist in moderate to large cities.) Here, hot was is applied to the skin and then, after cooling, is pulled off, taking excess hair with it. One treatment does not remove hair permanently, but treatments over a period of time *may* retard hair growth.

Someone like Mark, who has extensive hair on his back and limited funds, might try this method instead of the more expensive electrolysis. Waxing is not entirely painless and may cause an inflammatory reaction. Also, individual results vary widely.

There are, presently, two kinds of permanent hair removal.

Electrolysis is the best known. Here, a tiny electrode placed, via a needle, into the hair follicle discharges a high-speed electric current, destroying the hair root.

This method of hair removal usually works well, but there are some drawbacks. It is expensive, time-consuming, may be painful, and can produce scars, es-

pecially if it is done by an inexperienced technician.

For this reason, we don't recommend home-style electrolysis. You may not be able to locate each hair follicle exactly, and in addition, the do-it-yourself units usually don't have automatic shutoff devices that stop the electric current after a few seconds to help prevent scarring.

Shop carefully for a qualified electrologist. Your search might begin with recommendations from your physician or your county medical association.

A new method of permanent hair removal is Depilatron, which is similar to electrolysis, but is, reportedly, less painful and less time-consuming. A number of beauty salons offer the Depilatron method of hair removal. Like electrolysis, it can be expensive. Also, there has been recent scientific controversy about this method and the advertising claims of Depilatron are currently under investigation by the Federal Trade Commission. It may be best to avoid this method until a ruling is made.

QUESTIONABLE BEAUTY AIDS

I saw an ad for some device that would make me lose a lot of weight in an hour with no pills, no diet, and no exercise. Is this possible do you think?
                                        Sheila B.

I'm flat-chested and hate it! Would this cream I saw advertised really increase my bust size?
                                        Donna D.

Tell me the truth, do those bust developers that you see advertised in all the magazines REALLY work? Do they increase your bust like they say? If not, how do they get away with such ads?
                                        Mary Q.

Some beauty devices promise more than they could possibly give you: instant (and seemingly effortless) weight loss or a quickly blossoming bosom!

Many people—especially the young—would like to believe such promises.

Being a smart consumer, however, means using common sense and recognizing some basic facts:

1. True weight loss is never instant nor does it happen without diet and exercise, generally. Some "instant weight loss" devices come with diet recommendations and, in most cases, if you simply followed the diet itself, you would probably lose weight eventually. Keep in mind that there are *no* miracles or shortcuts to weight loss. It takes time and effort!

2. Creams cannot really increase your bust size.

Such creams usually contain hormones and may cause an inflammation of your breasts (which may be harmful), but will not bring about a true increase in the size of your breasts.

3. Bust developers do not increase the size of your breasts. These devices, if used over a period of time, may increase your bust size overall, by exercising your pectoral (chest) and back muscles. This will perhaps lead to an increase in your all-around bust measurement (as it is measured around the torso), but will not increase your actual breast (cup) size.

A recent special study by Good Housekeeping Institute's Beauty Clinic confirmed that cup size was not increased at all by the use of several bust-developer devices. Their conclusion: Eternal hope rather than effectiveness accounts for the sale success of such products.

Don't let money-back guarantees cloud your skepticism. In some cases, the money-back guarantee time limit expires before the product has a chance to show whether or not it will be effective. In many cases, the manufacturer is betting that you will be too embarrassed, too lazy, or too eternally hopeful to return an ineffective device and demand your money back.

One fact to keep in mind as you scan the ads: If it sounds too good to be true, it probably is too good to be true!

It may be helpful, too, to keep all beauty aids—from plastic surgery to cosmetics—in perspective. These aids can help you to look more physically attractive—period. Looking more attractive may help to improve the quality of your life, but it will not change your life or the person you are. The growth and development of the person you would like to be and the life-style you would like to have is very much up to YOU!

CHAPTER SEVEN

Habits and Your Health

Oh, no! Not another sermon on smoking, drinking, and drugs! Argghh! I can't stand it!! I've heard SO many.

Kara S.

These things turn me off, man. It's up to the individual, you know what I mean?

Gary Y.

OK. Be honest. Do you share some of Kara's or Gary's sentiments as you start this chapter? Are you toying with the idea of skipping it altogether because you're heard all the old sermons and scare stories before?

As we discuss habits like coffee and cola drinking, smoking, drugs, and alcohol, and the effects that these habits may have on your health, we will try very hard to give you the facts—pro and con when possible—with no heavy judgments.

Let's face it: We all have habits that are part of our lives. We decide what our habits will be. Some may be beneficial, some potentially harmful. Some of the ones we know may be harmful, we may choose to do anyway.

It's true that we make our own choices. However, the best—and free-est—choices are *informed* choices. So let's share some information and ideas for a while.

Some of these ideas may make you want to reevaluate some of your choices. Some, on the other hand, may not affect you in the slightest. That's up to you. But it's important for all of us to look at our habits, whatever they may be, and see how they affect our lives and, perhaps, most important, see how these habits came to be.

As you read this chapter, you may discover a lot about yourself, not only about some significant habits and how they may be affecting you, but also some of the feelings behind these habits. You may also find ways to cope with and change some of these feelings—and habits—if you choose.

HOW DOES A HABIT BECOME A HABIT?

All my friends were smoking, so I decided to try it. I like it. I'm a nervous person, especially in social situations and smoking gives me something to do with my hands.

Terri M.

I love coffee! When I was little, my mom would say "No, you can't have coffee yet. Wait till you're grown up!" She let me have my first cup on my fourteenth birthday and I was so happy. Now I find I can't start my day without a cup of coffee!

Lisa R.

Don't laugh, but I think I'm addicted to chocolate! Sometimes I really feel like I crave it!

Bill T.

I'm basically shy and find it hard to talk to girls. In order to have any fun at all at a party, I'd have to get loaded.

Dennis C.

I smoke marijuana sometimes with my friends. I'm not a big doper or anything. It's just a kind of congenial thing you do with friends. Mostly, I do it because it feels good.

Judy P.

I see now that my drinking problem started in junior high. See, I was skinny and shy and didn't have any friends. Then this one group of girls took an interest in me. They helped me to fix myself up and feel more confident. They were also drinkers and I started drinking so I could really be part of the group. But I was different. Once I started drinking, I couldn't stop.

M.L.

My parents always fight. (They hate each other.) I've been living in pain all my life. No one knows I take drugs and alcohol. I always felt I'm divorced from the real world.

Desperate

We acquire our habits for a variety of reasons and with a myriad of feelings.

Smoking and drinking alcohol or coffee may have a positive meaning for you. Doing these things may symbolize growing up.

Some habits are socializing, friendship habits: talking with a friend over a cup of coffee, smoking a joint with some really good friends, or sharing some beer with your buddies.

In some cases, though, some of these same habits—like drinking and drug use—may be a push in the opposite direction, an attempt to shut out the world around you and feelings that are simply too painful to handle. Whatever the feelings and reasons behind a particular action, you may find that this activity works for you in some ways.

Smoking and/or drinking coffee or alcohol may help you to feel more grown-up and independent or less different and more accepted by others.

Use of drugs, which includes nicotine (cigarettes), caffeine (coffee, tea, colas, chocolate), and alcohol as well as marijuana, may feel good, too. And if you're trying to dull your senses and block out pain, alcohol and other drugs may work—for a while.

It may not surprise you that these habits are often found in various combinations. Those who smoke are more likely to drink and use drugs as well. Coffee drinking and cigarette smoking are also frequent companions. All of these habits may be ways some of us find to cope with feelings and to help make us feel better.

When something feels good and seems to help you to cope with life, it can quite easily become a habit, something you do on a regular basis. It may be very difficult, in some instances, to imagine what life would be like without that habit.

How would you cope without a cup of coffee to get you going in the morning? Or that cola to banish the midafternoon "blahs"? Can you imagine finishing a meal and not having a cigarette? Or going to a party and not drinking or smoking grass?

You might scoff at the idea of real addiction.

"After all," you may be saying, "I won't fall to the floor in fits if I don't have a cup of coffee or a cigarette or if I go to a party without any booze or pot. I might feel like something is missing, but I could stop any of these habits any time I want."

A lot of times we don't want to stop. (Who wants to stop what seems to be a good thing?)

Sometimes, though, we can't seem to stop a habit, or we can't do so quite as easily as we thought we could.

There are different levels of intensity to any habit. Maybe your habit is not really a habit yet, but still a matter of conscious choice. Seventeen-year-old Sarah says that she smokes pot "maybe twice a year and only with certain people and under certain circum-

stances. Lots of times, I'll go to parties or to someone's house and not smoke, even when others do. When I do smoke pot, it's because I choose to." Sarah is hardly a habitual drug user.

Peter, on the other hand, acquired a rather intense coffee habit during his freshman year of college. He drank great quantities of the beverage from morning until late into the night to help keep alert to study just a little longer. His roommate (who noticed his own cache of instant coffee disappearing alarmingly fast) kept a record of Peter's coffee consumption for a week and then presented him with the evidence: Peter was averaging ten cups of coffee a day. Astonished, Peter decided to quit his newly acquired habit.

"I got along without it for 18 years before," he says now. "I was just drinking it because it was there. It was a pretty easy habit to break and I'm glad I did. I was feeling kind of shaky and nervous before I stopped—and now I know why."

Patti, 18, says that she would like very much to stop smoking, but it just isn't that easy. She has vowed to quit many times. "But it's hard to get through a day without a cigarette," she admits. "I crave them! I practically go crazy if I can't have a cigarette after a meal or when I'm studying or talking with friends. When I try to quit, I feel really irritable. I'm hooked. I don't like that idea, but I am."

"Hooked" takes on a whole new meaning with Alan. He is, at 15, an alcoholic. Alan drinks from the time he gets up until he falls into bed. He has been thrown out of school on several occasions for being drunk. He has suffered some blackouts. His parents, relieved that "at least he isn't on drugs . . ." (although alcohol *is*, technically, a drug!), get mad when he gets sent home from school, but are not alarmed enough to seek help for him. "He could stop if he wanted to," his father contends.

But Alan can't stop on his own. "Once I tried to go without drinking for a while and it was terrible," Alan admits. "I got really sick to my stomach."

Obviously, there are differences among the teens we've mentioned here. The difference is not as much in what they drink or smoke, but how, to what extent, and under what circumstances they do it.

Some may think it is strange to compare marijuana, coffee, cigarettes, and alcohol. Yet these habits are not as different as one might think. All are drugs. Some are legal, even socially sanctioned. Some are illegal.

Many people get hung up on what drug you take. Some may feel that cigarettes, coffee, and alcohol are not as harmful as marijuana, for example. However, what should be of most concern is the intensity of a particular habit. Does this habit—in some ways—run your life?

WHEN DOES A HABIT BECOME A PROBLEM?

Some might consider use of any one of the drugs we have mentioned as a problem. It is true that, for optimum health, it may be desirable to avoid all of these habits. Many others might see no problem in *moderate* use of these substances. Caffeine, cigarettes, alcohol, and various other drugs are part of many people's lives—maybe yours, too.

What we would like to do is to help you to discover whether or not you have a habit that might be a problem for you.

Drug *abuse,* whatever the drug, can be a serious problem. Could YOU be abusing some substance? To find out, ask yourself the following questions:

1. Does your habit influence—for the worse—your relationships with others?
2. Does it put you in the position of breaking a law?
3. Does it expose you to medical hazards?
4. Is it creating a lot of personal problems for you?

Let's consider these questions one by one.

Does Your Habit Influence Your Relationships?

There are a number of possibilities here. See if you can identify with any of the following letters.

In my crowd, drinking is OK, but I don't know when to stop. I always get smashed out of my mind and barf! This is considered uncool. I went on a date with this guy I liked a lot and I got sick all over his car. He was really pissed off at me and now won't even speak to me. Some of my other friends don't like to be around me as much. One girl said I wouldn't be invited to any of her parties until I learn how to handle myself right.

Cece Y.

This guy I like a lot and have had a few dates with doesn't like to kiss me because he says I have bad breath from smoking. He won't let me smoke in his car or if we have dinner together either and sometimes tries to lecture me about it. I really like this guy, but it seems we're always fighting about my smoking.

Gina J.

I started smoking pot with my best friend about six months ago. Now that's about all we do when we're

together. We smoke a joint and just sit there, not saying much. It's OK. But I don't feel as close to him now as I did when we could really talk with each other. We used to go out and do things together. Now, even when we're together, we're kind of into ourselves. I miss my friend.

Kevin M.

These are just three examples. There are many others.

For example, does your habit—whatever it may be—trigger hassles with your parents?

If so, does this make the habit more—or less—desirable to you?

Think carefully about all the important people in your life.

How do your habits affect them, if at all?

Does Your Habit Require You to Break a Law?

Some things—like marijuana and other street drugs—are illegal for everyone, although some states have taken steps to reduce penalties for the possession of a very small amount of marijuana. At this time, though, probably a major argument against the use of marijuana is that it is illegal.

Some drugs—like barbiturates—are technically legal if prescribed, but are, all too often, acquired illegally and used under dangerous circumstances.

While alcohol and cigarettes are legal for adults, most states have laws regarding the minimum age you must be to purchase such items legally. Everyone knows that cigarettes are easy to buy from vending machines and liquor is pretty easy to get, too, with phony IDs, a careless liquor store clerk, the cooperation of an older acquaintance, or by shoplifting. However, in so acquiring liquor, you may be breaking at least one law, and maybe more!

Some drug, alcohol, and even cigarette habits are expensive enough that some young people may end up stealing to get what they need.

If *your* habit puts you in the position of breaking a law every time you acquire and/or use it, it can be a serious problem.

Does Your Habit Expose You to Medical Hazards?

Caffeine

I've been watching my weight for the past few months and have started drinking a lot of diet cola. I like one at breakfast to wake me up and then I drink them all day. My mom hates this. She says all that cola drinking isn't good for me. Is she right?

J. L.

I'm scared because during exams last week, I drank a lot of coffee. I usually drink only one cup at breakfast and that's it, but last week I had about ten cups a day to help keep me awake to study. Anyway, the last day of exams, I felt really jumpy and my heart was pounding! My roommate says it was probably just nerves, but I wonder if it didn't have something to do with the coffee?

Burt C.

My science teacher said that there's caffeine (the same thing that's in coffee) in cocoa and chocolate, both of which I love. Is caffeine good or bad for you?

Curious

Caffeine, which has been called Americans' favorite drug, is a powerful stimulant of the central nervous system. It is found in coffee (86–150 mg per cup), tea (60–75 mg per cup), cola drinks (40–72 mg per 12-ounce can), bittersweet chocolate (25 mg), and milk chocolate (3 mg).

In moderate doses, caffeine may be beneficial. It can give you a lift, make you more alert, and enable you to study, work, or socialize longer without feeling fatigue. It may help to alleviate some migraine headaches (since caffeine constricts cerebral blood vessels) and is also included in some pain-relievers.

Caffeine is also being used on an experimental basis to stimulate the breathing of premature babies with breathing problems and to help calm down hyperactive children. It may also be helpful to those suffering from nausea and/or diarrhea.

But excessive caffeine can cause a number of problems. A recent study by a team of British scientists revealed that *excessive* consumption of beverages containing caffeine can cause recurrent headaches, irritability, and gastrointestinal problems.

Another study at the University of Michigan found that "caffeine-ism" may cause symptoms like anxiety, depression, and headaches. An earlier Army study corroborated these findings, adding yet another possible symptom of too much caffeine: irregular heartbeats.

Caffeine and other ingredients in coffee may, in addition, cause the release of stomach acids, making coffee drinking inadvisable for those with stomach problems, especially ulcers.

Some current studies—still inconclusive—are examining the role that caffeine may play in complications of pregnancy, including miscarriage and premature birth, among other possible problems. Even though these studies are still ongoing and inconclu-

sive, many physicians may caution pregnant women to drink decaffeinated coffee or, preferably, no coffee at all during pregnancy.

For the rest of us, how much caffeine is too much? Any amount that would cause symptoms like those we have described.

Those conducting the University of Michigan study defined a "high user" as one who would drink more than 6 cups of coffee or 15 colas or 12 cups of tea, or someone who would drink, say, 5 colas and 4 cups of coffee a day.

Teens and young adults, who have been found to be the heaviest users of cola drinks, may have to be especially careful not to overdo caffeine consumption.

In some heavy coffee or cola drinkers, there may be very real "withdrawal" symptoms, including depression, drowsiness, and headaches, if the person tries to quit the habit. For this reason, it is advisable to ease off caffeine rather than stopping your consumption abruptly, if you tend to be a heavy user. Cut down gradually.

Cigarette Smoking

I like smoking a lot, but hear it can cause a lot of problems for you later in life. Is this true? What kind of problems can you have? Are these problems real or just exaggerated to scare us?

Cindy W.

I heard this really dumb rumor about smoking giving you wrinkles! This isn't true, is it? I can't see how this could happen.

Bonnie A.

Please give me a truthful answer. I'm scared to death. You see, I'm 20, four months pregnant with my first baby, and I smoke about a pack and a half of cigarettes a day. A friend of mine told me that I should stop smoking or my baby could be seriously harmed! This really upsets me. I hate to think of giving up smoking, but could I be hurting my baby?

Annie G.

It seems that everywhere I look, people are going on about teen-age girls smoking. This bugs me. A lot of people of all ages smoke! So why pick on us? Also, I hate all the scare stories. There are some good things about smoking. Why doesn't anyone ever talk about the advantages?

Upset

Especially for teens, there may be some social advantages to smoking.

A recent survey by the American Cancer Society

revealed that most teen-agers consider people their age to be smokers, despite the fact that only 30 percent of boys and 27 percent of girls smoke. Teen girl smokers were found to be (and to be considered) more outgoing and confident, while teen boy smokers had *less* self-confidence than their nonsmoking peers.

Smoking may also be seen by teen-agers as a symbol of independence, as a pleasant way to relax or finish a meal or to give awkward hands something to do. If there are some social benefits, why so much alarm about teens smoking?

There are a number of causes for alarm:

• Young people are smoking earlier. More than half of teen smokers begin the habit at age 12 or younger. Studies have shown that the younger you start smoking, the more likely it is that you will be a heavy smoker and suffer more potential damage to your health.

• The number of young women 12 to 18 who smoke has doubled in less than a decade. This rapid increase is creating particular concern as more links are discovered between smoking and increased threats to the health—and lives—of unborn babies.

• A report from the National Institute on Drug Abuse recently found that a much higher percentage of people who smoke cigarettes actually become hooked on tobacco than hard drug users become hooked on heroin. Many of us have not realized the addictive potential of cigarettes—until we try to quit.

• Smoking can shorten your life significantly. A habitual smoker may be giving up five and one-half to eight and one-half years of life!

• The link between smoking and cancer is well-established. Heavy smokers are 24 times more likely than nonsmokers to get lung cancer as well as cancers of the lips, mouth, pancreas, esophagus, and bladder.

• Medical evidence has linked smoking to other major health problems. Smokers have a two or three times greater chance of dying from a heart attack than nonsmokers. They also have many more strokes than nonsmoking counterparts and are 19 times more likely to become victims of emphysema, a crippling respiratory disorder that destroys the lungs' elasticity and leaves the victim gasping for breath.

• Studies show that smokers are more likely to get wrinkles sooner than their nonsmoking friends. Dr. Harry Daniell of Redding, California, found that the level of wrinkling in women who smoked heavily to be equivalent to that of women *20 years older!* This wrinkling pattern may be due to the fact that smoking causes constriction of blood vessels and may make the skin more susceptible to wrinkles. It has been found that smokers are much more likely to have severe wrinkling than even those nonsmokers whose profes-

sions require them to be outdoors and exposed to the sun constantly.

Although many of these above-mentioned health risks are well in the future and may be difficult to imagine right now, there are smoking-related health risks that may affect your life in the near future.

• A pregnant woman's smoking habit may have harmful, even lethal, effects on her unborn baby. Recent studies have found that women who smoke during pregnancy are almost *twice* as likely to miscarry or spontaneously abort. They are more likely to have a stillborn baby or to give birth to a smaller-than-normal child. There is still much debate about why this may be so. Some feel that nicotine and carbon monoxide from cigarettes may deprive the fetus of oxygen, retarding its growth. Others feel that smoking women may eat less than nonsmokers, depriving the baby of vital nutrients. Whatever the reasons, the babies of smoking mothers do tend to be smaller and are more likely to die at birth or soon after than babies of nonsmoking mothers.

A recent study in *Pediatrics* magazine also explored a possible link between smoking and the tragic Sudden Infant Death Syndrome, or "crib death," in which an apparently healthy baby dies for no apparent reason. In comparing mothers of SIDS victims and mothers of healthy infants, this study found a higher proportion of mothers who smoked before, during, and after pregnancy among the SIDS group.

Some studies that have followed smokers' babies for several years have found that detrimental effects may linger. One study, for example, showed that at the age of seven, the children of heavy smokers tend to be significantly shorter in height, have more difficulty reading and lower social adjustment ratings than the children of nonsmokers.

• Those who smoke may be more prone to stomach problems, including peptic ulcers.

• If you smoke, you have a greater risk of dying in a smoking-related accident. More than 25 percent of all U.S. fires are caused by smokers and so many automobile accidents seem to be smoking-related (the smoker takes his eyes off the road or hands off the wheel to light up or retrieve a dropped cigarette) that some car insurance companies offer discount rates to nonsmokers.

• All smoking injures you to some extent. If you're lucky, you may simply experience more than your share of illnesses every year, missing more work or school than a nonsmoker.

NOW FOR THE GOOD NEWS: If you stop smoking now, your risk of death—especially from heart and lung disease—will lessen until, after 10 or 15 years of abstinence, you will be at no greater risk than the lifelong nonsmoker.

Dangerous Drugs

Every time I have a fight with my father, I take some of my mom's sleeping pills to calm me down. Can these pills hurt me?

Wondering

You can buy any kind of drug at my school including "salads" of all sorts of stuff. Isn't this pretty dangerous? Also, I hear about people taking Quaaludes. Can these be dangerous at all?

Jay G.

A friend of mine bought what she thought was grass, but it was really bad stuff. She said it made her real paranoid and strange. Another friend said that the grass could have been laced with something called "Angel Dust." I've heard of it, but I'm not sure what it is. What is it?

Carol S.

Has it been proven that smoking pot is bad for your health? I have smoked it for about a year and like it. But I've heard so many different things about it being harmful, then not harmful. Could you tell me more about it so I'll know if I should quit or not?

Confused

My parents and teachers make me laugh when they talk about drugs and get so bent out of shape about things like heroin and LSD. To hear them talk, you'd think half the kids in the nation are junkies! They also think pot is bad, bad, bad! I know that pot is OK and I don't know any kids who are on heroin or LSD. I think those kinds of things pretty much went out with the sixties. What do you say?

Greg B.

It may well be true that the use of drugs like heroin and LSD may be down somewhat among teen-agers. It is true that the great majority of young people are not drug abusers in the stereotypical sense.

In recent years, in fact, there has been more and more concern about the problem of alcohol abuse among teen-agers, which has seemed to displace some of the concern over hard drugs that flourished in the sixties.

We all know, however, that drug abuse has *not* ceased to exist.

Drugs that seem to be frequently used—and often abused—today include barbiturates (downers), am-phetamines (uppers), cocaine, PCP ("Angel Dust") as well as marijuana.

Some of these drugs can be beneficial when taken in prescribed doses under medical supervision. Barbiturates, for example, may reduce tension and induce sleep. Amphetamines may be used medically to curb the appetite. When these drugs are abused, however, the results may be serious—even deadly.

• Chronic use of uppers may bring about acute psychosis. Abuse of uppers can also mask fatigue and cause you to overextend yourself, sometimes going without sleep for days. A serious overdose may cause convulsions, coma, and death.

• Barbiturates, which tend to depress the central nervous system (including respiration) may, in larger than prescribed doses, cause one to stop breathing altogether. The overdose is not always intentional, since the hypnotic effect of barbiturates may make a person lose track of how many pills he or she has already taken. Combined with alcohol, barbiturates can be lethal. Death can also result from combinations with other drugs. This is why those "drug salads" (random combinations of various drugs) are so dangerous.

Unfortunately, it is possible to become physically addicted to barbiturates eventually and abrupt barbiturate withdrawal may be fatal.

• Quaaludes, another type of downer, which may also be prescribed to help induce sleep, are also more and more frequently abused. What concerns many physicians about Quaaludes is this: While your tolerance level for the drug increases with habitual use, the lethal dose level remains the same, increasing the danger to your life over a period of time. Also, some preliminary studies indicate that Quaaludes may be harmful to unborn babies and should be avoided altogether by women who are pregnant. When laboratory animals were given high doses of Quaaludes in a recent study, they produced offspring with skeletal abnormalities.

• Cocaine is a powerful—and illegal—stimulant and can cause both addiction and tolerance in the user. It may also cause strong psychological dependence. Poisoning, due to a high rate of absorption, may result in practically instantaneous death. Another danger: Cocaine may be cut with other dangerous substances such as strychnine. So you don't always know what you're getting.

While there are some drugs that may be harmful in instances of abuse, there are other drugs that are always harmful, and if you value your health and your life, you will never use them. We're talking about "Angel Dust," or PCP.

• "Angel Dust," or PCP, is a highly dangerous

drug and is becoming something of an epidemic among teen drug users. It has been used legally as an anesthetic for large animals, but was long ago banned for human use. Although it non-addictive, Angel Dust's effects are unpredictable. You never know what it will do to you. And people who have used it say that it doesn't give you any real high, just a feeling of emptiness. The drug can cause confusion, bizarre behavior, hostility, dangerously high blood pressure and pulse rate, irregular heartbeat, and even death.

Death may come via a bizarre accident—like diving into a pool and never surfacing. (PCP users have a penchant for water, but are often so disoriented that they forget to surface—and often drown!) People under the influence of PCP have walked across freeways, been involved in fatal auto accidents, set themselves on fire or, in frenzies of hostility and confusion, have unwittingly killed others. San Francisco authorities say that, during the past year, at least five murders in that area may have involved PCP users. PCP was the known cause of almost 100 deaths last year and may have contributed to a number of other fatalities. Still, young people are taking this drug. The National Institute on Drug Abuse estimates that six to seven million teenagers and young adults have used or are using PCP.

This drug seems to be popular with younger teens. A federal study of drug users recently found that the average first-time PCP user is only fourteen and one-half years old.

Although some kids choose to take PCP (which is often sprinkled on mint leaves), others may become involuntary users (and victims) of the drug when they buy marijuana laced with PCP.

One of the leading experts on PCP, drug researcher Steven Lerner of San Francisco, has said that PCP "may be the biggest problem drug in terms of seriousness and potential consequences. People chronically exposed may never be normal again. . . ."

• In general, it is also dangerous to your health to: take pills from friends and/or in unknown mixes and combinations; combine any drugs and alcohol; (this includes aspirin, antibiotics, etc.), try to be your own doctor and medicate yourself with barbiturates and amphetamines, for example, without medical supervision; buy street drugs. You never know what's in them. Vic Pawlak, head of the Do It Now drug information foundation estimates that pills sold on the street are misrepresented from 50 to 75 percent of the time.

What about marijuana? Is it or isn't it a possible threat to your health?

There is still a great deal of controversy surrounding marijuana, its possible legalization, and the effects the drug may have on one's health. Probably the least debatable drawback to marijuana at the present time is that it is still illegal.

Beyond giving you a temporary sense of well-being, confusion, or distortion, what does marijuana do?

While we're not going to say that pot is completely harmless, we feel, on the basis of a number of studies that we have seen, that some of the old scare stories about marijuana may have been exaggerated. The old stereotype of the strung-out, half-crazed pothead does not really describe the typical marijuana user.

As far as we know, marijuana does not result in lasting mental or physical damage nor does it cause physical addiction, although some may become psychologically dependent on it.

There is some evidence that use of marijuana may accompany use of other drugs. But it does not seem to cause further drug experimentations. Studies have shown that a lot of habits may be interrelated. For example, a person who smokes or drinks is more likely to use marijuana and, perhaps, other drugs. A UCLA study found, though, that it was unusual for college students who did smoke marijuana to start regular use or addiction to other drugs.

Can marijuana cause brain damage?

Brain damage from habitual use of marijuana has not been demonstrated by the evidence we now have. Two studies—one by Harvard Medical School and the other by Washington University School of Medicine in St. Louis—found no evidence that even heavy use of marijuana triggers changes in the central nervous system or brain structure.

Can marijuana cause harm to unborn babies?

The effect of marijuana on unborn infants is still being studied and is, at this time, not well known. We do know that THC, a major ingredient of marijuana, can cross the placental barrier to the fetus in the first three months of pregnancy. What effects this might cause are still unknown, but it is a good idea to avoid use of marijuana during pregnancy.

Can marijuana smoking damage the lungs as much as tobacco smoking?

There is some evidence that smoking marijuana may have some of the detrimental effects that tobacco has, although marijuana is smoked less frequently and in smaller quantities, generally, and THC, its major ingredient, does dilate the bronchial passages. It has been difficult in studies to isolate the effects of marijuana on the lungs versus the effects of tabacco, since so many of those who smoke grass are also tobacco smokers. It has been reported that marijuana users who are concerned about the possible effects of smoking pot ingest it in brownies, cookies, or tea instead.

Can marijuana be medically *beneficial* in any way?

Some studies have found that marijuana may be of some benefit to those suffering from asthma, glaucoma, and the undesirable side effects of cancer chemotherapy.

Alcohol

Lots of kids at my school drink a lot. Some are even drunk in classes. My friends are getting into drinking a lot. I don't want to be a superstraight and out of it, but I'm scared of alcohol because my dad is an alcoholic. I have been hurt a lot by his drinking and I'm afraid of becoming an alcoholic myself. Is it true that if you're the child of an alcoholic, you're more likely to become one, too?

Upset

My boyfriend drinks like a fish. He can go through a six-pack of beer in an evening. He gets drunk about four times a week. He says he doesn't have a drinking problem and couldn't be an alcoholic because all he drinks is beer! I'm not sure about that. Am I silly to worry so much?

Gina

I like to drink pop wine and beer. Getting smashed a lot helps me feel better. When I'm drunk I don't care about school pressures or anything. I used to be on the honor roll. Now I don't care. When I drink, it doesn't even hurt me that I don't have a boyfriend. My parents don't know I drink, but my older brother found me sick in the bathroom one night and he said, "I know you're drinking. You'd better start getting your act together or I'll have to tell Mom and Dad!" He suggested that I go to Alcoholics Anonymous. I think he's crazy. I'm not an alcoholic, am I?

Shelley Anne G.

Alcohol is a drug. This drug is being abused more and more by teen-agers and young adults. This phenomenon is causing widespread concern.

The National Institute of Alcohol Abuse and Alcoholism has estimated that alcoholic beverage consumption among teen-agers has increased 700 percent in the past few years. They estimate that one out of 20 teens has a drinking problem, and one out of ten of these will become an alcoholic.

According to another recent study on teen-age drinking for the National Institute of Alcohol Abuse, 28 percent of the nation's teens are problem drinkers (for example, they have been drunk at least four times in the past year and have had problems with authority figures or peers at least twice in the past year on account of drinking). Another revelation from this report: Only 38 percent of American 13-year-olds don't drink at all.

A statement from the American Academy of Pediatrics Committee on Youth noted that society tends to get alarmed about light use of marijuana, yet does not consider alcohol consumption an abuse problem unless it is extreme. "Both attitudes are faulty and potentially dangerous," the report said, adding that while some teens drink because their friends do, many drink to relieve negative feelings like depression and anxiety. The report noted that "such self-medication paves the way for drug abuse and early alcoholism."

These statistics mean that alcohol *abuse* could be a serious problem now and in the future for many young people. They also belie the old stereotype of the alcoholic as a Skid Row bum. An alcoholic can be anyone. Beer drinkers are not immune. It's the alcohol, not the flavoring, that matters. And no one who drinks is too young to become an alcoholic. There are Alcoholics Anonymous members as young as nine.

Of course, not everyone who drinks will become an alcoholic. Some people drink moderately for years and are not alcoholics. Others claim that they became alcoholics immediately or soon after beginning to drink. It is difficult, if not impossible, to predict who will become an alcoholic.

"But many young alcoholics are children of alcoholics," says Vicki Danzig, a clinical social worker at Careunit Alcoholism Treatment Center at Glendale (California) Memorial Hospital. "If one parent is an alcoholic, you may have a 40 percent chance of becoming an alcoholic, too. If both parents are alcoholics, your chances are even greater."

Some theorize that this tendency to duplicate parental drinking patterns may be genetic predisposition. Others cite environmental influences and parental example as well as the very real pain involved in living with an alcoholic parent.

"One thing that really concerns us is that kids may blossom as alcoholics faster than adults do," says Marilyn Sachs, an alcoholism counselor at Careunit. "We're not sure why. The whole process may be accelerated by adolescent growth."

"Or by the pain of adolescence," adds Gary Gordon, director of the Careunit at Glendale Hospital. "Adolescence means a lot of pain and fear. When you find something that helps—even temporarily—to alleviate some of these fears, you can get really hooked."

Some other experts theorize that the tendency of many teen drinkers to combine alcohol with other drugs may make alcohol abuse a greater problem and possibility in the young.

How can alcohol abuse and/or alcoholism be a health problem?

• Alcoholism, a serious illness that makes you lose control of your drinking, is the country's most serious health problem after heart disease and cancer. On the average, it could shorten your life by 10 to 12 years.

• Health problems related to alcoholism may include malnutrition (due to drinking instead of eating) and damage to the brain, liver, pancreas, and the central nervous system.

You don't have to wait years for some of these problems to develop. Malnutrition can happen rather quickly, and even damage to vital organs is not unknown in young alcoholics.

"I'll never forget this little girl I met once who was a member of Alcoholics Anonymous," says Gary Gordon. "She was only ten years old—and a few weeks later, she was dead of alcoholic cirrhosis of the liver."

Nannette de Fuentes, a counselor with the Alcoholism Council of the San Fernando Valley and its Teenage Alcoholism Program (TAP) adds that "a recent study estimated that a youngster who starts to drink heavily at age 13 (three or more drinks, three or more times a week) can develop cirrhosis of the liver by age 23!"

• Suicide and accidental deaths also figure prominently into fatality statistics for alcoholics.

"Alcoholics have a suicide rate two-and-a-half times greater than the general population," says Gary Gordon. "And the accidental death rate for alcoholics is seven times higher."

• Fetal Alcohol Syndrome in newborn babies is a tragic disorder that has been linked to heavy drinking during pregnancy. These babies may be mentally retarded with heart, face, and body defects. A study at Boston City Hospital found that 74 percent of infants born to women who had 10 to 15 drinks a day suffered one or more symptoms of FAS. Scientists in Seattle discovered something even more alarming: In a group of 164 women who drank two ounces of whiskey a day during pregnancy, nine had infants with FAS. Thousands of babies a year are subjected to this very real prenatal child abuse. The National Council on Alcoholism recommends that pregnant women stay away from liquor altogether during pregnancy. Others may recommend only light consumption of wine or beer.

These facts, of course, don't necessarily mean that alcohol is the root of all evil. They're simply saying that *abuse* of alcohol, as abuse of just about any drug, may be health-threatening, even deadly.

"What we're saying is that young people must learn to drink *reasonably*," says Vicki Danzig.

Some young people—due to alcoholism—may *never* be able to drink responsibly and, to protect their health and their life, must abstain from alcohol.

How can you tell if you might be an alcoholic?

The following are some of the questions that young participants of the TAP program are encouraged to ask themselves.

• Have you lost time from school or work due to drinking?

• Has drinking made it difficult for you to get along with your family?

• Do you drink because you're usually shy with people?

• Has drinking affected your reputation?

• Have you ever felt unhappy after drinking?

• Do you crave a drink at a certain time every day?

• Do you ever want a drink the morning after?

• Is your drinking making it difficult to do well in school or work?

• Have you ever taken drinks to escape worries?

• Have you ever had a loss of memory after drinking?

• Do you ever drink alone?

• Do you ever drink to build up your self-confidence?

• Have you ever been sent to a hospital or jail as a result of drinking?

Other questions to ask yourself:

• Have you stopped caring about how you look?

• Do you sneak drinks?

• Do you eat irregularly while drinking?

• Do you stay drunk for long periods (like several days)?

• Do you get extremely depressed after drinking?

If you answered yes to any of these questions, your drinking may be a problem for you.

If you have a drinking problem, look into Alcoholics Anonymous (see listing in the Appendix).At A.A., you can receive help from those who understand you best—others who have battled drinking problems, too. Through group discussions and sharing in a personal way, you can discover that you can conquer and control a drinking problem. Most important, perhaps, you find that you are not alone.

Does Your Habit Become a Problem For You?

This is something only you can answer. A habit may cause symptoms or side effects that may be a problem for you, but not for somebody else.

Bill, who eats a lot of chocolate, may find that he is gaining undesired weight. His friend Mark may be able to eat great mounds of chocolate without weight gains.

Pam, an aspiring dancer, feels that her heavy smoking may be the cause of occasional shortness of breath during strenuous classes.

Jenny enjoys smoking pot and feels that it isn't harming her physically. However, she has found that her attempts to reduce some of her tensions are beginning to interfere with her performance at school. Good grades are important to her, she has decided. But lately she has been feeling too laid-back and mellow to spend as much time on homework assignments as she feels she should.

Don isn't a big drinker, but he has found that his occasional drinking has caused some problems: a fight with his parents when he came home a little drunk (and two hours late!) and a near-accident with the family car when he drove it while drunk a few months later. He is beginning to wonder if he enjoys drinking enough to take the risk of an accident or parental wrath (translate that into being grounded for two weeks!).

Since beginning art school, Amy has started drinking a lot of coffee. Lately, she has found her hands shaking by midafternoon, making it impossible to draw well. She is beginning to think that her coffee drinking is a problem for her and she is planning to cut down or quit altogether.

Other teens may find that habits that block feelings—including painful feelings—may be keeping them from growing emotionally. Feeling pain, anger, confusion, and rebellion may be an important part of one's growth to maturity and learning to deal with hardships and setbacks. A habit that keeps you from feeling may postpone this vital growth—or prevent it entirely.

It really is *your* decision whether to continue a habit, cut down, or quit after giving yourself a yes answer to "Is this habit adversely affecting my life in any way?"

You may feel that the habit is more important to you than the undesirable side effects.

You may feel that, although you enjoy the habit, you might want to cut down on it to minimize some of the potential problems.

Or you may want to get rid of a habit that is a problem for you.

Changing a habit, of course, is usually not as easy as saying "OK. I'll change."

There are special feelings and needs behind our significant habits. And, in order to change our habits, we have to face and deal with some of these feelings.

CHANGING YOUR FEELINGS— AND YOUR HABITS!

I started smoking because I'm sort of shy and smoking makes me look a lot more with-it to others I think.
Ben L.

Why do I drink? Because I get so self-conscious at parties. I feel like a real clod. If I get drunk, I can talk to people, and even if I do say something stupid, nobody holds me responsible for it. They might say "Oh, she said that because she was drunk!" instead of "Boy, did you hear THAT? What a dummy!"
Nancy F.

I used to drink when I was depressed—and then I got even more depressed than ever!
Brian A.

I often find myself feeling kind of low and not like doing much. Colas really pick me up.
Renee

I smoke pot to get a little relief from some of the tensions and problems of my life. . . .
Mike C.

Many of our habits help us to cope—at least temporarily—with our feelings. Some habits, as we have seen, may anesthetize your feelings and may interfere with emotional growth. Some of these feelings, though painful, are endemic to the human condition and it's important to learn how to cope with them.

- Fear of taking responsibility for your life—and your actions
- Feeling inferior, that you're not as smart, attractive or well-liked as other people
- Feeling hurt by special problems—the death of someone dear to you, a parental divorce, an alcoholic parent, or a major disappointment
- Worrying about other people liking or accepting you
- Feeling frustrated at being considered a kid by those in authority when you've grown up in so many ways
- Feeling so very much alone.

Whatever your feelings, learn to identify them and to ask yourself if there is some way you can change these feelings. This is necessary if you're working on a problem habit. If you try to change habits without dealing with the feelings behind them, you are more likely to fail to make the change and may end up feeling even worse about yourself.

Low self-esteem can be a huge problem, making you not only despair of your ability to cope with life, worrying about whether others will accept you, but also this low self-image may make you put a habit like smoking or drugs or drinking ahead of your own health and well-being.

"Is your drinking more important than *you?*" one young alcoholic was asked in a counseling session recently.

Her face crumpled. Tears slid down her cheeks. "Yes!" she cried. "I'm *nothing . . .*"

For tips on dealing with feelings—including inferiority, stress, loss, fear of the future—please see Chapter Four.

Coping with—and changing—your painful feelings is not a skill you will acquire overnight. It takes time. Be patient with yourself. And take one day at a time.

It's also important to know that even when you are more skillful at coping with painful feelings, there will not always be bliss. We *all* have pain in our lives. We *all* have moments when we may feel stupid, ugly, awkward, or very much alone.

So, if you still hurt at times, you're far from alone!

"Sometimes I hurt a lot," says 21-year Melody T., a recovered alcoholic. "But I know how to help myself. I have friends and people close who can help me, too. I feel that my life is so full. You know, when you're drinking, you're always just talking about the things you're going to do. Somehow, you never get around to them. Now that I'm sober, I'm actually *doing* some of these things that were only distant dreams not so long ago!"

HOW TO CHANGE A HABIT

Changing a habit—especially one you've had for a while—isn't easy. It takes time and, again, patience. If you try and fail to give up coffee or cigarettes or alcohol or other drugs, don't put yourself down. Just try again. And don't be embarrassed to ask for help.

With some habits, you may need help to change them. If you're an alcoholic or problem drinker, Alcoholics Anonymous and/or a hospital treatment center—like Care unit (located in selected hospitals across the nation)—may be able to help you. If you

have a serious drug problem, you need help from your physician and/or a special drug abuse program or facility. "Stop Smoking" clinics sponsored by the American Cancer Society and other groups for aspiring ex-smokers may help you if smoking is the habit you'd like to stop.

You can help *yourself*, too, to stop smoking or coffee consumption or moderate drinking—if you choose.

Here are some ideas that may help you:

Set Realistic Goals for Yourself. Don't say "I will never, ever have another cigarette [drink, cup of coffee, etc.]. Say, instead, *"Just for today,* I will try not to smoke [drink alcohol or coffee]."

Take Responsibility for Your Habits. No one *made* you do it. You chose it. So you can choose to change the habit. Knowing that you have power over your life—and your habits—can help a lot!

Tell Your Friends. Advertise your intentions to change. Friends often have great memories for this kind of thing and may be quick to remind you of your good intentions.

Cut Down Gradually. If you drink three cups of coffee a day, for example, eliminate one of them this week. If you drink colas from sunup to sundown, cut yourself down to one or two. If you smoke, try cutting down, too. Some people, according to the American Cancer Society, may find it helpful to carry one cigarette in case of dire emergency—for a while. Most, it seems, find that this dire emergency never comes.

Seek Alternatives. Ask yourself "What would I be doing if I *weren't* smoking [drinking, etc.]?" Maybe you'd call a friend. Take a walk. Do something kind—and unexpected—for someone else. Write a poem. Read a book. Answer a letter. Listen to a favorite song. Try a new craft or hobby. Plan for the future. Ask yourself what you'd like to learn to do in the future. Make a list of things you like about yourself . . . or of five people you can really count on. These are just a few suggestions. There are many things you can do—if you choose.

It all comes down to choices—YOUR choices.

We don't believe in hassles or lectures.

We *do* believe in information.

We feel that it's important for you to remember what we have shared with you about habits and health. You don't have to agree. Just think about it a bit.

Ultimately, however, the choice of keeping—or changing—your habits is entirely yours!

CHAPTER EIGHT

Mind Over Body

Since starting high school, I've been having terrible headaches. Could this be nerves—or what?

Sheila A.

I have terrible stomachaches when my parents fight and when things are really bad at home, I get a lot of diarrhea. Could this be related to my feeling scared about my parents fighting?

Jill H.

I'm worried about my best friend. She eats all the time, even half MY lunch sometimes! I get upset about that, but it scares me how she doesn't really know how much she's eating. She didn't used to be like this and she's gaining lots of weight. Why is this happening? Is it a disease? Or is she crazy?

Marilyn P.

I'm 14 years old, 5 feet 3, and weigh 77 pounds. Is that a good weight? My father bugs me to gain weight, but I keep saying "No way!" I really think I'm too fat and when he makes me eat, I just go into the bathroom afterward and make myself throw up. The only things that bother me at all are: I don't get my period anymore. (I had regular periods for a year and a half before I started my dieting.) Also, I'm really nervous and uptight. How can I calm down?

Puzzled

I have this terrible fear of cancer. Every time I get a pain I'm afraid it's cancer. My doctor won't pay any attention when I tell him that I'm scared.

Lisa C.

I'm a freshman in college and have had three colds the first semester. I've also been very homesick and scared about not doing well. (I'm doing fine, but still . . .) I also feel like sleeping a lot. I can hardly get up in the morning and I often take a nap after my classes are over for the day. Also, last week during midterms, I got stomach cramps you wouldn't believe. When I wrote to my parents about this, my dad replied, "Get down off your cross, sweetheart!" My mom just said (as usual), "Oh, it's just all in your

head!" If it's all in my head, why is my body such a mess???

Julie N.

"It's all in your head . . ."
"It's just nerves . . ."
"Forget it. It'll go away . . ."
"It's all psychological . . . that's all . . ."

How many times have you heard this and gritted your teeth as your headache pounded unmercifully or your stomach churned?

How many times have you wondered if symptoms like this might mean that you have a serious health problem?

How many times have you thought, "If this *is* just all in my mind, does this mean I'm crazy?"

Too often, people dismiss disorders that we call *psychosomatic* (caused, at least in part, by emotional factors) as imaginary and unimportant. But these disorders are real and they may be important. Contrary to popular notions, the pains and other symptoms of psychosomatic disorders are connected with the mind and the emotions, but are not imaginary.

How does the mind enter into these problems?

Feelings, especially emotional response to stress, may help trigger or aggravate certain physical conditions. It's virtually impossible to separate your body and your mind.

As we will see in the next chapter, a new special medical need like diabetes can, and often does, bring an emotional crisis with it.

In this chapter, we'll be taking a look at the reverse situation: when an emotional crisis or response pattern may bring on special health problems or physical symptoms.

What are some of the feelings that may give us physical symptoms?

Anxiety, tension, and depression—to name only three—are some of these and may all be related to stress. And no one is immune to stress. It's an inescapable fact of all our lives. We can see—and even expect—stress as we cope with exams, the breakup of an important relationship, the death of someone close, or hassles at home.

But stress can come from positive events, too. Winning an award, graduating from high school, going away to college for the first time, getting married and/or moving into an apartment of your own, getting your first full-time job, having a baby—all of these positive life changes bring stress along with the challenge and the joy.

Dr. Thomas H. Holmes III, who is a professor of psychiatry at the University of Washington, studied the relationship between the stresses that change may bring and illness. His 43-item stress rating scale covers everything from the death of a spouse (100 points) or close family member (63 points) to marriage (50 points), pregnancy (40), outstanding personal achievement (28), starting or leaving school (26), change in schools (20), a vacation (13), and minor violations of the law (11). Dr. Holmes found that if a person scores 300 change points in a year, he or she has an 80 percent chance of experiencing a change of health as well.

Your body may react to stress by becoming more prone to illness, like colds, or you may develop one of the more common health problems that may be rooted, at least in part, in stress—and how you handle this stress.

Migraine and tension headaches, gastrointestinal problems like gastritis and ulcerative colitis, compulsive eating, anorexia nervosa (compulsive starvation), hypertension (high blood pressure), and hypochondria can bring you very real pain—both mentally and physically.

HEADACHES

It's unusual if I don't get a headache every day at school. I'm very tense and try to do well in school. Could this make me have headaches? If yes, how come? I've had my eyes checked and they're fine. I think I have a brain tumor. What do you think?

S.Y.

I have frequent headaches, resulting in dizziness and occasional fainting. This headache has been with me forever. I can't remember when I didn't have it. It feels like pounding in the back of my head. I'm tired and sleep most of the day after school. I sleep about 16 hours a day. Help!

Dizzy

Why do emotions have an effect on your health? I'm 16 and get headaches every time something is bothering me or when I'm holding my feelings in. I might be mad at someone or sweating an exam. How can I prevent such headaches?

Lynda

I started started migraine headaches when I was 13. I'm now 18. My mother and grandmother also had them. What's strange about my headaches is that I get them in times of stress and at times when I'm relaxing—like on weekends. I also feel really giddy before one and weak afterward. Is this a common thing? I wonder if I ought to see a doctor about these headaches.

Cheryl W.

There are many types of headaches and not all of them are tied in with emotions.

Some, for example, may result from illness: colds, flu, a sinus infection, or dental problem. Others may come from allergies, eye strain, high blood pressure. Still others may result from something *you* do—like skipping a meal, drinking or smoking too much, or becoming fatigued. Only in rare instances does a headache signal a brain tumor, although this is a possibility that occurs to anyone who gets headaches regularly.

If you are plagued with regular headaches, however, it's important to see a physician. He or she may help you to identify the type of headache you're having and its possible causes. If you're like most chronic headache sufferers, your physician's examination and tests are likely to reveal that there is nothing organically wrong with you.

What, then, can cause chronic headaches?

A combination of physical and psychological factors can combine to bring pain and suffering via tension (caused by muscular contraction), psychogenic (depression), migraine headaches.

Tension and depression headaches are, of course, rooted in both the emotions and muscular responses to these feelings.

Tension headaches, which may be felt at the front and/or sides of your head or at the base of your skull, can be caused by stress-induced anxiety, which causes you to tense your shoulder and neck muscles. As your headache throbs, you will probably also feel muscular tightness in your neck and shoulders. These headaches, which can be fairly constant, may be relieved by aspirin or other analgesics and rest.

Psychogenic headaches stemming from depression and anxiety may involve tense muscles in the face, head, and neck, and/or a pattern of pain that may feel like a band circling the head. These headaches are more likely to strike early in the morning or in the evening and on weekends. They are the result of long-standing depression. Other signs of depression may be present. For example, in her letter at the beginning of this section, ''Dizzy'' describes another symptom of depression: sleeping too much. Sleeping 16 hours a day is an urgent signal that something is wrong in her life.

Sleep patterns, researchers have found, can help one to tell the difference between tension and depression headaches. The person with tension may have trouble getting to sleep at night. The depressed person, on the other hand, may fall asleep readily, but his or her sleep pattern may be fitful—with awakening during the night or early in the morning.

Pain-relievers are only part of the answer in combating a psychogenic headache. It's also important to deal with the feelings behind the physical pain. You may do this with the help of a professional or maybe combine professional help with support from family and friends.

With both tension and depression headaches, it's vital to attack the source of your pain, not just the symptoms.

Migraine headaches are something else again. They can be extremely painful and cause physical symptoms like nausea, blurring of vision and, in some forms, temporary paralysis.

There are several different types of migraine headaches, but all are classified as *vascular* headaches. That is, they are triggered, not by muscular tension, but by changes in blood vessels. Contrary to widespread opinion, the blood vessels that change are *not* in the brain, but *around* the brain.

What happens when a migraine strikes?

For reasons as yet unknown, there is a change in the concentration of a substance called *serotonin*. This causes the blood vessels in the brain area to experience changes, too. In some people who suffer from migraine, these blood vessels will *constrict* first, causing a phenomenon known as an "aura." This is characteristic of the *classic migraine*. The person may see flashing lights or colors, spots before the eyes, blind spots, or may experience extreme sensitivity to light and visual distortions—with people or objects growing smaller or larger. Mood changes may accompany the aura or may occur even without an aura. The migraine victim may feel giddy and euphoric. Then the pain hits.

The pain of the migraine headache, which comes when the blood vessels dilate (swell), can be intense. It is usually felt on only one side of the head, centered in the temple or the eye. Unlike muscular contraction pain, which is steady, the pain of a vascular headache throbs with each heartbeat initially before it becomes stabilized. This pain may continue for several hours—or even a day or so.

The victim, sensitive to light and noise, will crawl off to a dark, quiet room to fight pain, nausea, and a variety of other symptoms.

These other symptoms depend on the type of migraine one has. There are two major classifications of migraine: classic (with an aura) and common (with possible mood changes preceding the headache, but no aura).

Within these classifications are some other types of migraines. Among these are the *ophthalmoplegic migraine,* involving paralysis of an eye muscle; *hemiplegic migraine,* which causes temporary paralysis of one side of the body; *basilar artery migraine,* a hemiplegic migraine with a few extra symptoms like loss of balance and dizziness; *cluster migraine* (rare in teen-agers, this type of headache is most common in men), which doesn't last very long, but keeps coming back again and again; and *ophthalmic migraine,* where the victim gets the migraine aura without the headache. He or she may have hallucinations and changing moods and, perhaps, pain in another part of the body.

Beyond these physiological facts, what causes migraine headaches? What can predispose you to have migraine?

Despite the fact that much remains to be discovered about these headaches, there are certain common factors in migraine attacks.

Your personality may be a factor. Are you intelligent, ambitious, hardworking, and a bit of a perfectionist? If so, you have the classic migraine personality. This description is, of course, not invariably true, but some doctors who specialize in treating headaches claim that they have never seen a migraine victim who is not intelligent.

Your heredity may be a factor, too. If both of your parents suffer from migraines you have a 70 percent chance of doing so, too. Did one parent have these headaches? Your chances are 45 percent. Sixty-five to 80 percent of all migraine sufferers have a family history of these headaches. Some researchers theorize that there may be a migraine-prone gene at work here, giving you a physical, genetic predisposition. Others contend that migraines may be learned or acquired from your environment. You may imitate your parents or experience migraines as a reaction to an atmosphere of tension and high expectations. Whatever the reasons behind this phenomenon, migraines can, indeed, run in families.

Stress can figure prominently in migraine attacks. The headaches may come in times of stress or in the letdown period after a stressful time (the weekend after final exams, for example, or on the first day of a long-awaited vacation).

Hormones may also influence your headaches. Some women experience increased migraines just before or during menstruation or in response to the synthetic hormones in birth control pills. For this reason, women who begin to suffer migraine-type headaches while taking birth control pills should consult their physician and, possibly, switch to another form of birth control.

The hormonal changes of pregnancy, on the other hand, may cause a temporary halt of migraines and most women find that they have fewer migraines as they get older. These headaches may even stop altogether after menopause.

Certain emotions—like anger and frustration (particularly if these feelings are repressed)—may be a factor in migraines.

What you eat may also bring on a headache. The chemical *tyramine,* which is found in most cheese, many citrus fruits, freshly baked bread, lima and navy beans, pork, vinegar (except wine vinegar), onions, and nuts, has been pinpointed as a possible migraine trigger. Chinese food (which contains the food additive MSG) and chocolate may also cause problems. Some feel that alcohol, along with the other substances mentioned here, may stimulate the blood vessels and should be avoided if you suffer from chronic migraines.

Your life-style may also be a factor. Do you live in a city with heavy traffic and gasoline fumes? Do you often spend time in crowded, smoke-filled rooms? Do you lead such a hectic life that you may miss meals? Do you get only irregular and insufficient sleep? Do you get too little good physical exercise? If so, you may be risking a migraine headache.

What are the treatments available for victims?

There are prescription drugs—from the *ergotamine* family—that help to constrict the swollen blood vessels. These drugs, which may be taken by mouth, by inhalation, by rectal suppositories, or by injection, are most effective if taken during the aura or at the first hint of pain.

Researchers at the University of Kansas Medical School's Headache Clinic have recently revealed that the drug *amitriptyline* (originally used to treat depression) may also help to prevent—or interrupt—migraine headaches.

A great deal of research is being done in non-drug treatment methods, too. Most notable, perhaps, is the technique of biofeedback.

Here the patient, hooked to the electrodes of a biofeedback machine, learns to relax by listening to the sounds emitted by tensing and relaxing muscles, and learning to control other functions at will. Many migraine victims learn, via biofeedback, to concentrate on raising the temperature in their hands. Some feel that warm hands mean relaxation, while cold hands mean you're uptight. Concentrating on warm hands, then, may mean relaxing. It may also mean sending more blood to your hands—and away from your head.

This may sound like a strange form of treatment, but the initial studies look promising and biofeedback may become a common alternative in migraine treatment.

Perhaps one of the best methods of treatment for all headaches—tension, psychogenic, and vascular—is stress management. You can learn to manage stress by making a conscious effort to relax when you feel yourself tensing and by expressing feelings instead of bottling them inside. Exercise is a great help in managing stress. So is getting some order into your life. Establishing regular sleep patterns, rather than keeping irregular hours, is essential.

What about the insomnia that may be common in those who suffer from tension and migraine headaches?

Taking time to relax fully before bedtime and keeping your bedtime constant may help. Avoid eating for two hours before going to bed. A warm bath may also ease tension and help you to relax.

What if you *still* have trouble sleeping?

"It's better to get up and read or write letters than to lie in the darkness desperately seeking sleep that will not come," says Dr. Samuel Dunkell, a psychiatrist and author of the book *Sleep Positions: The Night Language of the Body.* "Usually, after about fifteen minutes, you'll feel sleepy. Your tension will have been relieved by focusing on something besides the fact that you can't sleep. This may make it possible for you to fall asleep quickly."

By making changes in your life-style and in your sleep patterns as well as seeking your doctor's help, you may discover that, even if your headaches are chronic and severe, there is hope.

STRESS AND YOUR STOMACH

When I'm nervous and especially right after eating, I get this pain in my chest. I'm scared because I think it might be pain in my heart, but my parents say it's just indigestion. Why do I get like this?

Worried

I have this problem that's not only embarrassing, but also rather inconvenient. I always get diarrhea at the worst possible times—before exams or just before a date with a new girl. Is this due to nerves?

David C.

I have a serious problem and I'm scared. I've been having bad stomach cramps and diarrhea and sometimes I notice blood in my stools. Could this be cancer? I'm scared to tell my parents because they're in the middle of getting a divorce and have their own problems.

Betty H.

The gastrointestinal tract—most notably the stomach and intestines—may also be affected by stress. Some of us, in fact, are so good at burying our feelings that it may take a stomachache, diarrhea, or more alarming symptoms to tell us just how tense, frightened, or angry we feel.

Physical symptoms may range from relatively mild gastritis to more serious conditions like ulcers and ulcerative colitis. Often only a physician can tell the serious from the minor, so if you do experience frequent gastrointestinal problems, it's a good idea to consult your physician.

The following descriptions are not included so that you can diagnose and self-medicate your condition, but simply to give you an idea how stress can affect your stomach—and how important it is to seek help and treatment early.

One of the most common stomach problems that may be stress-related is *gastritis*. The stomach secretes acid in response to two stimuli: first, food in the stomach and, second, under the influence of the central nervous system. Stress, anxiety, and tension can cause this acid to be released in an empty stomach. This excess acid may then begin to digest the lining that protects the stomach wall. People who have less than adequate stomach linings to begin with may be particularly prone to problems. So can junk food addicts who favor colas or greasy fried foods. (These foods add even more acid to the stomach.)

What symptoms are you likely to feel with gastritis?

You may have a hollow feeling in your stomach, pain, and heartburn. Many people—like "Worried"—mistake this stomach pain for heart pain. The fact is, your stomach is located high in the abdomen and the pains of gastritis may be felt in the chest area and even the esophagus (if excess acid comes up into the esophagus).

Gastritis may or may not be the beginning of an ulcer. If allowed to progress, it may actually begin to eat away some of the stomach lining.

How can you help yourself if you have a problem with gastritis?

• To a limited extent, antacids may provide temporary relief.

• Don't eat foods that may irritate the condition.

• Don't eat too fast. Don't gulp down or skip meals.

• Eat foods like milk and ice cream that are alkaline, to help neutralize the stomach acid.

• See your physician for diagnosis and further treatment.

• Examine your feelings and the stress points in your life. It does little good to load up on medicine that will only relieve your symptoms. To help remedy the condition and keep your problem from becoming worse, it's necessary to identify and find more workable ways to cope with (or eliminate) major stresses in your life. You may need special help to do this. Or you may find that good exercise, meditation, and/or talking about your feelings with a family member or friend may help you to calm down.

The same "calm down" advice might work for those stricken with "nervous" or "pre-exam" diarrhea. This condition can come from nervousness or poor diet or, frequently, a combination of the two. Teen-agers and young adults are common victims. Here, food rushes through the colon so fast that the colon doesn't have time to absorb the water.

Another possible stress-related condition is *irritable colon* (also called spastic colon), or *colitis*. Here, the abdomen may be distended. There may be pain, alternate bouts of diarrhea and constipation, nausea, heartburn, perspiration, and a feeling of faintness.

With colitis, it is important to avoid spicy foods as well as alcohol, coffee, or tea and foods high in fiber (also called roughage).

Learning to manage your feelings—whether these are fear (before exams, a special date, or ?), anger, or general anxiety—is probably one of the most effective ways to combat these stress-related intestinal ills.

There are some young people, however, whose problems have gone beyond inconvenience to become serious, even incapacitating.

Ulcers, which may occur in anyone (even small children), are often a by-product of stress.

Researchers are finding that it may now be possible to identify those with a predisposition toward a certain kind of duodenal ulcer. Dr. Jerome Ratter, a medical geneticist, told a recent meeting of the National Commission on Digestive Disease that there is a large hereditary influence involved in acquiring ulcers. Those who are predisposed to ulcers may be identified by measuring the level of pepsinogen, an enzyme, in the blood. Now research is focusing on factors in the environment that may cause a person who is already physically predisposed to ulcers to develop one.

An ulcer can happen in the wake of chronic gastritis or excess stomach acid. The acid, having attacked the stomach lining, now eats its way to and, in some cases, through the stomach wall or the wall of the duodenum (the beginning of the small intestine). This is a serious problem and demands care from a physician.

Both stomach (gastric) and duodenal ulcers (which are more common) produce similar symptoms: a burning sensation in the chest and upper abdomen. This may be aggravated by spicy foods, coffee, or alcohol and may be alleviated somewhat by antacids and milk.

Early medical treatment of an ulcer is essential. This treatment may include a special diet (with frequent small meals of easy-to-digest foods), medication, and rest. If stress is not curtailed, the acid will continue to pour into the stomach and the healing process may be delayed.

If left untreated, an ulcer may cause bleeding in the stomach or intestines and the victim may even vomit blood or have blood in the stools (the stools will look black). If the stomach or duodenal wall is perforated (broken through), the results are serious.

Even if you have had an ulcer in the past and are now free of symptoms, you still need to be careful. The ulcer *can* recur. Avoiding excessive cigarette smoking, coffee, alcohol, aspirin, and continued stress may help to keep you free of this condition.

Another potentially serious condition found primarily in young people is *ulcerative colitis*. Here, ulcers develop in the colon (large intestine) and the wall of the colon becomes diseased and inflamed. Ulcerative colitis may be caused by many factors, but the stress factor may play a major role in causing—or aggravating—this disease.

Symptoms of ulcerative colitis may include cramps, blood (and sometimes pus) in the stools, and diarrhea. Or the disease may first manifest itself via *painless* rectal bleeding.

At its worst, ulcerative colitis may cause severe pain and abdominal cramps as well as bloody mucous diarrhea, which may be dangerous due to loss of blood.

If this disease occurs in the upper bowel (ileum), it is called *regional enteritis*.

Treatment of ulcerative colitis may involve a combination of medical and psychological therapy as well as steroids and other drugs. For particularly severe cases, surgery may be necessary.

A correct diagnosis can be made only by a physician. While you can help yourself to manage stress in your life, your physician can help relieve some of your distressing symptoms with appropriate medical treatment.

STRESS AND EATING DISORDERS

I'm 17 and have a problem: I'm a compulsive eater. I can almost inhale a whole cake or loaf of bread and hardly realize it. Once I start eating like that, I can't seem to stop until the whole thing, whatever it is, is gone. This usually, but not always, happens when I'm upset. Sometimes the binge comes out of nowhere. I'll be into a new diet (I'm about 25 pounds overweight) and feel good about it. Then, all of a sudden, if I get mad or upset, I'll find myself eating like a crazy person again!

Molly

Have you ever found yourself eating a lot—even when you're not hungry?

Do you tend to eat normally in front of people, but binge in secret?

When you feel like blowing up and telling someone off or crying, do you eat instead?

Do you find yourself eating a lot *before* an event that scares you—like a first date or a job interview?

These are just a few examples of stress eating, which can be a problem for all ages, but may hit especially hard in adolescence when there there are so many changes and so many pressures.

Compulsive eating may come from a number of feelings including fear, anxiety, anger, and even rebellion.

Lucy, for example, found that her fear of dating would trigger eating binges. Until she sought counseling, she didn't understand that she was using food to make herself unattractive (overweight) because she feared having to make decisions about her sexuality.

Sharon has found that anxiety—worrying about friends, school, the future, you name it—can cause her to overeat.

Jeff, who is considerably overweight and taunted by the other guys in his ninth-grade class, tries to dispel the hurt he feels every school day by seeking the solace of his favorite foods.

Nina, whose svelte mother takes great pride in her physical fitness and abhors fat, locks herself in her room with cakes, cookies, and pizzas. She seems to use eating as a rebellious act. "I might lose weight if only Ma would get off my back about my weight," Nina grumbles.

All of these teens—and maybe you, too—use food as a tranquilizer, a way to deal with stressful feelings. This isn't a surprising response to stress, although many people may react to such feelings in an opposite way, finding it impossible to eat. Food, of course, is necessary to physical and emotional well-being. When we were children, it was often held out to us as a reward when we were good and a comfort when we were hurt. So it may be easy, in moments of stress, to revert back and try to recapture those long-ago good feelings: the candy that said "You're a good girl (boy)" or the just-baked cookie that meant love to us or that peanut butter sandwich that spelled security.

While these feelings may not be difficult to understand, there is a dark side to this eating pattern. While eating may function as a temporary tranquilizer, it may eventually bring more stress into your life. A number of compulsive eaters are overcome by guilt feelings after a binge and also suffer further stress that comes from being different, from being a fat person in an essentially slender world. The stress of being considered unattractive by others is very real, and particularly acute in adolescence.

How can you deal with the problem of compulsive eating?

A group like Overeaters Anonymous or Weight Watchers may help a great deal. But first and foremost, YOU must accept responsibility for your eating and your life.

Taking responsibility for your eating may mean identifying trouble times or situations and trying to find alternate ways to deal with them. For example, if you're tense after classes each day and feel the urge to overeat, try jogging or some other form of vigorous exercise instead. Not only is exercise non-fattening, it's also a great tension reliever. Make up a list of alternate activities and choose one from your list the next time that the familiar craving for food hits you.

Taking responsibility for your life means realizing that food does not control you. Neither do other people—unless you let them. A number of compulsive eaters may be rather passive and not inclined to express feelings like anger. So all that anger is turned inward and you may do hurtful things to yourself. It's important to remind yourself that you have all kinds of options, including the choice of being nice to yourself. You wouldn't dream of hurting a friend who happened to be suffering from stress—right? You can choose to be a good friend to yourself, too, and to try to change both the stresses and the hurtful ways you may be coping with pressure. (For more tips on managing eating habits, see Chapter Five.)

I just threw up, but I wasn't sick. I made myself do it. I also take laxatives and diet pills to lose weight. There are times when I don't eat for days and when I do eat, I feel so guilty about it that I make myself throw up. I wasn't even fat to begin with. I have lots of friends, a high average in school and a semihappy family. (My dad is never around.) Please help me find out what's wrong!

Messed Up

My best friend is starving herself and has been since last fall. She has lost about 40 pounds. She's 5 feet 4 and went from 120 pounds to about 80. She looks disgusting, is always cold, and hasn't had her period for months. She tricks people into not making her eat, takes laxatives constantly, and gets annoyed when anyone tries to help her. She's a real achiever: a straight A student and a school officer. Whatever she wants, she gets. She's always talking about food, but never eats. It's annoying!

Concerned

"Messed Up" and "Concerned" have described quite vividly a problem that has touched the lives of an increasing number of teens: anorexia nervosa.

Anorexia nervosa, a psychosomatic disorder of the gastrointestinal system, which is most common in girls and which may cause the victim to literally starve herself has puzzled physicians for years. There is still controversy about its exact causes and best method of treatment, but many experts agree that the condition seems to stem from psychological problems and conflicts.

There are certain traits that victims of this disorder tend to have in common. The typical anorexia victim is a middle-class female in her teens, a high achiever both in her studies and in outside activities. She may be considered a model child by her parents: polite, considerate, and no problem—until anorexia strikes. Her family may include a protective mother and a more-or-less absentee father whose love may be conditional, that is, based on the girl's achievements.

When anorexia strikes, the young girl's behavior may become more and more bizarre. To get an idea of what it is like to live within the nightmare of anorexia nervosa, we asked a teen named Karen to share her experiences with us.

"A year ago, I weighed 148, which is heavy for my height (5 feet 7)," says Karen. "I decided to really diet this time. I was sick of being teased by my family. I cut down more and more on the foods my body really needed. It got to the point where I was eating only enough to keep me moving. I would eat the same thing every day and would exercise vigorously all the time. I couldn't settle down, except for homework, which I did well. Everything had to be perfect. The homework had to be 100 percent correct. The house had to be spotless. Just everything! I changed from an outgoing, humorous person to a shy, withdrawn crybaby. I started sleeping a lot. At first, my parents yelled at me to eat. Then I wouldn't because they were mean. Later, they begged me with tears in their eyes, telling me how much they loved me. This time I really wanted to eat, but I couldn't. All I wanted to do was die so I wouldn't cause any more problems. I stopped eating altogether for about three weeks straight. Then my doctor put me in the hospital."

Other behavior characteristics of a person with anorexia nervosa include: an obsession with food and cooking (while not eating), occasional binges punctuated by vomiting at will, heavy use of laxatives, and a completely distorted body image. An emaciated anorectic will look in the mirror and think she looks great—or even a little chubby!

Leslie, an anorectic patient who spent a number of weeks in a Los Angeles hospital, confesses that "I worry about getting fat. I exercise and try to keep real active. It makes me mad. I lost all that weight and I don't want to gain it all back!" Leslie weighed 63 pounds (at 5 feet 6) when she was admitted to the hospital. She now weighs 80 pounds.

Anorexia victims, who often stop menstruating, lose up to 50 percent of body weight and maybe even die, seem to be increasing in numbers.

"We're seeing something of an epidemic of anorexia nervosa and we don't really know why," says Dr. R. G. MacKenzie, director of the Adolescent Unit at Children's Hospital of Los Angeles.

As the incidence of anorexia nervosa grows, there is some controversy over which treatment methods work. Some advocate psychotherapy and others, behavior modification. Still other medical experts contend that behavior modification without backup therapy may be useless. Some programs combine behavior modification with psychotherapy, often involving the whole family in the treatment.

The program at Children's Hospital of Los Angeles follows this latter concept.

"First, we help the patient and her family to accept the diagnosis and consent to treatment," says Dr. MacKenzie. "We hospitalize the victim for about a month. We don't force her to eat. That's her decision. We emphasize weight gain. If the patient gains weight, she gets certain privileges. Family therapy—which will go on for a minimum of six months—starts during the hospitalization phase of treatment. There are private sessions combined with family group sessions. We emphasize the fact that we're here for *everyone's* purposes, that the child with anorexia is simply expressing problems shared by the family. This takes a lot of pressure off the patient. Also, there are special rap groups here where teen-agers with anorexia can share feelings and ideas."

Dr. MacKenzie believes that early treatment for anorexia nervosa is essential. "We urge doctors and families to look for classical anorexia behavior patterns and not wait for extreme weight loss to occur before seeking help," he says.

HYPERTENSION (HIGH BLOOD PRESSURE)

My doctor just told me that I have high blood pressure. What does this mean? I thought that was just something that old, fat people get. Is it dangerous?
                                                    Gavin O.

Hypertension, or high blood pressure, can strike at any age, including childhood, adolescence, and young adulthood.

High blood pressure means an increased stress on the walls of the blood vessels. This can be serious if the pressure becomes so great that it actually causes a break in the vessel wall and bleeding into surrounding tissues. If this occurs in the brain, it is called a *stroke* and can be most serious. Bleeding into the del-

icate tissues of the brain can result in paralysis and even death. The higher one's blood pressure, the higher the risk of stroke.

Some people are more likely to develop hypertension than others. For reasons not fully understood, blacks suffer a much higher incidence of high blood pressure. So do people who are obese and those with serious ailments like kidney disease. High blood pressure can run in families. (If your family has a history of high blood pressure, you should have yours checked regularly.) We know, too, that people who eat a lot of salt may be at a greater risk of developing hypertension.

While high blood pressure may occur for a number of physical reasons, stress and anxiety may also be a major factor influencing your blood pressure. The blood vessels are regulated by the nervous system. Given the body's "fight or flight" response to severe stress, tension, and anxiety, these blood vessels may constrict and high blood pressure results, especially in someone who may already have a preexisting tendency toward hypertension.

How do you know if you have high blood pressure?

You won't know unless you have your blood pressure checked.

Many victims of hypertension have no symptoms. Others experience dizziness, headaches, and nervousness, symptoms often associated with high blood pressure. But it is possible to have one or all of these and not have high blood pressure.

So a reading of your blood pressure by a physician or other health care professional is essential. This is a painless procedure.

Two readings—systolic and diastolic—are taken in a blood-pressure examination.

In a blood pressure reading of 120/80 (considered normal for young adults), 120 is the systolic. This means the highest pressure achieved with cardiac output. This may be affected by tension and anxiety. (If you had a bad day, for example, your systolic might at 150.)

The diastolic reading is the low pressure as the heart is filling up once again with blood. This is usually considered to be the most significant reading, as it reflects the true estimate of the dynamics of the body regarding blood pressure.

Although the blood pressure reading for those in the mid-twenties or younger should not—as a rule—be higher than 120/80, there are significant variations of normal.

Athletes, for example, have wide pulse pressure with a strong cardiac output. Wide pulse means that the person has an efficient cardiac output requiring fewer heartbeats to circulate the blood. Consequently, an athlete's blood pressure might be 110/50.

Children and very young teen-agers whose vessels have not aged may have a 90/60 reading.

When does a reading cause concern? Generally, if you have a diastolic of 90 or greater as well as a systolic of 140 or above.

If you have high blood pressure, your physician will investigate possible causes. If you show no evidence of a disease that might be a factor, he or she may advise you to cut your salt intake, avoid taking birth control pills (which may elevate blood pressure) and, possibly, he or she may suggest that you take diuretics. A diuretic will cause you to urinate more frequently and thus help to remove salt and fluid from your body. If you're overweight, this, too, may be contributing to your hypertension. Losing weight may also mean a drop in your blood pressure.

A POINT TO REMEMBER: If you do have high blood pressure, you *must* be under the care of a physician.

You can care for yourself in important ways, too, since hypertension can be tied to stress. Taking time out from your hectic daily schedule just for you, to listen to music or just stare at the ceiling or whatever, can help to alleviate some of the stress you may be feeling every day. Learning to say no when you want to and taking care not to overload your already busy schedule are important preventive measures, too. You need time to just *be*.

HYPOCHONDRIA

I get headaches in math class (which I hate) a lot. My teacher calls me a faker and my doctor says there's nothing wrong with me, but what they don't understand is that my headaches are real!

L.T.

I worry a lot about my body. Some say too much. I get real upset over every pain I have because a 14-year-old body isn't supposed to have that much wrong with it. Am I wrong to be worried?

Jennifer

I miss a lot of school. I have colds, problems with cramps, and headaches. My parents are concerned, but my principal is mean. He said this is all in my head and I could use some counseling!

Mad

It is unfortunate that the word *hypochondria* is often linked with "hysteria" and that *hypochondriac* has come to have the rather unfortunate connotation of "faker" or "troublesome complainer/attention seeker."

The fact is, the person who suffers from hypochon-

dria *does* suffer. The pain is real. The physical pain—a headache or a stomachache, for example—is psychosomatic (coming from emotional stresses), but is far from imaginary.

What kinds of stresses may be factors in hypochondria?

• Your body and life changes. Changes—whether positive or negative—are stressful, and in adolescence, you have to cope with an unprecedented number of them. Your social relationships are changing. So is your body. With all of the rapid physical growth and development going on, you can't help being extra conscious of your body right now.

• Your relationship with your parents is changing. As you become more and more independent, illness may be the one instance where you may feel that it's OK to go back and be a child again—temporarily. Some parents who want to bind their children to them are all too happy to cooperate and label you as "sickly," fostering your dependence on them.

• Your life at school is changing, too. Friends take on new meaning in your life. Schoolwork may be more challenging than ever—or dreadfully boring. Either way, you may find school stressful and seek to escape. Illness may furnish such an escape. This illness may start in your mind, perhaps unconsciously, but the physical symptoms are real.

• Your feelings are also changing. Although you may long, at times, to return to the comfort and security of childhood, you are growing toward independence. Sometimes being separate means getting angry and hostile to create distance from those you love most. It's easy to feel guilty about this and to try to swallow angry feelings. You may bottle up emotions in order to avoid antagonizing others. Your friends are so important right now. Do you dare tell them how you really feel? Would they like you even if you do have angry feelings at times?

With all the stresses in your life, it's not surprising that your body may suffer.

"I feel that hypochondria is a misused term, especially with adolescents," says Dr. Lonnie Zeltzer, a staff physician at the Adolescent Unit of Children's Hospital of Los Angeles. "For example, we have seen a number of Job Corps women, ages 16 and up, who are dealing with adolescence and who are not used to talking about their feelings. So stresses are internalized and the autonomic nervous system reacts with stomachaches, headaches, muscle aches, low back pain, chest pain, and feelings of being tired, weak, or nervous. We work to teach these young women more appropriate coping so that they don't have to use their *bodies* to talk with those around them. The pain is a message, a way of signaling the individual that something is going on. We work with people to try to decode the message. Why is pain there? What's going on?''

More and better pain-killers are not necessarily the answer.

"Frankly, I'm dismayed when I see a physician who just gives out pain pills, transquilizers, and so on," says Dr. Zeltzer. "This just reinforces the idea: 'Something's wrong with me . . . I'm getting pills!' This may increase your anxiety. You must discuss the feelings behind the pain. If you find yourself being sick with all kinds of colds, headaches, and the like or have a lot of injuries and accidents (which may also be related to stress), it's time to step back and say 'Something is going on with me. Let me see what I can work out and what I need to talk about.' But *don't* label yourself as different or crazy or anything else. Your pain is very real and you just have to find the message behind it.''

Sometimes we need help to decode our pain messages, but we hesitate. Somehow, seeking help for a problem that is, at least in part, psychological is more difficult than going to a doctor with a physical complaint.

"Teen-agers may have a great fear of being crazy or of being *thought* to be crazy," says Dr. Marilyn Mehr, a clinical psychologist at the Adolescent Unit. "It may be helpful to know that everyone goes through this. Accept your psychological needs as well as your physical needs and ask for help when you need it. It may be easier when you see counseling as necessary for healthy, strong people who want to grow.''

Growing may mean accepting responsibility for your health: asking for help when you need it and helping yourself when you can.

It may help a great deal to realize that feelings must be expressed in some way.

If you can't express them in a way of your choosing—talking or writing, for example—these feelings will choose their own way to come out.

If you let anger build up, for example, it may burst out in a temper tantrum, in a throbbing headache, or stomach cramps . . . or even trip you up in an accident!

In the long run, then, it may be much less painful to say ''I feel angry'' than to find yourself yelling ''Ouch!'' or moaning ''Oh, my aching head!''

It's important, too, not to put yourself down for feelings or characteristics that you consider to be negative. We *all* get angry. We *all* have flaws and failings. Having compassion for your faults and accepting feelings like anger as normal may reduce stress in your life considerably. (For more suggestions on handling stress, see Chapter Four.)

A certain amount of stress, however, is inevitable. So it's important that your body be ready for it. Regular aerobic exercise (see Chapter Five) will not only help you to work off some of your tension and frustration, but it will also increase your body's capacity to handle stress when it does come.

With a physically fit body, the knowledge that outside help is available to you when you need it, and the conviction that YOU have the power—if you take it—to prevent many feelings from hurting you physically, you will be well-equipped to handle the stresses that will always be a part of your life, stresses that nobody can ever quite escape.

CHAPTER NINE

Young Adults and Special Medical Needs

"I'm angry. This is really messing up my life."

"I'm scared. What will happen to me?"

"I really feel out of it."

"What I want to know is . . . why me???"

"Sometimes I feel on the verge of giving up."

The statements above were made by young adults who were suffering from a variety of ills—from mononucleosis (first statement) to diabetes (last statement).

There is, quite obviously, a difference between mono, a curable, short-term disease, and diabetes, a chronic, controllable disease. But both mean that you may have special medical needs, and these may, indeed, have an impact on your life.

Any kind of illness may be hard on you as an adolescent. You're so conscious of and concerned about your body. When something goes wrong, it's easy to get scared—and to feel very much alone. If you're like most young people, you want to be active and may resent any illness that you may feel keeps you from doing what you want to do, either temporarily or permanently.

You may also feel that a special medical need is keeping you more dependent than you would like to be on your parents, and your parents may—even with the best intentions—tend to foster such dependence.

You may hate feeling different, yet when you have special medical needs, you may be intrinsically different. You may have to take medications and be on a special diet. There may be certain procedures you have to follow that make it necessary to have detailed plans for simple things that other teens may take for granted, like slumber parties and field trips, which point up the fact of your difference even more.

Maybe you don't have a special medical need yourself, but you may know someone who does: a college roommate with mononucleosis; a cousin who has asthma; the girl next door who has scoliosis (curvature of the spine); and a boyfriend/girl friend with diabetes. If someone you know and love has a special problem, it's natural to be concerned. We have received a number of letters from teens concerned about those they love, asking questions like:

"My boyfriend is a diabetic. Is it true that he'll die young?"

"My sister has asthma really bad. What causes this? Can she ever get better?"

"A classmate of mine is epileptic. If she would have a seizure at school, how could we help her?"

So this chapter is for everybody—for those who may have either temporary or chronic medical problems and for those who may know and love someone who does. We hope we can help you to better understand some of the common medical problems that adolescents can have and, most important, to learn how to *live* with these special needs.

Of course, space does not permit us to talk about every possible affliction that may beset young adults. So we'll simply discuss some of the more common medical problems. We will not be discussing necessarily the most common causes of *death* in young people (in case you're curious, accidents and suicides kill more teens and young adults than any disease). Cancer, for example, is a common cause of death, but it is not especially common, on the whole, in the teenage population.

So we're focusing on medical problems that are most likely to be part of your life, either directly or indirectly. Some are temporary. Others are chronic. Some of the problems may be relatively minor. Others may have serious consequences. All may cause pain, upset, a feeling of being different, and may impinge on your life in a number of ways.

What problems are we talking about? All kinds, including mononucleosis, urinary tract infections, bed-wetting (nocturnal enuresis), allergies, asthma, anemia (iron-deficiency and sickle-cell), hypoglycemia (low blood sugar), diabetes, scoliosis, Osgood-Schlatter disease, and epilepsy.

We hope that this information will give you new insights into special medical needs: your own or those of someone close to you.

INFECTIOUS MONONUCLEOSIS

Is there really a disease called the "kissing disease"? If so, what is it and do you really get it from kissing? What are the symptoms? Is it serious?

Concerned

I'm 20 and a college student. I have just been diagnosed as having mono. My doctor was most emphatic about my getting a lot of rest. He said something about complications if I don't take proper care of myself. What complications can happen? Is there something I can do for myself besides just resting?

Doug W.

Infectious mononucleosis is a very common problem among young adults, especially college students.

A lot of research has been done on the disease that most young people call "mono" and it has been found that it is caused by a virus. How this virus is spread, however, is still subject to debate.

It's true that, in the past, mononucleosis was often called the "kissing disease," but that has proved to be something of a misnomer. You can have close contact with a victim of mono and not get it.

Some evidence suggests that people who are fatigued and exhausted may be predisposed to the disorder. This may explain why it has such a penchant for college students around exam time.

What are the symptoms of mono?

These may vary a great deal, but the most common tend to be extreme fatigue and the need for a lot of sleep. Of course, if you're exhausted to begin with, it may be difficult to tell whether your problem is simply fatigue or mono.

However, when you're tired, you can usually pull yourself together and function pretty well when you want or need to so so. If you're a victim of mononucleosis, on the other hand, you may not be able to function even if you want very much to be awake and alert.

Other symptoms of mono may include swelling of the lymph glands (especially those in the neck), headaches, and a very severe sore throat. There may also be a skin rash and, in some cases, enlargement of the liver and/or spleen.

It is important to have this condition diagnosed by a physician, which he/she will do via a physical exam and a blood test.

How is infectious mononucleosis treated?

With lots of rest and a good diet. These simple instructions are important. If a victim of mono doesn't get proper rest, avoid contact sports (if so directed by the physician), and eat well, enlargement and possible rupture of the spleen could result.

How serious is this?

While rupture of the spleen would mean emergency surgery, one can live a normal life without this organ. (But who *needs* complications like that?)

Many teens with mononucleosis may risk such complications by resuming normal activities too soon. It's sad but true that mono seems to strike at times when you don't really have time to be sick—like around exam time or graduation. Yet, sufficient rest is vital to complete recovery.

How long could mono keep you sidelined?

This can vary a great deal. Some are only out of step with their normal schedules for a week. Others may take a month to recover. It's a highly individual matter. Your body will usually let you know when it's ready to function at full capacity again.

URINARY TRACT INFECTIONS

I have pain and burning when I go to the bathroom and a friend told me that this is a urinary infection. How do you get it? (I heard it may have something to do with sex, but I don't have sex!) How do you get rid of it?

Alice D.

Is it true that bubble baths can give you infections? What kind of infections?

Wondering

I started having sex about 10 months ago. I'm 19 and have been having one urinary infection after another. Is this tied to sex? I feel like it's almost a punishment or something for having sex! How can I keep this from happening again and again?

Renee

Urinary tract infections are common in young adults, most often in young women. Quite frequently, these may be young women who are having their first sexual experiences.

But sex is not the only factor in urinary tract infections.

Bubble baths may cause irritation of the urethra and, as a result, a urinary infection.

Careless wiping after a bowel movement can be another causative factor. The rectum is close to the urethra (urinary opening) in the woman and it is easy for bacteria from the rectum to invade the urinary tract. This may be especially likely if you have a habit of wiping toward the vagina (forward) after a bowel movement. Wiping away from the vagina and urethra (backward) will minimize this risk.

How can sexual activity increase your likelihood of developing a urinary tract infection?

During intercourse, the man's penis—while thrusting—may touch areas near both the woman's rectum and urethra and may thus spread bacteria from rectum to urethra. For some sexually active women, this may mean almost continuous urinary tract infections.

How can you avoid such problems?

Use Good Hygiene. Bathe or shower regularly, taking care to wash the genital and the rectal area.

Urinate as Soon as Possible After Sex. This can help to wash out any bacteria that may be present in the urinary tract.

Drink Water After Sex. Some urologists recommend drinking water after sexual intercourse. This will be flushed rapidly through the kidneys and thus further urination will help to wash any remaining bacteria out of the urinary tract before the bacteria have a chance to multiply.

How do you know if you may have a urinary tract infection?

In some cases, it may be difficult to distinguish a urinary tract infection from a vaginal infection. However, with a vaginal infection, you will usually have a vaginal discharge as well as painful or burning urination.

Symptoms of a urinary tract infection include pain and burning on urination and greater frequency of urination (not as a result of drinking a lot of fluid), blood in the urine (when you're not having your menstrual period) and, in some cases, a concurrent kidney infection with pain in the lower back.

If you have such symptoms, don't just wait and hope that they will disappear. See a physician. A urinalysis will reveal whether or not you do have a urinary tract infection. If you do, your physician may treat the condition with antibiotics.

NOCTURNAL ENURESIS (BED-WETTING)

I'm 14 and still wet the bed. My mom is so mad at me and calls me a baby. I can't help it! I'm so embarrassed and avoid things like slumber parties for obvious reasons. Why do I do this? What can I do to stop? Please help me!

Embarrassed

I'm almost 16 and wet the bed sometimes. I'm so ashamed, I could die! I've thought about asking my doctor about this, but I'm too embarrassed.

Crying

It's easy to feel embarrassed or to feel like a baby, if you have a problem with bed-wetting (medically termed *nocturnal enuresis*). It may be some consolation, however, that you are far from alone. This condition is not uncommon in teens and young adults.

Another note of optimism: Nocturnal enuresis is *not* a sign of emotional immaturity and it can be treated.

What causes this condition?

Recent research has found that nocturnal enuresis is related to a specific stage of sleep. The fourth stage (deep sleep) may be *so* deep for some people that muscle control of the bladder may be lost, causing urination during sleep.

What can you do if you have this problem?

First, don't be embarrassed to ask your doctor for help. This problem is not uncommon and it can be treated.

What forms of treatment may be used?

One of the most common medical approaches to nocturnal enuresis is a drug that, when taken before bedtime, causes the level of sleep to be more active, preventing the sleeper from going into such a deep fourth stage. It has been clinically proven that these drugs, by elevating the sleep level, decrease the incidence of bed-wetting.

There are some commonsense ways you can help yourself, too. Don't drink fluids or cut down on fluid intake in the evening. And don't forget to urinate just before you go to bed.

ALLERGIES

Since coming to college in the Midwest this fall (I'm from California) I feel like I've got a cold all the time! I'm beginning to think I might have an allergy. But I've never had any problems with allergies before. What could be causing this?

Puzzled

I've always had bad trouble with allergies. When I was younger, my mother took me to an allergy doctor. He ran some tests and told me all the things to stay away from and not eat. But there's some things you can't help like pollen, dust, and my grandmother's banana pudding!

Sneezy

Allergies afflict people of all ages, causing a variety of uncomfortable symptoms including nasal congestion, sneezing, nasal dripping with throat discomfort, redness and watering of the eyes, itching, hives or skin rashes, nausea, diarrhea and, in some serious types of allergies like asthma (which we will discuss in detail a little later on), respiratory disorders and difficulty in breathing.

What exactly *is* an allergy?

It is a reaction by the body against a substance that it recognizes as foreign. Such a substance is called an *allergen.* In response to an allergen, the body forms antibodies and releases certain chemicals that, in turn, cause the allergy symptoms. While many people are able to adapt to allergens, many remain sensitive to common substances that may be completely harmless to those without allergies.

Allergies may run in families. If both parents have allergies, you have an 80 percent chance of being allergic, too. Even if only one parent is allergic, you still have a 50 percent chance of developing allergies.

There are many different kinds of allergies.

Environmental allergies mean that you are allergic to certain pollens, plants, flowers, weeds, grasses, molds, dusts, or tobacco smoke.

Food allergies are quite common. The allergens may be common foods like chocolate or eggs or, perhaps, unusual foods like macadamia nuts. Reactions may include sneezing, bronchial congestion, skin rashes, diarrhea, and constipation.

Drug allergies happen when people are extremely sensitive to certain drugs—often aspirin, sulfa drugs, or penicillin. Reactions range from mild itching to severe shock.

Cosmetic allergens range from eye makeup to shampoo. People are often allergic to the oils in some of these products and may suffer reactions like rashes after use of the product.

Animal allergies are also fairly common. Here people may be unusually sensitive to the dander (skin and hair) of a pet dog, cat, or horse. While a clean, brushed animal may trigger fewer allergic reactions, some people cannot be around allergen animals at all.

Contact allergies mean that you have an unusual sensitivity to certain metals such as gold or silver. You may experience redness or itching of the skin when you make contact with the metal in a piece of jewelry.

Hives, incidentally, may be classified as a sign of an allergy, but, especially in teens and young adults, may be a sign of extreme stress and nervousness as well.

How do you know if you have an allergy and what the allergen might be in your case?

The answer is not clear-cut.

You may—like "Puzzled"—suffer what you may think of initially as prolonged cold symptoms after moving to another area of the country. It may be helpful to know that certain geographic areas have different allergens. So if you have grown up in the East and go to college on the West Coast, you may find yourself with a long-lasting "cold" that may prove to be an allergy.

Some people, too, may find that a stressful situation, illness, or injury may lower the body's resistance to allergies. Other people may have very mild or seasonal allergies that are often mistaken for colds.

However, if you have more than an occasional problem, if your symptoms are chronic and stressful, you are probably fairly sure *already* that you have allergies. You may not know what may be triggering these reactions, however.

By going to a physician who specializes in allergies or to an allergy clinic, you can get skin tests to help determine your specific allergy or allergies. Here, prepared solutions of common allergens are injected under the skin at different sites to see if any reactions occur. In this way, your specific allergy may be determined.

However, if you have only an occasional problem or already know what your specific allergen is, it may not be necessary to go to the expense and time of having such tests. Some allergies disappear as you grow up; others may be with you for a lifetime.

How are such allergies treated?

There is some debate about this.

Some physicians feel strongly that patients should have immunization or de-sensitization shots. This series of injections, which may go on for years, usually on a weekly basis, helps to build up protection against an allergen and make allergy symptoms less severe. However, these shots not only require a regular, long-standing time commitment, they may also be expensive.

Many physicians advocate treating allergy symptoms with drugs like the antihistamines. This form of treatment may be especially helpful for the patient with occasional allergies.

You can help yourself in specific ways, too. Probably the most important part of managing an allergy is avoiding—as much as possible—your specific allergen. This may mean working with your family to keep your home as dust-free as possible or parting with (or keeping a distance from) the family pet or avoiding offending foods (however much you may crave them!).

Of course, in living a normal life, you can't possibly avoid all allergens, but by using common sense, you can keep from exposing yourself unnecessarily to substances that may cause you misery.

ASTHMA

I first got asthma at the age of two. I'm now 15. I've heard things about its causes, but nobody has really talked to me about it. Is asthma an allergy or tied to the emotions or inherited?

Sue A.

Asthma may mean an occasional wheeze or, in its most severe form, may kill.

While asthma is usually considered to be a severe form of allergy, recent research by Dr. Elliott of the State University of New York at Buffalo reveals that viral infections may play a major role in triggering asthma attacks in young children. Underlying the reaction to the virus, he says, is a genetic predisposition to a defect involving the airways in the lungs or the bronchial tubes. He adds, however, that when asthma develops after early childhood and before middle age, it may, indeed, be caused by an allergy. As an allergy, asthma may run in families.

What happens during an asthma attack?

The lung tissue begins to secrete a substance that causes the air passages of the lungs to become blocked. The tiny bronchial tubes will squeeze shut, making the victim fight desperately to breathe. The victim may experience a sensation of tightness in the chest, shortness of breath, wheezing, or rapid breathing.

The attack may be brought on by a specific allergen or by stress. This stress may involve a specific situation in the young person's life or may be the result of ongoing family problems. Because of this, some physicians may treat severe asthmatics with a combination of drugs, psychotherapy, and family counseling. In especially severe cases, the asthma victim may even be removed from the home. Asthma can be an extremely serious lifelong problem for some.

Anyone with asthma should have a regular physician who will prescribe and monitor drugs needed and who can help the patient and his/her family to monitor the environment (removal of dust and animal hair from the home, for example). For some, such environmental management may cause rapid improvement. For others, management of asthma may not be as simple.

Specific drugs may help somewhat to alleviate symptoms in some victims. However, there is no one perfect drug yet and what works for you at one time may cease to help later on. Some new drugs like Cromolyn are helpful to some, but not to others. Cortisone-type hormones may bring relief, but, when taken over a long period of time, may have some undesirable side effects. Small doses of certain cortisones that are inhaled show considerable promise and seem to be relatively free of the side effects that large doses of cortisone drugs may have. For those with especially severe cases, Beclomethasone (also inhaled) may be effective, according to a recent report in the *Journal of the American Medical Association*.

A person with severe asthma may be instructed to drink lots of fluid to help unplug congested lung tissues and may also be taught a series of deep-breathing exercises to be used at the first sign of an attack.

A trip to the doctor's office or to the hospital may be necessary in the event of a severe asthma attack, however. Injections may be given to bring relief. For some, a period of hospitalization may be necessary.

There are some young people who are so severely afflicted with asthma that they are afraid to laugh, have attended school only irregularly, have been in and out of hospitals for years, and who live with the constant reality that the next attack could bring death.

There may be hope for those with such severe symptoms, too. Each year, approximately 128 young people between the ages of 6 and 16 receive intensive treatment at the National Asthma Center in Denver, the world's largest residential asthma treatment center and hospital for children and the only full-scale research facility in the Western world that specializes in asthma. Here, where the emphasis is on learning to control one's own disease, young people receive intensive medical care and counseling to help cope with their fears and problems. While officials at the center say that asthma cannot be cured, they are finding that 95 percent of their young patients (all of whom have been severely afflicted with asthma) leave the center to live normally, often for the first time in their lives.

No matter how mild or severe one's case of asthma may be, teamwork is essential. Your physician, your family, and your environment are all important in the unified effort to help make treatment effective. But your efforts—most of all—can be crucial in controlling this disorder.

ANEMIA

I've been sort of tired lately and was wondering if I might be anemic. Can anemia be caused by heavy menstrual periods? How can I find out if I'm anemic and what can I do about it?

Barbara F.

I've been hearing a lot about sickle-cell anemia the past couple months. What is it? Can anyone get it? What are the symptoms?

Tom W.

Thanks to certain television commercials, the word *anemia* is often used to describe everything from depression to the legendary "tired blood" claim. We do not, obviously, support such television diagnosis.

Anemia is a very specific problem that must be diagnosed by a physician (via a blood test) rather than by symptoms alone, since some victims have no unusual symptoms.

There are many types of anemia, and while it is beyond the scope of this book to cover every type, we will discuss two forms that are seen commonly in teenagers and young adults: iron-deficiency anemia and sickle-cell anemia.

Iron-Deficiency Anemia

This type of anemia is often mislabeled "tired blood."

When you have this condition, your blood is not tired, but is lacking sufficient iron supplies to manufacture a constant resupply of red blood cells. When the body lacks sufficient iron, the number of red blood cells may decrease, causing so-called iron-deficiency anemia.

There may be many factors that cause the body to lack iron. Among these may be a heavy menstrual flow. While actual blood lost during menstruation does not have to be replaced, lost iron must be.

One of the best sources of iron is a good, well-balanced diet (see Chapter Five). However, many young adults favor junk foods, which may do little, if anything, to help replenish the body's nutrients and iron supplies.

It is quite common, then, to see an active teen with regular menstrual cycles (and often a heavy menstrual flow) and who favors a predominantly junk food diet, develop iron deficiency anemia.

How do you know if you have it?

You may feel fatigued. But it is also possible that you will have no symptoms. A simple blood test is the only reliable way to tell if you may have this form of anemia.

It is encouraging to see a majority of family planning centers—most notably Planned Parenthood—test for anemia routinely as part of annual gynecological exams. Such routine testing may help to alert more young women to this special problem—and help them to correct it.

If you have iron-deficiency anemia, what can you do about it?

For some, diet alone may correct the anemia, while others may require additional iron supplements, taken under a physician's supervision. Don't try to diagnose your own condition and don't attempt to treat yourself with over-the-counter iron supplements. You and your physician together need to work out the best method of treatment for you.

Sickle-Cell Anemia

Sickle-cell anemia is an inherited disease, most often seen in blacks, where there is a genetic defect in the structure of the red blood cells and, as a result, a decrease of healthy red blood cells in the body.

Due to a structural defect, the red blood cells are shaped like sickles or half-moons, instead of being round, and are not able to carry on the functions of the normal cells—specifically, that of oxygen-carbon-dioxide exchange in the lung tissues. Because these blood cells have an unusual shape, they cannot pass through the rounded blood vessels easily and may become lodged in them, causing congestion in whatever part of the body that this occurs. This congestion can become very uncomfortable, with leg, abdominal, or chest pain, impaired circulation, and possible skin ulcers.

The disorder is a serious one and may become even more critical in instances where the oxygen level of the blood is affected, for example, when anesthesia is given or when an infection occurs in the body. For this reason, it is vital to know if you do have sickle-cell anemia or if you may be a carrier. It is estimated that 8 to 10 percent of all American blacks may be carriers of the sickle-cell trait.

If you are black, we strongly urge you to be tested for this trait. In many cities, there are testing centers for sickle-cell anemia and even some mobile vans that enable medical personnel to do free testing in certain neighborhoods. The test for sickle-cell anemia is a simple, but important, blood test.

You may not have the disease yourself, but you may be a carrier. If you conceive a child with a person who is also a carrier, it is possible that the child will have sickle-cell anemia. It is important to know the possibilities—and the risks—in advance.

It is also important to know if you may have the disease, since it does require the care of a physician.

HYPOGLYCEMIA (LOW BLOOD SUGAR)

Something strange happens to me during my second-period class (10:00 to 10:50) almost every day. I start to feel really hungry and faint, and sometimes I also tremble and feel sweaty. I can't understand this since I do eat breakfast (coffee and a sweet roll) every day. What's the matter with me?

Scared

What exactly is hypoglycemia? It seems that everyone has it! Is it just the latest fashionable disease to have? What causes it?

Mark P.

Hypoglycemia, or low blood sugar, has been discussed and self-diagnosed a great deal during the past few years.

The fact is that true hypoglycemia (caused by disease or factors besides poor dietary habits) is relatively rare. As mentioned earlier, Dr. Rachmiel Levine, a noted metabolic specialist, says that he sees only five or six cases of true hypoglycemia a year.

Hypoglycemia—like diabetes—involves a problem with the body's metabolization of a kind of sugar called glucose.

The body needs glucose for all its functions and is able to obtain it from almost every food substance. The pancreas, which lies near the stomach, breaks nutrients down into glucose, and a constant level of this substance is maintained. The pancreas secretes an enzyme called insulin, which enables the body to utilize glucose in a number of ways.

However, if the function of the pancreas is impaired—most notably in diabetes—the body is unable to correctly regulate its use of glucose.

Someone with hypoglycemia-like symptoms (feeling faint, dizzy, or shaky) is probably *not* a diabetic. Here, the level of insulin is high and the blood sugar (glucose) level is low.

How does this happen?

It could be your diet. If you—like "Scared"—eat a high-carbohydrate, sweet roll and coffee breakfast, your pancreas will secrete a high level of insulin in anticipation of more food to follow. When that food doesn't follow, you may experience a drop of blood sugar and the symptoms of hypoglycemia.

If you're basically healthy (do not have organic hypoglycemia), more careful eating habits may remedy the situation. A more nutritious breakfast—with protein instead of a high concentration of sugar and carbohydrates—may help to correct the condition.

If you're suffering symptoms of hypoglycemia, eating or drinking something with a high carbohydrate level (like orange juice) may help to alleviate the symptoms themselves. Orange juice has a high level of carbohydrate which is quickly metabolized by the body. You can feel better quickly with orange juice (especially with sugar added), but this benefit is temporary. For long-lasting beneficial results, eating protein rich foods is best.

If, despite the fact that you are eating a good breakfast and following a prudent diet in general, you continue to have symptoms of hypoglycemia, see your physician for further evaluation.

DIABETES

My boyfriend is a diabetic and he says that he probably won't live to be 30. (We're both 15 now.) Is this true?

Kay L.

I have diabetes and I feel like a Martian. Taking shots and stuff like that makes me feel dumb. My sisters laugh at me and call me a "dipabetic." What should I do?

Mad

I'm a diabetic and am supposed to stay on this special diet, but I cheat. All of my friends can eat whatever they like—candy all day if they want. But I can't. Life is terrible since I got diabetes.

Sharon B.

I just found out that I have diabetes. I wish I was dead. My friends and parents treat me like a cripple. I've also read stuff about all kinds of complications connnected to diabetes, and frankly, I don't see any reason to go on living.

Lisa M.

Diabetes mellitus (the inability of the pancreas to produce insulin and thus convert food into glucose, the body's major energy source) afflicts almost one million young people. It is estimated that one in every 1,000 people 17 years old and under has diabetes.

This chronic metabolic disorder comes in two basic varieties: Juvenile-onset diabetes usually begins in childhood or adolescence and, because there is usually very little or no natural insulin production, requires regular injections of insulin. The other variety, maturity-onset diabetes, usually strikes adults in middle age and is less severe, often involving *impairment* of the functioning of the pancreas, which may still continue to produce some insulin. For this reason, older people who have this kind of diabetes may be able to control the disorder by diet and oral medication, although some of those with more severe cases will take insulin injections.

What causes diabetes in a young person?

Heredity may be a strong factor. Diabetes can run in families. Recent research has indicated that, especially in juvenile diabetes, serious infections may also be a factor. Some researchers believe that this type of diabetes may result from damage to the pancreas by viruses like those causing mumps or hepatitis. There is also a new theory that a virus may attack the pancreas in young people with a genetic predisposition to diabetes. In short, there is still a great deal to be discovered about the causes of this disease.

We do know, however, that diabetes, particularly if it is not well-controlled, may lead to a number of direct and indirect complications, including diabetic coma (and possible death), kidney disease, and blindness, to name only a few. So early detection and good control of the disease are vital.

How do you know if you may have diabetes?

Symptoms may include sudden excessive thirst and a surge in appetite (without a weight gain), weight loss, fatigue, frequent urination, irritability, and confusion. If you have a combination of these symptoms with or without a family history of diabetes, please see a doctor.

If diabetes is suspected, the physician will test your blood and urine to discover whether there is excess sugar in your urine and bloodstream and to determine how your body is able to absorb and utilize sugar.

If diabetes is the diagnosis, it may be tough to take at first.

True, there are certain procedures that must be followed. Daily insulin injections are essential for those with juvenile-onset diabetes. So is a sensible diet and exercise regimen. A diabetic must eat meals regularly and right on schedule. The young diabetic must also learn to adjust the amount of insulin taken, depending on how much exercise he or she will be getting on a particular day or what foods may be consumed. Also, certain illnesses—like colds or flu—may increase one's need for insulin.

It is also important to know the symptoms of insulin reaction (too little sugar in the body) and approaching diabetic coma (too much sugar). Most diabetics keep a source of sugar—candy, a sugar cube, or injectable glucagon—readily available in case of need.

It may be important to wear an ID bracelet or necklace giving your condition, name, doctor, and instructions for emergency treatment. This may save your life if, for example, you are injured in an accident, for there are certain drugs that diabetics should never be given. It may also be a lifesaver if you lapse into a coma away from home. This may not be particularly likely, but it could happen and when it does, diabetics may, all too often, be mistaken for drunk. So it's vital that people be able to determine what your problem may be—if you are unable to tell them.

This may look like an incredibly long list of *musts*—right?

Many teens rebel. It's tough to be different and to have to do so many things: to eat meals regularly, test urine, take shots. It may be difficult, too, to assert your independence when you are dependent on a drug for your life and when your parents may be concerned and even overly protective. However, making the decision *yourself* to know and regulate your disease can be, quite literally, a lifesaver.

Taking responsibility for yourself may give you a new feeling of independence. You may find that careful planning of your day may allow you not only to regulate your diabetes but also to organize your work and play time better. You may find, too, that little things like taking your own supply of sugarless diet drinks to a party may not set you apart in an extreme way. Some of your diet-conscious friends may be doing the same thing (or eyeing your diet drink supply!). You may find, too, that by following the rules, you'll really start to feel better.

Following your physician's instructions for management of the disease may, in the long run, give you more freedom. If you are in control of your diabetes and free of complications, there is no reason why you can't lead an active, normal life.

Diabetes is not the death sentence it was half a century ago. With good management of your diabetes, you may have a normal life span. In fact, by keeping your weight down, your body trim and well-exercised and your diet balanced and nutritious, you may even live longer than people without diabetes who eat junk foods, get overweight and don't exercise—and otherwise abuse their bodies!

SCOLIOSIS

I am supposed to get a brace at the end of July for my back because I have a curvature of the spine—scoliosis—and I'm scared. I know I'll feel like such a jerk running around with a thing like that on my body!
Scared

I had a problem with scoliosis when I was 14 (I'm now 17) and had an operation in which a rod was put in my back to straighten it. I'm so glad I had it done. Since getting scoliosis, I've found out some interesting facts: like it usually occurs in teen-age girls. So it should be talked about more with teens!
Deb P.

I'm so scared, I don't know what to do. I was looking in the mirror today and saw that my shoulders aren't level. I know this can mean you have a curvature of the spine and that would be awful! I couldn't face it. I recently saw the movie Looking for Mr. Goodbar *where the main character has to sleep on a table in the living room for a year in this really GROSS cast!!! And even that doesn't make her well! I'd rather die than go through all that. Is there some way I could fix this myself without going to a doctor????*

Desperate

Scoliosis is a correctable deformity in which the spine will curve to one side instead of growing straight. It is especially common in girls (who outnumber male victims four to one) in the growing years between 10 and 16. There is some evidence that this condition may be inherited, although certain diseases (rheumatoid arthritis, cerebral palsy, polio) and spinal injuries may also be factors. Most cases of scoliosis have no easily discernible cause, but we know that this condition afflicts about 10 percent of young adolescents to some degree.

Early symptoms may include shoulders that are not level, uneven hips, and prominent shoulder blades. An S curve to your spine may also be observed if you have a friend or family member look at your back as you bend over. In a number of school districts across the nation, there are special screening programs to detect scoliosis in its early stages.

Contrary to the bleak, frightening and, in many

ways, inaccurate picture of scoliosis portrayed in the film *Looking for Mr. Goodbar,* scoliosis does not have to be a horrendous affliction, especially if it is diagnosed early.

When there is less than a 20-degree curvature of the spine, no treatment at all or only simple exercises may be required. The physician, however, may watch the curvature over a period of time to make sure that it is not increasing.

If the curvature is more pronounced, the teen may need to wear a Milwaukee brace for a period of time and do special exercises. The brace, while it may *look* cumbersome, doesn't have to interfere with your normal activities and may help a great deal to move your spine back into a normal position.

Only in relatively rare instances, with more severe cases, is surgery and casting required. Here, as Deb indicated in her letter, an adjustable rod is surgically implanted to help straighten the spine.

Treatment for scoliosis—whatever the method may be—will keep the curvature from progressing and causing serious deformities in later life. So if you notice any indications of scoliosis, don't be afraid to tell your parents and your doctor. Treatment now will be of lifelong benefit, and the earlier you seek help, the less help you're likely to need.

OSGOOD-SCHLATTER DISEASE

I've been having a lot of swelling and pain in my knee and lower leg. I'm active (co-captain of our varsity basketball team) and hate having this pain. What could it be and what can I do to get rid of it?

Rusty C.

I'm 13 and have Osgood-Schlatter disease in my right knee. The doctor told me I can't run, jump, or do any kind of flips or take gym class for two to three months. What I want to know is what can I do to keep from getting bored and what causes this disease anyway?

Mandy

Osgood-Schlatter disease, a disorder of the mineralization of the leg bones, is quite common, especially in active young people between the ages of 10 and 15.

This condition, which can cause swelling and tenderness around the knees and pain in the lower leg, may be caused by irregular deposits of calcium in the tendon, knee, and tibia during the growth, development, and calcification of bones in the early teens. It is a *temporary* condition that is usually self-healing.

To facilitate healing, a physician will usually recommend that you stay away from vigorous sports and

exercises involving knee bending for a certain amount of time—from several months to a year. This doesn't mean, however, that you can't still be active. Just limit your activities to ones that don't put stress on the knees such as swimming.

Those with unusually severe cases of Osgood-Schlatter disease may require casts to help healing, but usually a relatively brief period of rest is enough. While this period of reduced activity may seem to go on forever, it may be some consolation that, once healed, you'll be as good as ever—as the following testimonial from a teen named Beth shows.

"I'm 16 and two years ago I had Osgood-Schlatter disease bad enough to have a cast on my knee for two months," she writes. "But now I'm going strong. I'm a cheerleader, a majorette, and am on the girls' basketball team. I just wanted to tell other teens to follow their doctor's instructions and take care. You'll be OK, too!"

EPILEPSY

I'm 14 years old and have epilepsy. I'm afraid to ask my doctor some of these questions, so I'm asking you. What IS epilepsy? (I know what it is kind of, but want to know more.) Is it hereditary? Will I have to take pills all my life? Is it true that it's harder to get a job if you're an epileptic? If so, why?

Want to Know

I'm 15 and my boyfriend is 16. I found out that he has something called "temporal lobe epilepsy" and gets stomach pains because of this. I don't understand and he doesn't want to tell me about it. Could you please tell me what it is? (In English, if you know what I mean!)

Anne A.

Epilepsy is an often misunderstood disorder of the central nervous system that, due to uncontrolled electrical discharges in the brain, will cause seizures.

Seizures may not be the epileptic's major problem, however. Lack of public understanding—and a number of myths—may be the greatest problem that epileptics of any age may face.

It is important to know that epilepsy is *not* a mental illness or a sign of mental retardation (although some retarded young people may have seizures). It is not contagious nor is it, strictly speaking, hereditary, although a tendency or genetic predisposition may be found in certain types of epilepsy.

There are a number of possible causes of epilepsy. The disorder may be caused by head injuries from accidents, birth injuries, infectious illnesses, brain tumors, or other diseases. Some causes may remain a mystery. Research into more causes and treatments of epilepsy is being done at the present time.

There are also a number of different types of epilepsy. The most common may fall into three general categories:

Grand mal seizures cause the victim to experience a blackout and convulsions of the entire body for a minute or longer, then, feeling tired and confused, he or she may fall asleep.

Petit mal seizures may be mistaken for a period of staring or daydreaming. The victim, usually in the 6- to 14-year-old age group, will stare, blink the eyes rapidly, or have minor twitching movements before resuming normal activities.

Psychomotor or temporal lobe seizures may involve staring, abdominal pains and headaches, chewing and lip-smacking movements, picking at clothing, pacing, buzzing and ringing sounds in the ears, dizziness and, in some cases, sudden feelings of fear or anger, followed by a desire to sleep and, later, amnesia about the whole attack.

In many cases, these seizures can be controlled. While there is no cure for epilepsy, it is estimated that 50 percent of those with the disorder may achieve complete control of seizures with anticonvulsant medication and can lead essentially normal lives. Another 30 percent gain partial control of seizures through medication.

There are some epileptics, in fact, who have not had a seizure for ten years or more, and according to a recent study at Washington University in St. Louis, some (though not all) of these patients may even be able to stop taking medication after a certain number of seizure-free years. Most epileptics, however, do face a lifetime of medication and some will continue to have seizures. The need for continual medication, fear of having a seizure, and a feeling of being different may plague many epileptics, but this can be especially painful emotionally in adolescence.

You may rebel at having to take medications.

You may feel smothered and angry when your parents remind you about your medications or show unusual concern.

You may feel ashamed about having epilepsy and may feel afraid to tell anyone.

You may be terrified of having a seizure at school and may be mortified if you do. Some kids, it's true, can seem pretty cruel and callous about other people's pain. Often, however, such a reaction may be due to fright, ignorance, and embarrassment.

You may feel embarrassed about being different in rather obvious ways. It can be particularly tough when everyone else is getting a driver's license and you're stuck, trying to make excuses about why you don't have one yet. While those with epilepsy may get driver's licenses in most states, you must submit written proof from your physician that you have been free of seizures for a certain period of time (two to three years in many states). If you have to wait for this time to pass, it may be difficult.

You may worry, too, about your future. Many epileptics go to college and do well and many have excellent jobs. Others, however, are still victims of the old myths regarding epileptics.

Discriminatory employment laws and practices regarding epileptics are now being challenged legally. And victories have already been won in other areas. It is now possible for epileptics to marry and have children. Until quite recently, this was forbidden in some states, due to a common misconception that epilepsy is, invariably, hereditary.

The future, then, looks brighter all the time, but the present may be difficult at times. There is still so much secrecy and fear surrounding epilepsy. Perhaps now that courageous people like actor John Considine and long-distance runner Patty Wilson are attempting to educate the public by taking the risk of talking about their epilepsy—and their feelings—the public will discard some of the hurtful myths and understand that a person who happens to have epilepsy can live a full, essentially normal life and has as much to offer society as anyone else.

Such understanding will help us to treat epileptics the way they want to be treated—just like anyone else.

Proper education will also help us to deal properly with a grand mal seizure when it happens. In such a case, says the Epilepsy Foundation of America, make sure that the victim is in a safe place and loosen tight clothing. DO NOT force a hard object between the victim's teeth or give him or her anything to drink. And stand by until the person has fully recovered and is able to go about regular activities.

"We're seeing more and more young people who get epilepsy as a result of head injuries from accidents involving cars or motorcycles or skateboards," says Gloria Schwed, a social worker for the Los Angeles County Epilepsy Society.

It is important for those who do not have epilepsy to understand what it is and is not for *themselves,* since epilepsy can happen to anyone, anytime.

LIVING WITH SPECIAL MEDICAL NEEDS

I'm a diabetic and have been for ten years. I get so tired of hearing "Did you have enough to eat?" and stuff like that. Most of my friends don't know I'm a diabetic, so I can't really talk to them about it. Are there any suggestions you have to make being a dia-

betic less aggravating? I'm 16 and on the verge of giving up!

N. P.

Anyone can have a special medical problem. But this may be especially hard to cope with if you're a teen and if your problem is *chronic* and not likely to change. Besides whatever discomfort that your physical condition may bring, there will be trying times emotionally.

There will be times when you'd like to throw your medicine out and pretend that you don't need it.

There will be times when your parents seem to nag or overprotect you or *take over* your illness instead of giving you the space and the responsibility to care for yourself.

There will be times when you may feel guilty about the time, expense, and emotional strain that your special needs may put on your family, times when you try to reassure your parents.

And there may be times when you find yourself almost enjoying the attention and special privileges or considerations you may get because of your condition, times when you may use your illness as an excuse to get out of doing things for yourself that you *know* you can do.

There will be other times when you may feel enraged at being different, times when you cry and rage about the unfairness of it all. You may feel like screaming "I hate this! I just hate it! Why me?"

And there may be times when you fear the future and what it may bring.

The fact is, though, that not one of us knows what the future will bring. Most teens who will die this year will do so in accidents.

Discovering that you have a chronic disease like diabetes or epilepsy does not mean that your life is over, either literally or figuratively. Part of living fully with (or despite) a special medical need means accepting your feelings of rage, denial, rebellion, and depression as entirely normal. If you've ever wondered "Why ME?" you're far from alone. It may help a great deal if you can express these feelings to an empathetic physician, social worker, counselor, and/or friends and relatives.

Once you begin to accept your feelings, it may be easier to get past the negative ones, to accept your special needs, and to take responsibility for your own care as much as possible. Control of your condition—even in little ways—may give you a new feeling of power in your life. When you have a chronic medical need, it's easy to start feeling that things are constantly being done *to* you rather than doing things for yourself. It may help you to achieve a real sense of independence if you can assert your right to be in-volved in your own treatment and to manage your own life as much as possible.

Keeping your condition—whether it's asthma, diabetes, epilepsy, or something else—stable and in control will free you to do many other things and see past your special needs to some of your special *potential* and possibilities.

And there are so many possibilities. People with special medical needs can—and do—live full and happy lives.

Actor John Considine has epilepsy. Actress Mary Tyler Moore has diabetes. Hockey star Bobby Clarke learned that he had diabetes when he was 15—and it hasn't slowed him down a bit! Noted film director Martin Scorsese *(New York, New York)* grew up having asthma, and because he was not able to participate in strenuous sports, he spent his free time at the movies, developing an interest that would grow into a successful career.

Kitty O'Neill is one of Hollywood's foremost stunt-women, who earned the title "fastest woman on earth" when she drove a three-wheeled, rocket-powered vehicle down a race course in Oregon, hitting speeds up to 512.710 mph. There are people, however, who would call Kitty O'Neill handicapped. But Kitty, who has been totally deaf since birth, does not think in terms of limitations. She's too busy looking for new challenges.

There are a number of teen-agers and young adults with a variety of special medical needs who are also facing challenges with courage and determination.

There is Lanton Kame, 18, of Tecopa, Calif., who, due to a birth defect, has only one hand. But Lanton recently won the Most Valuable Player award on the Death Valley High School basketball team, played defensive end on the varsity football team, and chalked up an impressive batting average on the school's baseball team.

There is Patty Wilson, 16, of La Palma, California, a champion long-distance runner who also happens to have epilepsy. Her seizures, ranging from grand mal to petite mal, are controlled to a certain extent by medication and have not kept her from her news-making runs. Last year, she ran 1,500 miles from Southern California to Portland, Oreg., in 42 days. Among her future plans: a 2,000 mile jaunt to Juneau, Alaska, and a 3,000 mile cross-country run to Washington, D.C.

It took some soul-searching before Patty decided to talk to the press about her epilepsy. "But I think it would help other people who have epilepsy if they know," she told reporters after her latest run. "If they see me running and know I have epilepsy, they might say 'Wow! Maybe *I* could do something like that!' "

There is 18-year-old Esther Barriga of Presidio,

Tex., who lost a leg to osteosarcoma (bone cancer) two years ago. After treatment at the University of Texas M.D. Anderson Hospital and Tumor Institute, Esther returned to her normal routines, wearing a leg prosthesis. She dances, drives, plays basketball and volleyball, enjoys horseback riding, and recently began college studies at Sul Ross University.

Esther admits that, immediately after her operation, she was very depressed. "At first I was too upset to try to walk," she says. "But eventually, I had to get around, so I began to walk more and more and now I hardly ever need my crutch! I don't give people a chance to feel sorry for me. And I don't want to live the rest of my life feeling sorry for myself either. Every morning when I wake up, I smile and say to myself 'Hey! I'm alive!'"

There is Nancy Anderson, 23, of San Gabriel, California, who, at the age of 17, sought help for her diabetes at the City of Hope National Medical Center. It was there that she made the decision to become a nurse and to help other young people to cope with diabetes.

"I first found out that I had diabetes when I was ten," Nancy says. "At first, it was kind of a novelty. But when I got into my teens, there were problems. Like N.P. who wrote to you about her diabetes, I got pretty tired of hearing things like 'Have you eaten?' My parents were very concerned about me. For example, when we would go into a restaurant, my mom would always make sure the chef knew I was diabetic! I would get furious about that. It got to the point where I felt like giving up trying to take responsibility for myself. My feeling was 'If my parents are going to live it for me, I'm not going to live it.' I felt that my parents sometimes would use my diabetes to keep me from doing things I wanted to do."

Nancy and her parents eventually came to an understanding and she began to take more responsibility for herself.

"But, until I was 17, I wasn't controlling my diabetes very well," Nancy admits. "I was approaching a real crisis. I couldn't relate well to my doctor. I felt rotten. My feet were swelling, and with my diabetes out of control, my mouth would get dry and I couldn't sing. That's what really bothered me, since I had been doing a lot of singing at church, at weddings, and in school musicals. I also began to read about the complications of diabetes and I was starting to get really scared."

It was when she was 17 and frightened that Nancy discovered the City of Hope, which has a metabolic unit specializing in the care of diabetes.

"It made all the difference," says Nancy. "I had a doctor—Dr. Wishner—who really cared about me and who motivated me out of love, not guilt, to take care of myself. I learned a new and easy-to-live-with diet there and a social worker helped me to deal with my feelings about diabetes."

What were Nancy's feelings about her condition?

"I was feeling bitter," she says. "I was thinking 'Heck! I hate this! I *hate* having to test my urine all the time and plan everything. I really don't like it!' It was important for me to be able to say 'I don't like having diabetes!' And to talk about feelings that are always there, like wondering if a man I would love would want to marry someone with a chronic condition. These feelings of insecurity come and go and it helps to be able to share them with someone and to learn that these feelings are *not* bad. You have to learn to live with these feelings or you may destroy yourself."

Nancy's strong religious faith has also helped her to cope.

"I feel that God has blessed me with so much and in so many ways," she says. "I have a wonderful family and lots of talents and interests. I feel that I was allowed to have diabetes because I could cope with it."

As a young nurse, Nancy has helped many other people learn to cope with diabetes, but she is also exploring many other areas as well. A talented singer, she has made several national tours with musical groups. She takes acting and dance classes. She has friends and an active social life. She loves to jog and ski and, not long ago, took a canoe trip down the Colorado river.

"At the City of Hope, I learned a new feeling of freedom as I learned to control my diabetes," she says. "Having diabetes is a big responsibility for a young person. But then, taking responsibility is what growing up is all about! Life isn't easy for anyone, but you can do anything, I believe, if you want to do it enough! Controlling my diabetes frees me to do ALL the things I love to do!"

Although Nancy talks freely about her diabetes when asked, she doesn't see diabetes as the central focus of her life and she doesn't feel compelled to tell everyone she knows that she is a diabetic. In short, she refuses to be defined by her special medical needs.

"I'm a person who happens to have diabetes," she says gently, but firmly. "I am—first and foremost—a person. I want people to know me that way—as me . . . just *me*."

CHAPTER TEN

You and Your Sexuality

I'm confused. People talk about sex. And then they talk about sexuality. My friend says that everyone has sexuality, even if they don't have sex! I always thought that the two words meant pretty much the same. Is sexuality something everybody has? Even old people and kids?

Wondering

Sexuality, which includes sexual *feelings* as well as actions and how you feel about *yourself* as well as others, is a major part of who you are all your life—from infancy to old age. All too often, however, people see it only in a limited sense. Some see sexuality as a synonym for sexual intercourse. But there is so much more to it than that. Sexual actions are only a *part* of your sexuality.

Others may define sexuality in terms of sex roles. They may be very concerned about being masculine or feminine according to traditional societal standards and may be afraid of any feelings or actions that may seem to contradict society's images of how a man or a woman should be. A young man may hide tender feelings to protect a macho image. A young woman may feel guilty about having strong sexual desires or may take great pains to hide her intelligence. Both may be sacrificing personal honesty to maintain old stereotypes.

Caught up in roles, where "sexuality" may be seen in terms of "sexiness," people may relate to one another as sex objects, foregoing the friendship that may give love and sex new meaning and bypassing the tenderness that may exist in a friendship. Indeed, someone who defines himself or herself in terms of traditional sex roles may have trouble maintaining close relationships with the same or the opposite sex, afraid to show tenderness in a friendship or honest friendship in a sexual relationship.

Some people see sexuality as a separate entity in their lives. It isn't. Your sexuality goes far beyond labels and stereotypes, far beyond sexual relationships, far beyond what sexual actions and options you may choose. The fact is, despite the choices you make regarding sexual activities, you are an innately sexual being—just like everyone else.

There is nothing bad or strange or mysterious about your sexuality. It just *is*. Like you. How you choose to express yourself sexually, on the other hand, may involve value judgments.

Sexuality is shared equally by males and females. No one sex is more sexual than the other. People feel tenderness and passion and love. People feel strong sexual desires. People have all kinds of sexual fantasies. People—of all ages—can feel sexual sensations.

Accepting your sensations, your fantasies, your desires, your feelings—from tenderness to passion—as normal and natural can help you to feel more at ease with others and with yourself.

Your sexuality is you—the man, the woman, the person.

FANTASIES AND FEELINGS

Is it healthy for a 14-year-old girl to have a yearning for a man's body in a sexual way? My mother said you shouldn't have this feeling until after you've already had sex. Is that true?

Upset

I'm 17 and really like this one girl. She wants to be a virgin until she marries. I respect that. But I have all kinds of horny fantasies about us making love. Also, I have to admit, I have lots of daydreams about me and other girls, too. Does this mean that I ought to be dating a lot of other people? I really care about my girlfriend and think about marrying her when we finish school. But these fantasies about all the others bother me. Does this mean I will probably be unfaithful to her?

Greg Y.

I have sex regularly with my boyfriend (we're both 18), but often (even during sex sometimes) I'll have sexy fantasies. Sometimes I imagine that I'm making love with a certain movie star or handsome stranger. At times, too, I imagine I'm with my boyfriend in a place other than his car or dorm room—like a beach or a cabin in the woods or something. Is this silly?

147

Our sex life is good, yet I love the fantasies, too. I just wonder if I ought to be having them.

Virginia L.

I'm really scared. I like to think sexy thoughts just before drifting off to sleep. Usually, I have these thoughts about men, but last night I was kind of half-way asleep when I realized that I was dreaming about kissing my best girl friend and touching her breasts. My girl friend is a wonderful person and pretty, too. I like her a lot, but, after all, she's a GIRL! Could this mean I might be a homosexual? I can't understand this since I really do like boys and dream about them 99 percent of the time—honest!

Gail N.

Fantasies play a part in everyone's life.

Mary likes to fantasize over newspaper want ads, picking the job, the apartment, and the car she would most like if she were 21 and on her own, instead of 14. She feels that dreaming about her life as it may be in a few years is a pleasant diversion from time to time.

Jim has fantasies, as he jogs, of running in and winning the Boston Marathon. He notes that when he fantasizes, it's somehow a little easier to run.

Julie says that she has fantasies about her wedding day—who the groom might be, what she will wear, what the setting will be (it changes from church to mountaintop to public park with great regularity), and who will attend. She feels that such occasional fantasies make being 13 a little easier.

We fantasize about all kinds of things—from jobs, cars, fame, success, future homes, changed life-styles, you name it! So it's not really so unusual that most of us fantasize about sex as well.

Young people who are not yet sexually active may have very vivid feelings and fantasies about sex. This is perfectly normal. Married and/or sexually active people fantasize about sex, too. And this is also normal. Some people—both young and older, sexually involved or not—may feel guilty about such fantasies, however. Maybe you're among them.

You may feel that the sexual urges that these fantasies seem to show are, somehow, wrong for someone who is young or single or a virgin or female. The fact is, these feelings and fantasies are entirely normal for everyone. Some, though, may fantasize more—and more freely—than others.

It's normal and OK to have sexual fantasies before you're ever sexually active, after you've started having sex, and even when you're actually having sex. Some married people and those in other types of long-term relationships find that occasional fantasies may make sex even more intense and interesting.

Some people may feel guilty about sexual fantasies because they may feel that to think about something may be practically the same as doing it. There are some religions that teach this, but for most people who suffer guilt pangs, such feelings are not consciously tied to religious beliefs.

Feeling is not acting! Neither is fantasizing. Our feelings and fantasies just are. They can't really be judged. You may never act out most of your fantasies. Maybe you wouldn't want to. But these fantasies themselves may be enjoyable. Many feel no need to translate them into actions. They simply enjoy the fantasies for what they are. Others wonder if they shouldn't try to turn some of these fantasies into reality. Whether or not one chooses to do this is a very personal choice, one that is best made after careful consideration.

"Think about it and maybe even talk it over with someone you trust," suggests Doris Lion, who does marriage, family, and sexuality counseling in Los Angeles. "Think about the possible consequences of your actions. Would acting on your fantasy be worth the consequences? Maybe . . . or maybe not. Would such actions be congruent with your own values? Or would you rather keep—and enjoy—the fantasy while deciding against the action due to consequences or your own values? What you do about your fantasies should be a *choice,* a choice based on responsible thinking."

Sometimes, we may have fantasies that we feel are distrubing. An example of this would be Gail's fantasy about kissing her best girl friend. So-called homosexual fantasies can cause a lot of guilt in young people, especially those who may have strong feelings against homosexuality (which may be based, in part, on fear).

Fantasies about those of your own sex are not necessarily an indication that you may be gay. As we will see in the "Sexual Preferences and Homosexuality" section of this chapter, few people are absolutely—feelings and all—heterosexual or homosexual. The majority, while preferring to express their sexuality with members of the opposite sex, are capable of feeling warmth, love, and even desire, at times, for those of the same sex. One may or may not choose to act on such feelings. But to have these feelings, or even to act them out, especially in adolescence, does not mean that you are a homosexual. It's important not to label yourself in any way as a result of your fantasies. These fantasies simply exist. They don't define you, no matter what your primary sexual preferences may be.

Could fantasies ever become a problem for you?

"Perhaps, if you find that your fantasy life is getting rather excessive," says Ms. Lion. "What is excessive? Well, if constant fantasies are creating a great deal of guilt or are interfering with other activities in your life, you might want to talk with someone you trust about this.''

In sharing your feelings with someone, you may find that your fantasies are not so unusual or way-out. Or you may discover how to improve the quality of your *real* life. Or you may learn to enjoy fantasies as a *part* of your life.

Fantasies may fulfill a function in your life, no matter where you are in terms of sexual involvement. They may be a safe way to channel sexual feelings when you don't feel ready to be—or can't be—sexually active. Fantasies may add variety and zest to an existing sexual relationship. However and whenever they happen, fantasies are OK—and very normal.

MASTURBATION

Is masturbation, in both males and females, normal? Is it habit-forming?

Anonymous Please!

What do you think about masturbation? I am worried that it may harm me in some way. Is it better to have sex or masturbate? I wouldn't feel right about having sex, but I read somewhere that masturbation is harmful and only bad people do it. Now I'm scared.

T.C.

I am 15, female, and wonder if masturbation is wrong at my age. It bothers my conscience when I masturbate. As a true Christian, I'm wondering if masturbation is wrong in the eyes of God. Will it affect my physical and/or mental health in the future and if I ever get married?

Melissa

I'm 19 years old and get an urge for intercourse quite often. So I masturbate and pretend that I'm having intercourse. Is this normal? Should I try to get someone to have intercourse with instead? The person I go with is very religious and does not believe in premarital intercourse. I tend to share those beliefs or, at least, I thought I did!

Confused

Masturbation is a natural expression of sexuality for males and females, young and old. It means sexual stimulation of oneself—in some instances, to the point of orgasm. It is estimated that about 97 percent of males and well over 90 percent of females have masturbated by the age of 21.

Contrary to old wives' tales, masturbation will not make you sterile, blind, insane, give you acne, or take your virginity.

It can offer release from sexual tensions, particularly if you are not sexually active in other ways. Of course, many married people and others with satisfying sex lives may masturbate as well.

Masturbation is being seen, more and more, as a healthy release, even by a number of church groups, which have modified the traditional religious stand that masturbation is sinful and bad.

Among the benefits of masturbation: release of sexual tensions, growing to learn what you enjoy, and experiencing orgasm.

Orgasm, a normal sexual experience, means reaching a height of sexual excitement. For the male, this usually means ejaculation. Women, of course, don't ejaculate, but have feelings of intense excitement and, perhaps, a throbbing feeling in the genitals followed by the same sense of relaxation and peace that a man may feel after ejaculating. Orgasm may occur when you're fantasizing about sex or masturbating, or when you're having some sort of sexual contact—from petting to intercourse—with someone else.

I am a 15-year-old girl. I masturbate. Lately, it seems as if I use it as a crutch to make me feel better when I feel depressed and upset. I don't understand my actions. I now have a terrible guilt complex and I hate myself. And that makes me masturbate more! I feel so terrible and guilty all the time!

R.T.

I've tried to stop masturbating so much and get into hobbies, but I can't seem to stop. I masturbate several times a day and can't seem to keep my mind on anything else.

Worried

After my brother went away to college, I got a room to myself. I find myself masturbating about twice a day. I always do the same thing in the same way: I put Vaseline on my cock and in a roll of toilet paper (to make it like a vagina). I like to thrust my cock in and out of this roll. In fact, I've come to depend on this. It's the only way I can come. My hand isn't enough. Could this harm me now or later?

Brian J.

What all the above letters seem to be asking is "Can masturbation ever be harmful to me?"

The answer is yes—in some instances.

First, if you are extremely religious and/or your values and beliefs are making you feel extremely guilty about masturbation, this may be a problem for you. The self-hatred that may be a by-product of extreme guilt may drive you to masturbate even more. And so you're caught in a cycle of misery.

How can you deal with this?

You may want to talk about your feelings with your physician, clergyman, counselor, or someone else you can trust to listen and who may reassure you that you are, indeed, quite normal.

It may help to remember, too, that masturbation is healthy and normal. But whether or not you do masturbate is very much a matter of personal choice. If you do choose to, this doesn't make you bad. If you choose not to do so, due to your personal beliefs, that doesn't make you strange. It's up to you.

Masturbation is not physically harmful unless you choose to masturbate with objects that may be irritating (soft drink bottles, for example).

However, we do advise against becoming extremely dependent on props and objects. If you come to rely solely on props—as Brian does—during masturbation, you may find it difficult to become turned on or to have an orgasm when circumstances change, for example, when you're having sex with another person. So it's best to vary your masturbation techniques.

Many teens wonder if you can masturbate too often. How often is too often? That's a good question—and one that's difficult to answer. We feel that setting rules is not really constructive. However, masturbation, though healthy, normal, and pleasurable, is not meant to take the place of other things in your life. If, like R.T., you find yourself using masturbation as a crutch to avoid problems, facing feelings, challenges, or encounters with others, or if it's causing you to turn inward and to become less able to share and to function in other ways, you may want to reevaluate its place in your life and make some changes.

A number of teens may feel especially guilty about mutual or group masturbation, which is quite common in teens, especially young adolescent males (although we've heard from a number of girls about such experiences, too).

This type of masturbation may take a number of forms.

It may mean masturbating in the presence of a friend or friends, or it may mean touching each other in erotic ways. Among boys, especially, some of these group masturbation sessions are almost competitive games to see who can ejaculate fastest and farthest.

Although some form of group masturbation may seem like a good idea at the time to some teens, they may be plagued by guilt afterward, wondering "What made me do that? Does it mean I'm a homosexual?"

Especially in early adolescence, such group masturbation is quite common and is not considered abnormal. As your own body is developing, you may have an intense curiosity about others, wanting to see if others are developing in the same ways and if they have the same feelings you do. Finding out that others may look, feel, and respond much like you do may help, in some cases, to reinforce your own positive feelings about yourself and your ability to function sexually.

Testing this ability to function sexually and, in some instances, to give pleasure to another person may be somewhat less threatening with people of your own sex—if you happen to be quite young and/or still a bit uncomfortable with the opposite sex.

But remember: it's important not to label yourself. Participating—or *not* participating—in group masturbation is very much a matter of personal choice. Some do it more than others. Some never try it at all—and that's also OK. Whatever choices you may make are really no reflection of your present or future sexual preferences.

Most people who participate in masturbatory games with those of the same sex during the adolescent years are not—and do not become—homosexuals. They will go on to enjoy relating sexually to the opposite sex.

A certain percentage of men and women, however, will find that they will always prefer their own sex physically. However, it is likely that their teen experiences did not make them homosexual. They simply are homosexual.

SEXUAL PREFERENCES AND HOMOSEXUALITY

I'm 14 and worried. I like to hug and kiss my friends—even the girls. Does this mean I'm queer?
                    Margie

I have a crush on my English teacher. Not so unusual, you're saying? Yes, except she's a woman and so am I. I really love and admire her. I also like boys, but my parents don't let me date yet (I'm 14). Do you think I might be a Lesbian?
                    Gina P.

I have a brother who's gay and my father can't cope with it. He seems to think he's doing this to spite him and he doesn't have to be this way. I disagree. I think my brother couldn't be any other way even if he wanted. My brother's a great guy and I hate to see him hurt. Is Dad wrong?
                    Kristy E.

I need help really bad. I'm 18 and in love with this boy who is also 18. I happen to be a boy. He doesn't know that I like him. I feel stupid and I don't dare tell anyone. It's really embarrassing. What makes me like this?

                                    M.O.

Sexual preferences are a major part of our sexuality. Few other aspects of sexuality may be so controversial—or so potentially painful.

We have never heard a young person complain or cry about his or her *heterosexuality* (which is, after all, strongly reinforced by society), but we have seen a great deal of anguish about homosexuality, either real or imagined.

Many teen-agers worry about homosexuality. Perhaps they worry because of group masturbation or fantasies. Perhaps such concern comes from having warm feelings for a member of the same sex. Or maybe a particular teen has stopped wondering and *knows* that he or she prefers those of the same sex. But it can hurt to be different and it can be frightening, too, to feel that your sexual preferences may expose you to scorn or hatred from some people if these preferences were to become known. Most teens who worry about homosexuality are *not* homosexuals, however.

"The fear that you might be a homosexual is one of the most common fears of adolescence," says Dr. Sol Gordon, a noted sex educator and director of the Institute for Family Research and Education at Syracuse University. "Many teens fear being homosexuals, yet don't really know what a homosexual is. My definition of a homosexual—and I think a lot of people share this definition—is 'someone who, *as an adult,* has constant, definite sexual preference for persons of the same sex.' "

If right now you have problems relating to the opposite sex, you may be shy, not gay.

Crushes on teachers or others of the same sex may be no cause for concern either. We admire and love many people, especially in adolescence. Everyone has idols and secret crushes. Admiring someone else may help you to discover more about what you would like to grow to become. It can be a positive step in your growth toward maturity.

Close friendships with those of the same sex are vitally important, too. Closeness with a best friend can be a great mutual comfort at a time in your life when you face so many changes. In friendships, people express affection in many different ways. Some express their feelings with thoughtful acts or gentle teasing. Some can say how they feel. For others, a touch or hug or kiss says "You're special. I care."

It may help to know, too, that although most of us have a definite sexual preference one way or the other, very few people are 100 percent heterosexual or 100 percent homosexual.

The Kinsey Institute has devised a scale to rate sexual orientation. An extreme heterosexual, someone who has never responded emotionally or physically to someone of the same sex, would be a "zero," while a "six" would be the other extreme—someone who is and has always been exclusively homosexual. A Kinsey study over a decade ago revealed that at least 60 percent of American men and 30 percent of American women have had at least one overt, intentional homosexual experience by the age of 15. Other studies have placed these figures even higher.

So a high percentage of the American population would be neither a zero nor a six, but somewhere in between. They would include people who are almost exclusively heterosexual, but who have had a minor homosexual experience; people who have had experiences with both sexes, but who prefer the opposite sex; people who have no special preferences; and people who prefer those of the same sex, but who are not exclusively homosexual.

When you see the wide variation of sexual preferences, you may see why labeling yourself or others in black-and-white terms can be confusing and hurtful.

What about the men and women—an estimated ten million in the United States—who do prefer the same sex primarily? Why do they have these preferences?

How we develop sexual preferences is still being studied and so the so-called causes of homosexuality are still very open to debate.

We do know that you find your gender identity—seeing yourself as a male or female—by the age of two. Most of us see ourselves by our anatomically correct gender. (Those who see themselves as the opposite sex are called "transsexuals" and are quite different from transvestites who are either heterosexual or homosexual and who see themselves as the correct gender even though they enjoy dressing in the clothing of the opposite sex.) Homosexuals see themselves as the correct gender. They simply grow up to prefer physically friends of their own sex. Some experts feel that this preference may be set by the age of five. Some others feel that firm preferences may come somewhat later.

We know that some people may not come to terms with their true preferences for years. Some homosexuals, in fact, may marry and have children before coming to terms with the fact that they are, primarily, homosexual. Some mental health experts feel that sexual preference may, in fact, be learned behavior and, as such, can be changed. Some therapists believe that sex preferences *may* be changed in instances where the individual is highly motivated and wants very much to change. Even then, however, we're not sure whether such therapy may change one's actual sexual orientation or, simply, sexual *behavior*. That is, you may learn to behave in a different way, but will your real feelings change? This is still open to debate.

A lot of therapy these days is aimed at helping gay people to understand and accept their feelings. Many wonder, to begin with, *"Why* am I this way?"

There are many theories about what can predispose a child to become homosexual. Domineering or retiring mothers and/or domineering or retiring or absentee fathers have all been indicted in various studies.

Dr. Evelyn Hooker of UCLA, probably the most famous researcher in the area of homosexuality, began her studies of the matter more than 20 years ago by disproving the prevailing idea that all homosexuals are sick. (The American Psychiatric Association and the American Psychological Association recently echoed her contentions by removing homosexuality from the official list of mental illnesses.)

Dr. Hooker contends that it is impossible to generalize about the family relationships of young people who grow up to prefer those of their own sex, but she has said that, in some cases, some early experiences may influence sexual preference.

Surprisingly to some, being approached and/or molested by a homosexual is not one of the factors that Dr. Hooker mentions. This may be because, although this is something many people worry about, such occurrences are relatively rare. (Most child molesters are heterosexual.)

Instead, Dr. Hooker has written that unpleasant experiences with the opposite sex or puritanical parents who put too heavy an emphasis on the evils of heterosexual behavior may make a young person feel guilty and anxious just thinking about the opposite sex. "The child may see homosexuality as the lesser of two evils," Dr. Hooker has said.

At this time, however, we have no way of knowing for sure whether homosexuals are born with their preferences or whether they learn such preferences and, if so, how and by what age.

The morality of homosexuality is also still a controversial matter. Although, technically at least, homosexuality per se is no longer considered a mental illness by health professionals, there are a number of people who consider homosexuals to be flagrantly immoral, citing biblical passages decrying homosexuality.

The religious view of homosexuality may also be in a state of flux, however. Some clergymen interpret some parts of the Bible as political expediencies of that time.

"Biblical society was much different from ours," says Reverend Robert H. Iles, executive director of the Marcliffe Foundation, a counseling-education service in Altadena, California. "It was a small, opposed minority whose survival was dependent on becoming more plentiful. Today, the opposite may be true. Most

sex today does not result in procreation. Many people of all preferences are choosing to be childless. Our attitudes and way of life are very different today."

Some theologians are putting new interpretations on the whole concept of sin and sexuality, seeing acts—both homosexual and heterosexual—without caring as sinful, while seeing relations between two people—whatever their sex—who love each other as moral.

Reverend Iles objects to the tyranny of labels. *"Homosexual* is an adjective to explain behavior," he insists. "The people who practice this behavior are individuals. Many live quiet, happy, dignified lives in long-term, deeply committed relationships. Some are famous. Some are brilliant and talented. Most are very ordinary people leading quite ordinary lives. Few match the old myths and stereotypes that people tend to have about homosexuals."

Joan, a beautiful, 24-year-old model, and Deena, an equally lovely airline flight attendant, have lived together in a committed love relationship for three years. "My choice is to live fully, the best way I can," says Joan. "My preferences aren't right for everyone, but they are for me."

"I'm at peace with myself, too," adds Deena. "But it has taken a lot of pain to get there. It's tough to be different. I'm not out to recruit anybody and I don't know anyone who is."

"Finding your sexual preference is such an individual thing," says Carl, a 24-year-old management trainee for a computer firm. "I would never try to force my feelings on another. It's hard enough to accept one's own feelings—whatever they may be."

Kerry, a 21-year-old college student hoping to become a veterinarian, has fresh, vivid memories of the agony she experienced trying to find—and to accept—her feelings.

"I always loved and idolized girls, but never heard the word *homosexual* until I was in my teens," she says. "Then I heard some kids joking and using the word at a slumber party. Later, I looked the word up in a dictionary. At first, I was relieved. There was a word to describe my feelings for girls. Then I started feeling cheated and mad. Why me? I wanted to scream and cry and I got very depressed about the fact that I was different."

Kerry's agony over the next two years included heavy drinking and drug-taking in an attempt to anesthetize the feelings she considered to be so wrong. Then one day, the silent anguish became unbearable, and in tears, Kerry took the risk of sharing her feelings with her mother.

"My mom is a beautiful lady," says Kerry. "She put her arms around me and said, 'It's your life. Do what you want to do. I love you very much and I will not hold you back, disgrace, or degrade you in any way.' Mom's understanding helped me to start to cope with my feelings, but it was still some time before I could come out and say—even to myself—'I am a Lesbian.' "

Before she came to accept her homosexuality, Kerry dated guys and even had sex with several of them. "But it wasn't normal for me," she says. "I began to realize that what's normal for others is not normal for me. I started being honest with the right people and began to feel good about knowing who I was."

At first, however, she had some doubts. "I thought maybe I was going through the usual adolescent phase we all read about," she says. "Yet, I knew somehow that this wasn't a passing thing. It hurt to feel different. I felt anger at being cheated of a so-called normal life and I was scared to open myself up to others, afraid that they'd reject me or hurt me or tell everyone."

Kerry's life today is not without pain and complications. Her mother and sister accept her as she is. So do her closest friends. Her father and two brothers, however, know nothing of her sexual preference. "They would disown me," she says sadly.

Some of Kerry's fears are fairly universal.

"I fear loneliness, not finding someone special to love," she says. "I fear being hurt in a relationship—like anyone else does. I'm a real person. I love swimming, animals, horseback riding, and music. I laugh and I cry. I feel joy and pain, love and hate like anyone else. I don't push my ideas on others. I've learned to love who I am, and the people who matter most to me accept me as I am. My straight friends are great, understanding that it's silly to think I'd attack them or something. That went out with werewolves and full moons! But a lot of straight people do fear that in homosexuals and it keeps them from seeing us as people and from trying to understand those of us who are different."

What if, like Kerry, you know that you are different, that homosexuality is a preference, not a passing phase?

Counseling—with a well-trained, empathetic professional—may help you to sort out your feelings and to try to change them if you are so-motivated, or if you don't wish to change or sincerely feel that you can't, counseling may help you to accept who you are.

As a member of a minority group, self-acceptance will not always be easy. Although public opinion about homosexuality is changing somewhat in metropolitan areas, many people will feel strongly that your feelings and life-style are abnormal, sick, and even illegal. As a result, you may feel guilty, frightened, and lonely at times.

"You're not alone. Lots of people have experienced what you're feeling," says Kerry. "It can be scary to be different, but when you start accepting yourself and start learning to channel your feelings in a constructive way, you can be happy. I'm not saying that you won't ever know heartache or hardship. Everybody experiences this. But if you love and accept yourself, you'll feel a new sense of peace."

Growing in self-acceptance and in your capacity to relate to others in a nonexploitative way, to give and receive love, is vital, no matter which person you choose to love.

"The real question is not whether you're gay or straight, but how you manage your relationships," says Reverend Iles. "The ability to give and receive love and the capacity to have a truly intimate relationship are so important. True intimacy is very rare and is the greatest challenge we face in life. Being heterosexual (or homosexual) won't guarantee this. It's who you are and how you feel about yourself that matters. Do you love yourself enough to allow another to give to you (as well as you giving to them)? Whether you love men or love women is, in the final analysis, not as important as the fact that you are able to love."

RELATING TO OTHERS

Sexual Games People Play

I have just one question for you: How do you know if you're being used? My boyfriend talked me into having sex with him. He said he loved me before. Now he says I'm a good kid and isn't too interested in seeing me unless it means we'll have sex. I'm really hurt that he doesn't seem interested in me as a person anymore.

Sarah H.

I have a really serious problem with my girl friend. I'm very turned on by her and she leads me on like crazy, but let me make a move and she starts in on something like "You men are all alike! Animals!" It makes me feel terrible. I'm not an unthinking animal. I really respect her. It's just that she teases me and drives me almost crazy and then puts me down for getting turned on! It's kind of painful for me physically and mentally. I really like this girl.

Rick G.

I'm 15 and confused. It seems like everyone else is having sex. If you're a virgin, guys call you "queer" and girls think you're pretty weird, too. I don't feel right about having sex, but yet I'm tempted to go ahead and get the loss of my virginity over with so that people will get off my case!

Geri

I love this guy, but he won't have sex with me or even go to base three! I think he's just a big chicken. All the kids at school are teasing me because we haven't hit third base yet, but I keep telling them it's not me, it's HIM that's chicken. Help!

Anonymous

Having nonexploitative, sharing relationships may be especially difficult in an atmosphere of sexual game-playing. Such game-playing may abound in adolescence. There can be a lot of peer pressure—for both boys *and* girls—to be sexually active.

Boys may bombard girls with some old, historic lines: "If you really loved me, you would," "What's the matter? Are you frigid? A Lesbian?," and so forth.

Girls may play their own traditional games, using sex as a bargaining ploy, with lines like "I will if you promise to . . ."

Some girls, too, may try to pressure guys into sexual activity. The letter from "Anonymous," who was protesting to her peers that it was her boyfriend who was chicken, is not particularly unusual.

Although most studies would place teens who are *not* having sex in the majority of the teen-age population (or at least 50 percent of it), male and female virgins, all too often, may feel like a minority of one at times.

Both guys and girls may feel pressure to perform sexually. They may also find a certain amount of self-affirmation in the fact that other people desire them, that they can—and do—evoke excitement in others.

Some girls who may feel that sex is not right for them yet may still enjoy seeing guys get turned on. They may tease boys physically simply to get attention, not realizing, perhaps, how difficult they may be making life for the boys.

And some guys are not above lamenting that, if they don't have instant sexual satisfaction, they will be stricken with intolerable pain or felled by a mysterious and incapacitating malady. The truth is that "blue balls," or ache in the groin (which is caused by engorgement of the genitals with blood due to prolonged sexual excitement without release), may be uncomfortable, but is not intolerable and will go away after a while. In the meantime, though, a girl can work up a good case of guilt.

Out of such dilemmas, a number of stereotypes and clichés have arisen, things like "It's always the guy who wants to have sex. Men are animals!" or "It's the girl's job to put him down and hold the line."

Such stereotypes make men and women combatants and may make honest communication and sharing between the sexes virtually impossible.

So can preoccupation with scoring.

"Did you score???"

"We got to third base . . ."

Comments like these make sexual activities sound like a baseball game. Game-playing aside, it's important to know why you're on a particular base (stage of sexual activity) and what this means.

In such a pressure-filled atmosphere, however, it may be difficult to make a free choice about your sexuality, about what you will—or won't —do at this time. Yet free choices are what nonexploitative sex is all about.

When we talk about sex, incidentally, we don't mean just sexual intercourse, but any form of sexual contact—from kissing and petting to actual intercourse.

It's true that one step can lead to another and that many teens enter into physical relationships without really understanding what such involvement may mean.

It's important not only to know the physical facts about sex—how to give and receive pleasure and how to prevent unplanned pregnancy and VD—but also to know what's right for you, right now.

Are You Ready for Sexual Involvement?

What do you really think about virginity? Are you still a virgin if you do everything but have intercourse? Are you still a virgin even if you don't have a hymen? Is it healthy to be a virgin after a certain age?

Margaret

How old should a person be before making out with a guy? Before having sex? My friends and I have a lot of different ideas about how old is old enough.

J. S.

My boyfriend and I really love each other and we're finding it more and more difficult to keep from having sex. I would really enjoy having sex with him, but I'd like it to be right. Do you know what I mean? How can you tell if you're ready to have sex and make sure it will be a good experience?

T. G.

In one way or another, the question of virginity is a major concern to many teens.

There are some young people who plan to remain virgins for a while or until marriage. In the midst of all sorts of talk about sexual freedom, however, some of these teens may need a little reassurance that it's all right to be a virgin. As a free—and certainly acceptable—choice of many, virginity is definitely OK.

It's important to know what's right for you and to stand by this. Some people may tease you and urge you to grow up, but making your own decisions is a very grown-up step. Taking the risk of being different from a lot of people you know may take an extra measure of maturity. If there are times when you begin to feel like the last virgin on earth over the age of 14, take heart. A lot of people who claim to be having fantastic sexual adventures may simply be bragging.

"People who boast about their sexual activities are almost always lying," observes sex educator Dr. Sol Gordon.

There are other young people who wonder whether they are or aren't virgins. Many girls—and guys, too—may wonder whether the presence of a hymen (a thin ring of tissue around the opening of a woman's vagina) is the ultimate proof of her virginity. (A virgin is someone—male or female—who has not had sexual intercourse.)

If you try to determine a woman's virginity by the presence of a hymen, it can get pretty confusing, and it's easy to guess wrong. The hymen may or may not be present in the female virgin. The hymen can be stretched or broken in a number of nonsexual activities, particularly athletic pursuits involving the legs and pelvic muscles. Some women are born without hymens. Yet, if they have not had sexual intercourse, these women are virgins, despite the lack of physical evidence. Some women, on the other hand, who have had intercourse may have flexible hymens that have stretched, but not broken. Despite the presence of the hymen, such a woman is not a virgin. And still other women have done everything but have actual intercourse and are still virgins—at least technically.

Some of these technical virgins—both female and male—may be quite sexually experienced. "Making out," which may involve kissing and petting (fondling breasts and genitals), oral-genital sex, and other forms of sex play just short of intercourse, may be carried to orgasm in some cases and may sometimes lead to an essentially unplanned act of intercourse and/or pregnancy (more on this in Chapter Twelve).

It's difficult, if not impossible, to say how old is old enough for such sexual involvement. Chronological age may or may not be a major factor, although some well-known sex educators, Dr. Sol Gordon among them, personally feel that adolescents who are in high school and younger should be careful not to rush into sexual involvements.

"If a teen-ager in high school were to ask me whether or not to have sex now (nobody has so far!), I would say that it might be better to wait," says Dr. Gordon. "Most of these very young people having sex do not use birth control and that can be a problem. There were over one million teen-age pregnancies last year. Also, if you are still somewhat immature and lack perspective in your life, sex can introduce even more confusion. The experiences themselves may be in less than ideal settings and circumstances and may make for unsatisfactory, guilt-ridden encounters. As a result, many young people may label themselves prematurely as frigid or impotent or as having some other kind of sex problems, not realizing that first sexual relations at any age are not usually the greatest. However, you may have more perspective about this later on, when you're in college or working."

Of course, maturity levels vary so much that it's impossible to generalize about the immaturity of all adolescents under college age. Dr. Gordon agrees that the decision regarding when and with whom to have sex is, ultimately, entirely yours.

How do you make a responsible decision regarding sexual involvement? You might start by asking yourself a number of questions.

1. *Am I thinking about having sex to prove something to others? To myself? Out of fear of losing someone? Out of curiosity? How do I really feel about having sex right now?*

Some teens become sexually involved because everyone else seems to be. Others do so to define themselves as adults. Still others may have sex out of fear of losing a boyfriend or girl friend. Some begin sexual activities just out of curiosity, while others do so within the framework of a committed love relationship.

It's important to know how you really feel about having sex right now. If it doesn't seem right to you and you feel extremely guilty, it could be that being like everyone else, for example, might be small consolation in the long run. It's important, too, to realize what sex *cannot* do for you.

Sex cannot fill gaping holes in your self-esteem or make you instantly wise, mature, and adult.

Sex also cannot necessarily bind you to a person forever or make love, commitment, and intimacy grow where these qualities have never existed before.

Such expectations may only guarantee disappointment.

2. *What feelings do I have for the other person?*

Do you see your potential sex partner as a challenge, a conquest—or a person with feelings?

Do you like this person? Do you love him/her?

Can you be vulnerable and real with one another?

You can have sex with anyone. It can be fun. But sex may be most enjoyable with someone you know and care about, someone with whom you can really be yourself.

3. *How well do we communicate?*

Can you talk to one another openly and honestly?

Can you share what you're really feeling?

Being able to share your feelings about sexual involvement is vital. What will such involvement mean to him/her? To you? For example, does one person see having sex as an act of love and commitment, while the other sees it as an adventure, period? If your feelings about sexual involvement differ, can *both* of you live with such differences?

Differing concepts about what sexual involvement means, coupled with poor communication, can add up to a lot of hurt!

Can you make a responsible decision together, sharing the responsibilities for being involved and for whatever consequences may happen? Can you talk to one another about birth control and venereal disease, for example?

Can you tell each other if something hurts, is uncomfortable or distasteful to you?

Can you talk about your expectations—and your fears?

4. *Do I have enough information about sex to make a responsible choice?*

Studies have shown that college students who have the most accurate knowledge about sex are less likely to be sexually active. Those who know the least, on the other hand, tend to be the most sexually active.

Sexual ignorance may not only cause a lot of unplanned pregnancies, but may also result in some grief and disappointment when the people involved don't have enough information about their own bodies—and each other's bodies—to fully give and receive sexual pleasure.

5. *Are we willing to take full responsibility for our actions?*

Responsibility means reviewing all possibilities—and options—in advance.

Pregnancy and VD are two very real risks of sexual involvement.

What would you do in the event of an unplanned pregnancy? Could you be supportive of one another? What options would you have?

If one of you noticed symptoms of venereal disease, could you take the responsibility of telling your sex partner and suggesting that you both get tested?

Do you know how to prevent an unplanned pregnancy? Have you learned what the most reliable methods of birth control are and how they may be obtained and used? (See Chapter Twelve.)

More to the point: *Will* you take the responsibility of using a reliable method of birth control, of planning ahead to prevent a pregnancy?

"Birth control is like planning for sex and I feel that such planning is wrong. Sex should be romantic and just happen . . ." is a comment we have heard a lot— often from teen-age mothers.

There may be a number of feelings behind such a statement. Some of these teens may be victims of the old double standard, which sees the man as the se- ducer and the woman as the seduced. This old myth seems to say that, unless a woman is quite literally swept off her feet, she's no lady.

A variation on this theme is the romance myth that says that sex is romantic only when it is totally unexpected. Some victims of the "He swept me off my feet!" school of thought feel that they have to get drunk or stoned to make sex OK.

Others feel that just getting carried away by passion may justify the act. Still others believe that "planning for sex" by taking birth control precautions destroys the romantic aspects of sex.

This attitude is reinforced by society's mixed messages, vividly illustrated at a recent teenage health conference, "What's Happening," sponsored by Emory University.

Personal responsibility for sexual decision-making was the central theme of the conference attended by some 1,200 teenagers. Yet a number of conflicting feelings were evident.

While some teenage delegates answering a special questionnaire voted 342 to 12 in favor of birth control information being taught in high schools, other young people avoided or ignored birth control information at the conference because they didn't plan to have sex anytime soon. While some health professionals and counselors were urging personal responsibility for making choices about sexuality—and validating the whole range of choices from abstinence to sexual activity with use of reliable contraceptives, religious pamphlets decrying premarital sex, equality of the sexes and declaring that venereal disease is "God's curse" were also circulated widely.

Such conflicting attitudes and messages were neither new nor unique. They simply mirrored society's mixed messages.

The fact is, planned sex can be extremely romantic. In some cases, it may be much more so than the so-called spontaneous variety of sex. Taking birth control precautions to avoid an unwanted pregnancy and to help alleviate the fear of such pregnancy can free you both to enjoy sex.

Birth control is something that should be a mutual decision and should be discussed between the two of you *before* having sex, not during or after. Of course, seeking a reliable form of birth control means admitting to yourself and, possibly, to others that you're having sex or will have sex.

Can you do this?

If you're not ready to face this responsibility, you may not be ready to have sex. You may want to reevaluate some of your choices to see if your actions may be violating your true feelings.

6. *Are we friends?*

There's a lot to be said for having sex with a friend.

A friend will not put you down if you're clumsy, unsure, or scared.

A friend will enjoy sharing all kinds of experiences—some sexual and some not—with you.

A friend is not likely to say "You got pregnant? That's your problem!"

A friend will not brag and tell all.

A friend will ask "How do you feel?"

A friend will care about you—as a person.

When we're just learning about our sexual selves and are having our first sexual experiences, it really helps to have a sex partner who also happens to be a caring friend.

Sexual Involvement

I'm getting married in four months and my fiancé and I love each other very much. We have agreed that we'll wait until our wedding night to make love. I'm looking forward to it, but am a little nervous, too. I really don't know what to expect.

Sandra T.

I read somewhere that the first time a girl has intercourse, there is a discharge of blood from the vagina. I think that this would be pretty embarrassing. It is true or is it just a story to scare girls into waiting until they're married to have sex?

Rosalie M.

I'm not having sex now and don't plan to anytime soon. But I think about it a lot and about what my first time might be like. How can I make sure that my first time, whether it is my wedding night or not, will be wonderful?

W. G.

Even when you have decided that the time is right, you may still have a certain amount of concern and anxiety about sexual sharing. Some of this anxiety may be the result of some popular notions about one's first sexual intercourse.

One such view is that the first time, for a woman at least, may be painful and cause bleeding. This may or may not be the case, depending on how rigid the hymen (if it is present) may be, how gentle the male partner is, how relaxed the female partner is, and how much time and privacy the couple has.

How can all these factors make a difference?

If the woman has an intact and fairly rigid hymen, there may be some pain and minor bleeding (not a discharge) if the hymen is broken or torn the first time she has intercourse. (If you see a doctor to get birth control advice before having sex, he/she will probably notice if your hymen may be unusually rigid and may

then recommend that it be stretched or removed via medical methods—either dilation or surgical removal—before you have sex.) In cases where the hymen is flexible and stretches or is largely absent, there may be no bleeding or discomfort at all when the woman has her first sexual intercourse.

Whatever pain there may be for a woman may be minimized if the man is gentle and patient, not rushing things, and takes time to arouse her fully so that her vagina will be well-lubricated. Lack of sufficient stimulation and lubrication can cause discomfort during intercourse whether or not it is the woman's first time.

It helps, then, to be in a setting where privacy is assured and there is no need to rush.

There is another factor that may make first sexual experiences difficult: expectations that far exceed what is possible. We often grow up with the dream that the first time will mean passion and love, fireworks and champagne, soaring climaxes and complete fulfillment. Such expectations can lead to inevitable disappointment—as the following comments from teens show.

We were both scared and it wasn't much fun. Is this the way it will always be?

Sheri H.

My boyfriend and I just started having sex and I never get any pleasure out of it. What's wrong with me?

Jodi G.

My feeling after my first time was "Is that all there is?" I thought it would be absolutely fabulous. I was so disappointed.

L. S.

Of the whole experience, the only emotions I remember are those of fear of backing out, impatience that my partner took so long, relief that I wasn't in much pain and that I wasn't very upset. There definitely wasn't any kind of climax. Afterward, I couldn't help asking if he loved me. Of course he said yes. I said I loved him, too. We were both lying.

R. R.

Disappointment is a frequent reaction to first sexual experiences. The fact is, you can go through the motions of sexual intercourse with little preparation, but it takes time and personal growth to learn to make love with another person.

The first time, there may be some fear and anxiety for both partners. Some guys who are inexperienced don't know how to stimulate a girl or how to be gentle. And, lacking knowledge about one another physically (and sometimes themselves), the partners may be unable to deal with problems that can happen.

My boyfriend is just sick because we tried to have sex for the first time last night and he couldn't keep an erection. He thinks that there might be something horribly the matter and I don't know what to tell him. But I am a little scared that I might not be attractive enough for him or maybe he doesn't care about me deep down? What do you think it could be?

Tanya W.

I get excited really fast when my girl friend and I are going to get it on, but she takes so long! Yet she says she enjoys everything. Could she be putting me on about that? Or do women take longer to get excited?

Roger A.

Every time my boyfriend and I make love (which has been only three times so far), we're fine until he ejaculates. Then he loses his erection. He ejaculates real fast, too!

Aggravated

These letters point up the importance of patience—and some practical knowledge—when you're beginning to have sex.

For example, it is not unusual for a man or a woman to be uptight about performing sexually in the beginning. This anxiety may take several forms. A woman may not lubricate or, in cases of extreme anxiety, may experience spasms in her vagina that may make intercourse difficult if not impossible. A man may have problems getting or keeping an erection, particularly if he is feeling guilty and/or scared.

It is true, too, that young men are usually turned on much more quickly than women and may have a tough time trying to keep from ejaculating before the woman has had time to experience much pleasure. Control may come with more experience and with age.

To understand the difference in male and female responses, which can be the basis of a lot of misunderstandings between inexperienced sex partners, let's follow the pattern of a typical sexual experience.

People make love in many different ways, of course, but ideally there is some period of foreplay, which will help both to become aroused. The couple may kiss and stroke one another all over, including the face, breasts, and genitals. Some arouse one another by gentle stroking of especially sensitive areas like the woman's clitoris or the head and underside of the man's penis. Some combine this with oral stimulation. When a woman kisses, licks, or sucks a man's penis, this is called *fellatio*. When a man does the same with

a woman's clitoris, vulva, and opening of the vagina, this is called *cunnilingus*. We have received many letters from teens asking about oral sex. It is a normal option—either as foreplay to intercourse or as an act in itself—that many people enjoy a great deal. Some others don't enjoy it or choose not to try it. It's very much a matter of personal choice.

As the male becomes aroused (in teen-agers this may happen even without specific stimulation), his penis will become erect and some lubricating fluid may appear at the tip. This fluid may contain some sperm. This is why "pulling out" before ejaculation is not a good birth control method.

As the female's sexual excitement grows, her clitoris and labia may become swollen and engorged with blood and her vagina will become moist with lubricating fluids. This lubrication makes intercourse easier and certainly more pleasurable.

Many young people may rush into intercourse before the female is really ready. It generally takes a woman longer to become aroused than it does a man, but her arousal and pleasure are just as intense. In fact, a woman may be capable of having several orgasms in an act of intercourse whereas a man needs time to rest and recover, usually, between climaxes. However, it is not especially common for a woman to be multiorgasmic when she first begins to have sex. Having even one orgasm may be a challenge at first.

Orgasm occurs in the male when he ejaculates. Orgasm in the female is more difficult to describe, but involves the same buildup of sexual excitement and tension with climactic release. This may be felt all over the body and/or as a throbbing sensation in the genitals—among many other possibilities.

What happens *after* climax is important to know, for here again, men and women may differ.

After ejaculation, a man will lose his erection and feel a sense of peace and completion as well as a strong urge to sleep. The drop-off of his sexual interest may be rather abrupt.

A woman, on the other hand, takes longer to come down from her climactic high. She may feel energized and want to cuddle and talk. Or she may be a little sleepy and drowsy, too.

It's important to communicate how you're feeling. Out of consideration and general caring for their partners, many men fight their sleepy feelings to cuddle and converse. When possible, this is certainly preferable to falling into a stupor, turning over and snoring. A woman can feel rather shut out and rejected by this.

It may help for a woman to know, however, that a man's interest in sex will drop abruptly after climax. In fact, immediately after ejaculation, his penis may be extremely sensitive and it may be almost painful to him if you touch it. So, if he's not as amorous as he was a few minutes before, don't take it personally.

Some young women may worry about lack of feeling in themselves when they are just starting to have intercourse.

"My fantasies were so great and I would get so excited about the whole idea of sex," an 18-year-old college student named Linda told us. "But now that I'm having sex, I am really disappointed. I don't feel all I thought I would, despite the fact that my boyfriend is really considerate and takes a lot of time with me."

Linda and countless other women may simply need more time and experience before reality can measure up to fantasies, before they may be able to relax and enjoy sex. Better circumstances, including comfortable, private surroundings, may help, too. And a tender, considerate partner is vital.

Even with an understanding partner, some women—and men, too—may feel anxious. They may want so much to give pleasure and to be good sex partners that they practically freeze. When you're worried about how you're doing, it can be a real passion-killer.

A number of inexperienced couples may put themselves or each other down for failing to achieve great heights of sexual excitement in a simultaneous orgasm (when both the man and the woman climax at the same time). A simultaneous orgasm can be exciting when it happens, but, even with experienced couples who have excellent sex lives, it may not be particularly common.

Having orgasms at different times can be exciting, too. In fact, in this instance, you may be better able to *share* one another's pleasure.

Many young people, too, put a lot of emphasis on orgasm itself and, thus, a lot of pressure on themselves and each other. For example, "Did you come? Did you come?" is a frequent after-sex question usually, though not always, asked by a man to a woman. This question may be very well-meant, but may intensify feelings of performance anxiety in a person who may have a difficult time having orgasm. It can be a vicious cycle: The more you worry about having orgasm, the less likely it is that you will have one.

Some women get into the habit of faking orgasms. This can also be a vicious cycle: a woman has problems having orgasm (in some cases because she is not getting sufficient foreplay or stimulation suiting her particular needs from her partner), so she fakes orgasm. Her partner believes that she is being sexually satisfied and may make no effort to change his techniques or ask what else she might like. Instead of facing the fact that she is not being satisfied and exploring, with her partner, ways to change this situation, she is perpetuating it.

"It can be difficult to get out of the cycle," says one young woman. "After faking it for so long, how could I tell my boyfriend that I wasn't really satisfied? It's more difficult to face and discuss this as time goes on. I felt so guilty and was afraid he wouldn't love me anymore. I was afraid he'd think I was unloving and frigid."

Because such anxiety is so common in early sexual experiences, it is *so* important not to label yourself—or one another—as "frigid" or "impotent." Chances are, you're feeling scared, guilty, unsure—or a combination of the three.

You may wish to talk about such feelings with each other and, if need be, with a nonjudgmental physician or counselor.

It may be that you are violating some of your own values by having sex at this time and you may want to reevaluate your actions.

Or you may find that, by learning to communicate your desires and what you really enjoy to one another and by experimenting with new techniques and positions, you may make some exciting and fulfilling discoveries.

Or you may find that less-than-ideal circumstances or an insensitive, uncaring partner may be a major part of your problem, and you may choose to reevaluate your choices here, too.

It is also quite possible that you will discover that you simply need time to gain confidence and increase your capacity to give and to receive pleasure.

Sexual Growth

We expect so much of ourselves sexually right from the beginning. This isn't really fair.

Remember when you were just learning to ride a bicycle or to ice-skate? Remember how awkward, clumsy, and unsure you felt? Remember how many wrong notes you hit when first learning to play a musical instrument? Remember how much practice it took before you could drive a car well or type without having to look at the keyboard?

We don't expect to do all these things expertly the first time we try. Yet, all too often, we may expect such miracles when we have sex for the first time. People need time and experience to grow in their capacity to give and to receive sexual pleasure. As you grow you will make a lot of exciting discoveries.

• You may find that while sex is no substitute for true intimacy (a deep commitment to another person and the acceptance by that person of you as you really are), this intimacy can make sex infinitely more enjoyable.

• You may find that taking responsibility for your

actions can make you feel better about yourself and the other person. Mutual decision-making may deepen your commitment. Caring for each other enough to take steps to minimize the possibility of pregnancy or VD (see Chapters Eleven and Twelve) can make sex between you even better. In fact, when you are not worried about getting pregnant, catching venereal disease, or being betrayed by the other, you can relax and be very spontaneous!

• Your capacity to enjoy sex will increase—not diminish—with time. Some young people who may have heard, for example, that men reach a peak of physical strength and stamina in the late teens may feel that it's all downhill after that. No way. There is so much more to sexual sharing than physical stamina. As a man grows emotionally, he will be better able to share with a partner. And it is such a capacity to share feelings, pleasure, and vulnerability that can make sex beautiful. The same is true, of course, for women. For both sexes, sexuality grows and can become richer with time and maturity.

• You may discover, too, that there are many ways to make love, many of which have nothing to do with sexual intercourse, but have everything to do with sharing.

"Making love can take so many forms," says noted sexuality counselor Elizabeth Canfield. "Hearing a concert together is making love. Taking care of a loved one who is sick is making love. Working together on a project you really believe in is making love. Discovering a lovely flower together, having a good conversation, even sharing a disappointment or sorrow is making love. Love and intimacy mean having a great variety of shared experiences, both good and bad. That's what real commitment is all about. It can be fun. It can also hurt. It means committing yourself to struggle and to share."

However you choose to express your sexuality is very much up to you. However, sex is only a part of who you are and only part of a committed love relationship.

Growing to be your own person, capable of making your own informed choices, being sensitive to the rights of others to be themselves, and learning to take responsibility for your actions can greatly enhance your life in many ways—including your sexuality and your relationships on all levels.

With time and growth, so much of the pressure, fear, and uncertainty you may be feeling now will fade.

In its place may be joy in your uniqueness—your feelings, your fantasies, and your beliefs. There may also be new joy in sharing who you are with someone else and discovering another person in a myriad of ways: talking, touching, laughing, crying, liking *and* loving, discovering each other not only as lovers, but also as very special friends!

CHAPTER ELEVEN

The Truth About Venereal Disease

"Disgusting!"

"Dirty."

"Yik!!!"

"Terrible, just terrible."

"Nice people don't talk about it."

"I don't even want to *think* about it!"

Mention the words *venereal disease* and you may hear reactions similar to those above.

Actually, the name *venereal* comes from the Latin word *Venus,* the name of the Roman goddess of love. Today, a "venereal" disease is one that can be contracted from some type of lovemaking.

Note that we said *a* venereal disease. Although people talk about VD as if it were one disease, it is really a category used to describe a number of different diseases with one thing in common: They are all transmitted by sexual activity.

Not everyone who has sex will suffer from venereal disease, of course, but, as we pointed out in the last chapter, a major part of sexual responsibility may be in helping to prevent the spread of venereal diseases.

One of the best preventive measures is to know all you can about these diseases—how they are transmitted, their symptoms and treatment. This knowledge will not enable you to diagnose and treat yourself. VD generally needs to be treated by a physician. But such knowledge will alert you to signs that you need medical help.

It's easy to say "Oh, I wouldn't get VD. I'm not that kind of person!"

But it's impossible to generalize about the type of person who gets VD. Venereal disease is no respecter of age or social standing. *Nice* people *do* get VD. People who don't even have a lot of sex can get VD.

Venereal disease is, in short, a national epidemic. And teen-agers and young adults seem to be particularly vulnerable to it.

For example, in national statistics, the highest incidence of gonorrhea is in the 20- to 24-year-old age group. The second highest incidence is in the 15- to 19-year-old age group. In 1975, over a quarter of a million (266,613) cases of gonorrhea were reported in the 15- to 19-year-old age group nationwide.

So VD *could* happen to you.

It's important that you know the truth about VD, since there are a lot of myths around. We've had a lot of letters, calls, and visits from young people who wonder if it's possible to get a venereal disease from a toilet seat, a towel, or via germs in the air.

The fact is, some of the venereal diseases we will be discussing can be transmitted only through very close sexual contact. The organisms responsible for causing these particular diseases are quite fragile and, for survival, need a special type of moist, warm environment that may be found in the urethra of the penis, the vagina and cervix, the mouth, or the wall of the rectum. Some of the other venereal diseases may be transmitted by close skin-to-skin or hair-to-hair contact. But *no* venereal disease is transmitted through the air (like a common cold) or from contact with toilet seats or towels!

Another fact you need to know: Some venereal diseases, if left untreated, may cause serious damage to the body and, if occurring in a pregnant woman, may harm the fetus as well. We're not into scare tactics, but we do want you to know how serious some of these diseases can be. As we describe the common venereal diseases, you may find some of the facts hard to take. The descriptions aren't pretty. But the facts are important.

GONORRHEA

I keep reading about gonorrhea being like an epidemic among teen-agers. What causes this disease? Can you get it from anything besides sexual intercourse? I mean things like kissing or sitting on a germy public toilet seat? I really need to know!

Janet W.

My buddy told me yesterday that once you have the Clap and get treated, you're immune and can't get it again. I told him he was wrong. IS he wrong?

Randy

My Aunt Edna is always giving me and the rest of the family speeches about what this world is coming

to. (BORING!) But last week she finally said something that got my attention! She said something about a strain of gonorrhea that can't even be treated with penicillin. Is this true or is she full of you-know-what?
Debbie

Gonorrhea is chalking up some rather startling statistics.

• In 1977, over a million cases of gonorrhea were diagnosed and reported to the Center for Disease Control in Atlanta.

• Experts guess that these reported cases account for only a portion of the total cases of gonorrhea in this country.

• It is estimated that one out of every ten Americans had gonorrhea in 1977 and that someone was infected with the disease every 12 seconds during that year.

What is the disease behind these statistics?

Gonorrhea is caused by a bacteria called Neisseria gonorrhoeae. This bacteria is very sensitive and can only survive in the warm, moist environment of the human body.

So you cannot catch gonorrhea from a toilet seat. Nor can you catch gonorrhea from kissing. There must be sexual activity involving contact of the penis with the vagina, throat, or rectum.

What happens when you make sexual contact with a person who has gonorrhea and transmits this disease to you?

Once transmitted, the organisms will begin to multiply and symptoms may occur within two to nine days after sexual contact.

In the male, these symptoms may be quite obvious: pain or discomfort with urination or, perhaps, a slight tingling sensation at the tip of his penis. This will soon be followed by an uncomfortable, thick, yellowish-green discharge from the penis. Any male who has such symptoms should seek medical attention. Males are fortunate in a sense, though. When infected with gonorrhea, most will show definite symptoms.

This is not the case with women. Gonorrhea can be a silent disease in women, with 80 to 85 percent of those afflicted having no symptoms at all.

The 15 to 20 percent of women who *do* have symptoms may have a thick, yellowish-green vaginal discharge as well as vaginal or pelvic discomfort. However, since there are many other causes for vaginal discharges (and, indeed, a vaginal discharge does not usually mean that one has gonorrhea), the possibility that she may have this disease may not occur to the woman whose cervix is infected.

Gonorrhea may also be relatively symptom-free when it infects the throat (as a result of fellatio) or the rectum (as a result of anal intercourse, which means inserting the penis into the rectum instead of the vagina). Women and gay men may be the victims of silent symptoms in these instances. A sore throat may, in some cases, mean a gonococcal infection, but more commonly, it is a symptom of a viral or strep infection. Many people with rectal gonorrhea may also have no symptoms, although some may experience rectal itching or pain or mucus in the bowel movements.

The fact that many women (and some men as well) may become silent carriers of gonorrhea makes it very important for males who develop obvious symptoms of the disease to inform their sex partners about the possibility of infection. This is particularly crucial when that partner is a woman.

A woman who has no symptoms may not only unknowingly spread gonorrhea, but may also, if left untreated, develop serious complications. For example, gonorrhea of the cervix will spread through the rest of the woman's reproductive tract and into the Fallopian tubes. This infection of the Fallopian tubes can cause inflammation and constriction of the tubes and, ultimately, sterility.

Untreated gonorrhea in both men and women may also spread throughout the body, affecting the joints (especially the knee joints) and even the heart valves.

Gonorrhea can also have serious consequences for an infant who is born to a mother afflicted with the disease. At the time of delivery, the infection may be transmitted to the infant's eyes, causing blindness. Although most states have laws requiring that hospital personnel place a special solution of silver nitrate in the eyes of newborn babies to help prevent such a possibility, there are an increasing number of home deliveries these days where this practice may not be followed.

It is important to seek prompt medical diagnosis and treatment if you think that you may have gonorrhea or have been exposed to it. You can get no-cost or low-cost diagnosis and treatment at a variety of clinics, including those affiliated with your local health department. (We will be talking more about available help later on in this chapter.)

How is gonorrhea diagnosed?

If you have a discharge, a sample of this will be put on a slide and examined under a microscope for evidence of the bacteria. If you have no symptoms, a culture will be taken from any possible sites of infection (penis, throat, cervix, and rectum). Such cultures are not painful. The examiner will simply touch the site (for example, the os of the cervix) with a cotton-tipped applicator.

If you are a woman, don't let your menstrual period make you hesitate to be tested for gonorrhea. Studies have shown that one of the best times to pick up the gonococcal organism is during menstruation.

If you do have gonorrhea, what forms of treatment are available?

Penicillin is still the most common—and effective— treatment. It can totally cure the disease. If you are allergic to penicillin, however, there are other highly effective drugs that may be used. With early diagnosis and treatment, you can be completely cured and avoid suffering some of the serious complications of gonorrhea.

However, such a cure does not make you immune to gonorrhea. You can be infected again and again if you have sex with infected people. This is one of the reasons why the disease is now being reported in epidemic proportions.

It is true that a penicillin-resistant strain of the gonococcal organism has been identified recently. However, this strain has not spread at the rapid rate that health officials had initially feared. And these cases can be treated with drugs besides penicillin.

SYPHILIS

Is it true that syphilis will go away—even without treatment? I heard that somewhere. So why do people go for treatments?

R.G.

My fiancé and I found out that the blood test we have to get to obtain our marriage license is called a VDRL. A friend told us that it's to make sure we don't have syphilis. I think that's rather insulting. Why do we have to have such a test?

Marcy W.

Is syphilis about extinct? When you hear about VD these days, it's usually gonorrhea. Is syphilis less serious than the Clap?

Stan L.

Although syphilis is not as common these days as gonorrhea, it is still ranked third among reportable, communicable diseases, with 76,736 reported cases in 1976, according to statistics from the Center for Disease Control.

Like gonorrhea, syphilis is transmitted via sexual relations involving male or female genitals with the mouth, throat, or rectum. In some cases, the disease can be transmitted from an infected sex organ to an open cut in the skin of another person.

The organism that causes this disease is a tiny, microscopic corkscrew spirochete called Treponema pallidum. Unlike the gonococcal organism, the syphilis organism works very slowly. Ten to 90 days may pass before the symptoms of the first stage of syphilis appear.

Syphilis, a complex disease, has three distinct stages if it is left untreated.

The first stage, primary syphilis, appears 10 to 90 days after exposure. The most common symptom of this stage is usually a painless (though *sometimes* tender) sore that is ulcerated in the center and will appear on the penis, labia, around the rectum or, less commonly, in the mouth. This sore is called a *chancre*. The chancre may heal within a week or two, perhaps giving the victim the false impression that the disease has gone away. Unfortunately, this is not the case, unless the affected person has been receiving medical treatment. In untreated syphilis, the healing of the chancre simply means that the disease has gone into a latent or hidden stage. Here, the person may have no symptoms of the disease, but may still infect sexual partners.

Within a few weeks to a few months, the secondary stage of syphilis will appear. Here, the symptoms are quite noticeable. The patient may have flu-like symptoms—fatigue, headaches, chills, and fever—to begin with. But then comes the rash characteristic of secondary syphilis. This red rash covers the entire body—even the palms of the hands and the soles of the feet. There may also be whitish patches in the mouth. It is often at this stage that syphilis is first diagnosed, since such a rash is, certainly, hard to ignore.

How is syphilis diagnosed?

It may be diagnosed by examining any sores present (in the first or second stage) or by a blood test called the VDRL (which stands for Venereal Disease Research Laboratory). This is a screening test that is not only helpful in diagnosing suspected cases of syphilis, but is also a legal requirement in most states before a couple can get a marriage license.

Why does such a law exist?

It exists primarily to protect any baby who may be born to the couple involved. If a woman has syphilis during a pregnancy (especially during the critical third month), the child may be very seriously affected. That is why premarital blood tests (and good prenatal care) are so important.

If syphilis is not diagnosed and is left untreated in its second stage, it will go into another latent period. This may last for years before the third, or tertiary, stage appears. In this last stage, the disease invades the brain and nervous system, causing paralysis and even insanity.

Can syphilis be cured?

Yes . . . if it is diagnosed in the early stages (primary and secondary) and treated with effective drugs.

Here again, penicillin is the drug most often used. However, for those with an allergy to penicillin, other drugs may be used to cure the disease.

Since early treatment is crucial, it's important—especially if you have several different sex partners—to examine yourself regularly, checking for any sores on your genitals or around the rectum. Unfortunately, if a sore is painless and in the vagina, cervix, or rectum, it may not be noticed. The person will continue to infect sex partners for as long as six months until the second, more noticeable stage of syphilis appears.

So if you're sexually active and have a number of different sex partners, regular blood tests for syphilis may be a good idea.

OTHER VENEREAL DISEASES

Although gonorrhea and syphilis tend to be the most generally widespread and serious venereal diseases, other venereal diseases exist. Some are common in certain regions of the country and relatively rare in other areas. The following, however, are some of the more common varieties.

Nonspecific Urethritis (NSU) and Nonspecific Vaginitis (NSV)

For the past week, I have noticed a clear or kind of milky discharge at the tip of my penis, especially in the morning when I wake up. Also, it sort of burns when I urinate. Could this be some type of VD? Like gonorrhea? My girlfriend hasn't mentioned any symptoms she might have and I'm afraid to say anything about it to her. What could be the problem?

Gary D.

Although we really can't make a diagnosis on the basis of Gary's letter, he may be describing the symptoms of nonspecific urethritis (NSU), which is sometimes also called the Strain.

This disease, which affects the lining of the male's urethra, is a sexually transmitted venereal infection. Medical studies have shown that NSU is caused by certain organisms that share the properties of bacteria and viruses. Although many men who have NSU think immediately of gonorrhea when they notice a discharge, there are some significant differences between the symptoms of NSU and those of gonorrhea.

First, the incubation period of NSU is longer, usually two to three weeks.

Second, the discharge from the penis is clear to milky, and uncomfortable. The discharge of gonorrhea, on the other hand, may be thick and greenish-yellow, and urination may be painful.

Although it is possible that NSU symptoms will go away if you abstain from sexual activity and alcoholic beverages, it is best to seek medical help. It is usually impossible to accurately diagnose yourself, so it is important that you obtain a correct diagnosis of NSU and treatment—usually with antibiotics.

Don't try to medicate yourself with antibiotics you may have in your medicine cabinet. These may make an accurate medical diagnosis quite difficult. Besides, you may need to have antibiotics prescribed especially for treatment of this disorder.

What about your sex partner?

Women can develop a similar infection called nonspecific vaginitis. Here, too, the symptoms may be relatively mild: a slightly milky vaginal discharge that is uncomfortable and some vaginal discomfort. It is important for the woman, too, to seek medical help for a correct diagnosis and antibiotic treatments—usually with vaginal suppositories.

If both partners continue to have a problem with this disease—possibly taking turns reinfecting each other—both of them may be treated at the same time and sexual abstinence for the duration of the treatment may be prescribed.

Hemophilus Vaginalis

Please help me! For the past few weeks, I have been having an unusual discharge from my vagina. It has a bad odor and is sort of a grayish-yellow color. I've also had some vaginal itching. I'm so afraid that it might be some sort of VD. I'm afraid to see a doctor or tell my parents. I'm also afraid that my boyfriend might notice. What should I do?

Help!

The symptoms described in the letter above sound very much like those of a bacterial disease called Hemophilus vaginalis.

This infection is often, *but not always*, sexually transmitted and is caused by the introduction of a small organism into the vagina that results in irritation, discomfort, and a very noticeable discharge. Fortunately, this infection, like nonspecific urethritis, is limited to the area of infection and rarely spreads to other reproductive organs or to the entire body. Since this *is* a bacterial infection, antibiotics may be used to cure it. The treatment may be given in the form of vaginal suppositories and/or oral antibiotic medications taken on a regular basis for five to seven days. Treatment of the sex partner is vital.

Although the male partner may have no symptoms or only minor ones (slight discomfort or itching at the tip of the penis), he may carry the infection and, if not treated, may simply reinfect the woman again and again. So, for an effective cure, both partners must be treated.

Trichomonas Vaginalis

What is Trich? My girl friend went to the youth clinic last night because she had a discharge from her vagina and the doctor who examined her told her that she had this disease called Trich. Also, he prescribed some pills for me. Why should I take these pills? I don't have any problem. What's the deal?

Ted

Trichomonas vaginalis is another organism that is often—though not always—transmitted sexually.

Here, a small protozoan enters the vagina and begins to multiply, causing a painful irritation of the lining of the vagina and, possibly, the cervix as well as a yellowish-green frothy discharge. Sometimes there may be rather severe pain felt in the pelvic organs. While this may be rather similar to pain felt when gonorrhea spreads to the pelvic area, there are some important differences. Most notably, the woman usually has no discharge with gonorrhea. With Trichomonas, however, the discharge is copious and there may be rather intense itching.

What about the woman's male partner?

Often, he will have no symptoms, though some men may experience some discomfort or itching at the tip of the penis.

Trichomonas is quickly diagnosed by microscopic examination of the discharge and can be treated effectively with an oral drug called Flagyl, which may be taken in a dose of several pills at once or over a ten-day period and which may be prescribed for both the woman and her male partner. However, at the discretion of her physician or nurse practitioner, the woman may use Flagyl vaginal suppositories instead of the pills.

We can't emphasize too strongly that if the woman with Trichomonas has a regular sex partner (or partners) both (or all) must be treated to avoid reinfection.

Viral Venereal Diseases

I heard that some venereal diseases are caused by a virus. I know that colds are usually caused by a virus, too. So can you get VD in the same way you catch a cold? I'm afraid to ask my folks, and my girl friends will think I'm dumb. Can you tell me?

Marilyn M.

Some venereal diseases are caused by viruses, but are not transmitted in the air like cold viruses. These virus-caused venereal diseases—like other venereal diseases—result from close sexual contact.

What are these diseases?

We mentioned earlier that NSU and NSV are caused by organisms that share the properties of both bacteria and virus.

However, there are three other venereal diseases that are pure viruses: herpes progenitalis, condylomata acuminata (venereal warts), and molluscum contagiosum.

Herpes Progenitalis

Help! I noticed these little sores on my penis a few days ago. They seem to have clear fluid in them and they hurt and sort of itch, too. Could I have syphilis? I only have one girl friend and she doesn't have any sores. I really don't know what to do. I'm a college sophomore and wonder if I ought to go to the Student Health Center. However, now the sores seem to be going away. Should I just wait—or what?

Rick

Rick seems to be describing the symptoms of herpes progenitalis, which is caused by the same virus that can trigger cold sores in the mouth. (However, a cold sore in the mouth is *not* a signal of venereal disease.

When such sores appear on the genitals or around the rectum, the condition is called *herpes progenitalis* and is usually sexually transmitted.

In the past ten years, this kind of herpes has become quite widespread. In fact, according to a recent survey of physicians in private practice in the suburban areas of one large city, these physicians reported that they saw more herpes than any other venereal disease.

Why is this so?

There has been a lot of debate, but many experts feel that an increase in the practice of oral-genital sex during the last decade may be a major factor.

Even though cold sores in the mouth are *not* VD, this virus—if transferred to the genitals during oral sex—can become a venereal disease and can be transmitted, then, from one person's genitals to another's.

What are some of the symptoms of herpes progenitalis?

There may be tiny clusters of vesicles (filled with clear fluid) on the penis, labia, or even the anus. These may be extremely painful, especially when they occur on a woman's vulva. The sores will break and slowly heal with no treatment at all and may disappear within a week or two.

Unfortunately, however, this may not signal the end of the herpes siege. Once a person has an active herpetic infection on the genitalia, this can be transmitted to others.

And herpes can keep coming back, even without reexposure to the disease. Some puzzled young people have come back for treatment months later complaining that they have the infection again, in some instances after *months* of sexual abstinence! When the infection recurs, it may do so in a pattern that is identical to the previous outbreak, and it seems particularly apt to happen in times of stress, like around exam time.

While herpes is not really dangerous to an adult, it can cause serious—even fatal—problems for a baby whose mother has an active case of herpes progenitalis and infects her baby as it passes through the vaginal canal. So if you're a woman, particularly if you are pregnant, it is essential to get an accurate diagnosis and medical treatment for your condition. If you have an active case of herpes at the time of your baby's birth, your doctor may choose to deliver the baby via Cesarean section (removal of the fetus by means of incision into the uterus) to avoid possible infection.

When you have symptoms of herpes, please seek medical help. Sometimes an early case of syphilis may *look* like herpes. So an accurate diagnosis is vital!

If you *do* have herpes progenitalis, what can be done to cure the disease?

Unfortunately, there is no specific cure. Since herpes is a *virus,* antibiotics are ineffective, and to date, no anti-herpes vaccine has been developed. However, medical treatment can help to relieve the symptoms, alleviating the pain and discomfort and, perhaps, hastening the healing process.

If you have this disorder, there are also some self-help measures you may choose to take in addition to special medical treatment.

Soaking the sores in a bathtub (or basin) filled with warm, salted water or water mixed with Epsom salts or skim milk may help. This soaking should be done as often as possible—at least two or three times a day—for best results.

After soaking for 10 to 15 minutes, dry the affected area thoroughly. Since a towel might irritate the sores, you may wish to dry the area with a hair dryer or blow dryer, using a low setting.

Wearing loose-fitting clothing—without underwear if possible—may help, too. If you can wear a bathrobe, muumuu, or caftan while relaxing at home, this will let air reach the sores and will promote faster healing.

PLEASE NOTE: *Don't have sex relations while you have active sores!* Not only may this mean passing the virus on to another person, but it will also tend to slow your healing.

Since herpes is a virus, some people seem to have a natural immunity to it. Thus, if you have a problem with herpes and your regular sex partner never seems to get it, it could well be that he or she may have a natural immunity to the virus.

Condylomate Acuminate

I have these funny, skin-colored, cauliflowerlike things around my vagina and my boyfriend has the same on his penis. What are these things anyway? Could they be a form of VD?

Paula N.

Condylomate acuminate, or venereal warts, which look very much like the eruptions that Paula describes in her letter, are also caused by a virus. These may occur on the penis, around the vagina or the rectum (even in those who do not engage in anal sex). These venereal warts are sexually transmitted.

Although these warts are not dangerous, they are cosmetically unappealing and may spread rapidly to include a large area if they are not removed.

If you think that you may have venereal warts, you should have an examination to confirm this and then have them removed.

This removal may be done in one of several ways.

Some physicians prefer to use a medicine called Pedophyllin, which will gradually destroy the warts. This medication is applied by the doctor or nurse practitioner and, while effective, may require several visits before the warts are finally gone. (To avoid irritation of the skin while receiving this medication, wash it off with soap and water four to six hours after application.)

Besides this medication, there are two other ways that venereal warts can be removed.

One method involves the use of an electric needle (electrocautery), which will burn off the warts. This may sting for a second or two, but it is highly effective and often does not require any follow-up visits or treatment.

The third wart removal method is the use of liquid nitrogen. This chemical, when applied to warts, will burn them off. This method, too, will require fewer return visits and minimal discomfort.

It is important to remember that venereal warts are quite contagious and they will not go away by themselves.

Molluscum Contagiosum

I'm really scared because I have some bubblelike bumps on my inner thighs and near my vulva. They don't itch, but they're sure ugly and noticeable. What could this be?

Lucy E.

A round, smooth, bubble-like bump occurring on the genitalia and/or inner thighs may be a sign of *molluscum contagiosum,* another virus-caused venereal disease seen in teens and young adults. This venereal disease is not dangerous, but it is contagious and, like venereal warts, is cosmetically unappealing.

If you have such symptoms, seek medical help for correct diagnosis and treatment, which means removal of the bumps with a surgical instrument.

PLEASE NOTE: Such treatment is *not* a do-it-yourself project. If these bumps are not removed under sterile conditions, you may wind up with a skin infection.

It may be some consolation, however, that once these bumps are removed, they are gone for good—unless, of course, you are reinfected by another person.

Special Note on Hepatitis

Hepatitis is a disease of the liver. There are two types of this disease. Hepatitis A (also called "infectious hepatitis") has been most often spread via contaminated food and food handlers (who did not wash their hands after a bowel movement). It can be transmitted sexually if there is oral-anal sexual contact. Hepatitis B was once called "serum hepatitis" because it was often spread via transfusions of contaminated blood and by needle sticks. Now the virus has been isolated from the saliva and semen and thus can be spread sexually through certain sex practices.

So if you do know someone with hepatitis, it is best to avoid close physical relations, if possible. If you have had contact with an infected person, it may help to consult your physician and, at his/her discretion, receive an injection of gamma globulin. This injection may help to protect you from hepatitis if you have been exposed, but it is still no guarantee that you will not catch the disease.

So be forewarned.

Fungal and Parasitic Venereal Diseases

Tinea Cruris

I'm on the varsity basketball team and practice every day. For the past few weeks, I've noticed a scaling, itchy rash in my crotch. The coach says it's "jock rot" and told me to get some cream from the trainer, but now my girl friend has the same kind of rash. What's happening?

Alan

Alan seems to be describing a common fungal infection of the groin called *tinea cruris* or, more commonly, "jock itch."

Initially, this disease may be caused by a fungus that may develop on unwashed athletic supporters, which may be stashed in closed lockers. The fungus may then be transmitted from the supporter to the skin of the groin. This infection may then be transmitted—via skin-to-skin (usually sexual) contact—to another person, and in this instance, it would be classified as a venereal disease.

Tinea cruris is not serious, however, and may be treated with an over-the-counter drug like Tinactin, which will destroy the fungus when used as directed over a period of time.

Pubic Lice (Crabs)

What causes crabs? Do you get them from having sex?

Wondering

Pubic lice, or "crabs," are little parasites—visible to the naked eye—that may live and lay eggs in the pubic hair.

These parasites can be sexually transmitted during close physical contact when the pubic hair of the person who has the parasite comes in contact with the pubic hair of another. This usually happens, of course, during some kind of sexual activity.

Although pubic lice may cause intense itching, it is not dangerous and is easily cured.

One possible remedy is an over-the-counter drug called A-200. This is actually a type of medicated shampoo for the pubic area. Used according to instructions, it is quite effective.

There are other drugs—notably Kwell lotion and cream—that may be prescribed by a physician.

Whatever medication you use, be sure to repeat use of it within 24 hours and again one week later. This washing after one week will remove any residual eggs and keep the lice from recurring. Wait at least one week before having sex again.

It is also important to wash any clothes (like underwear and jeans) that may have been in contact with the infected area. Washing these clothes in very hot water will kill any of the parasites or eggs that may be clinging to them.

Scabies

Some kids I know went on a camping trip in the mountains and several came back with something called scabies. Is this something you get from sleeping in the wilds or is it some kind of venereal disease? (My older brother says it's a type of VD.)

Lorie L.

Scabies is a disease caused by a parasite called Acarus scabiei.

It can be transmitted in a number of ways. You can get it from bedding, blankets, or clothing that has not been laundered well.

The mite can also be transmitted from one person to another during close physical contact—usually during lovemaking—and in this instance, scabies *may* be a venereal disease.

However you acquire the parasite, the symptoms are the same. The mite will burrow under the skin, causing a red spot and sometimes even a red burrow line. There may be intense itching.

The mite may be killed by the cream Kwell, which is available by prescription from a physician. You will be given instructions on how and when to apply the cream, but, generally, the week-after follow-up treatment that is effective in curing pubic lice is also a good idea here. So is hot laundering of all clothing and bedding.

A Special Warning to Gays

Last week in our health class, we had a talk on VD by one of the people from the city health department. During the talk, he said that there are some kinds of VD that are seen especially in gay guys. Is this true? I was afraid to ask a question in class about this for fear the class might think that I was gay!

Jeff P.

There are some venereal diseases that are seen primarily in gay (homosexual) males.

Generally, these diseases are transmitted through the gastrointestinal tract and may infect gay males who engage in oral and/or anal sex.

It should be noted that the diseases we will mention in a minute are usually *not* venereal diseases. In many, if not most cases, they come from drinking contaminated water or eating contaminated food. But—among the homosexual population—they may *also* be sexually transmitted.

These diseases include hepatitis A and B, amoebic dysentery, bacillary dysentery (shigellosis), and typhoid fever (salmonellosis).

If you are gay and sexually active, it is good to be aware of these diseases. The symptoms of hepatitis include extreme fatigue, jaundice (the skin color becomes yellow-orange), a slight yellow coloring in the whites of the eyes, light-colored stools, and orange-yellow urine. The symptoms of the dysenteries and typhoid are fever and diarrhea (which is often bloody).

If you have any of the above symptoms, seek immediate medical help.

HOW YOU CAN HELP PREVENT VD

I just started having sex (with this girl who is a little older than I am) and everything is just great. But I worry a little about getting VD. I'm faithful to her, but I'm not absolutely sure she is to me. I really enjoy her and sex with her is just fantastic. How can I protect myself against VD?

Tom F.

Is it true that you can get treated for VD without your parents having to give their permission or even knowing? If so, where?

Carol K.

I guess you'd call me sexually active. I'm a 20-year-old guy who is active in sports at my college, and girls go for that. I have three girls I see a lot, but in any given month, I may have sex with about another five chicks (on the average). Anyway, I've got the Clap and the doctor wants me to notify my sex contacts (as he calls them). For some reason this bugs me. There are some chicks I just saw once and I don't know how to get in touch with them. I don't see why it's so important. If they have symptoms, they'll go to a doctor, right? And if they don't have any symptoms, that's fine, isn't it? So YOU tell me why I have to go through all this'

Annoyed

Helping to prevent VD is one of the major aspects of sexual responsibility. There are a number of ways you can act responsibly to keep from spreading venereal disease.

Learn as Much as You Can About Venereal Diseases. Know their symptoms and how they are spread. Read and reread this chapter.

Take Special Precautions When You Have Sex. In cases where venereal disease may be transmitted from the penis (for example, gonorrhea, syphilis, and NSU), a condom (prophylactic) may help to prevent the transmission of a venereal disease. However, it's important to remember that this condom must be worn *during the entire time of sexual contact.*

Also, urinating and washing the genitals after sexual relations may help to prevent VD.

If You Have Symptoms, Seek Help. Don't be afraid! County and city health departments, Adolescent Clinics, Free Clinics, and Youth Clinics throughout the nation offer low- or no-cost medical diagnosis and treatment for venereal disease. This care is *completely confidential* and may be given without parental consent or knowledge, in most states, to anyone over the age of 12.

The people who staff these clinics see all kinds of venereal diseases all the time, know how to treat them, and tend to be quite nonjudgmental.

If You Are Very *Sexually Active, Get Routine VD Tests.* Routine VD checks are important if you are sexually active with several partners (or many). You should have regular examinations, cultures for gonorrhea, and a blood test for syphilis. How often? If you are very active with multiple partners, you should have these tests every three months.

Know Your Contacts. To many teens, this may seem like an incredibly obvious piece of advice. But life-styles vary widely in all age groups—including young people. Some teen-agers and young adults may have life-styles that include multiple sex partners, one-night stands, and sex with people they don't really know. These are the people who are most likely to get—and to spread—VD.

If this is your life-style, make a habit of getting a phone number at least, even if you have no intention of seeing the other person again. This way, it will be possible to contact him or her in case you do develop symptoms of VD. Notifying contacts is an important way to stop the spread of venereal disease.

Notifying female sexual contacts is particularly important, since females, especially those with gonorrhea, may have no symptoms. They may not only continue to spread the disease, but may develop serious complications if they are not treated.

Contacting sex partners to tell them to be tested and/or treated for VD is not an easy thing to do. But it is the considerate thing to do. In the other person's place, wouldn't you want to know?

You may not always have to be the one to tell your contact(s) about the possibility of venereal disease. In some clinics, you may have the option of giving a staff member the names of your contacts and ways to reach them. The clinic will then notify these people (without mentioning your name) and ask them to come in for examination and treatment if necessary.

If the VD epidemic is to be conquered, prevention must play an increasingly major role. National efforts are under way to find new ways to prevent and cure venereal diseases, and to educate the public about these diseases.

Education is vital. The successful prevention of VD may be dependent on the knowledge and responsibility of all of us—young people included.

Whatever our individual life-style may be, we must educate ourselves to take responsibility in our own lives and to help inform others about the prevention, the symptoms, and the dangers of venereal diseases, as well as the availability of nonjudgmental medical help.

Most important, perhaps, we must educate ourselves to care.

CHAPTER TWELVE

Birth Control: An Ounce of Prevention

Why are so many teen-agers getting pregnant? My Aunt Sarah says that all these pregnancies happen because of sex education classes getting kids all eager to try sex because now they know about birth control, but I'm not sure about that. We don't have sex education in my school, but we sure have a lot of pregnancies! Two of my friends had to drop out of school on account of being pregnant. Neither of them knew much about birth control. One thought you couldn't get pregnant at certain times of the month and the other thought you couldn't your first time! I think they got pregnant out of plain ignorance. Do you think too much information or not enough is causing pregnancies?

Tracy D.

News stories and studies about teen pregnancies abound.

The statistics can be startling:

• More than one million American teen-agers become pregnant each year. Social scientists are calling teen pregnancy an epidemic.

• Pregnancy statistics are dipping into younger age groups. An estimated 3,000 13-year-old girls had babies last year and Planned Parenthood clinics across the nation are seeing an increase in pregnant 12-year-olds!

• According to Planned Parenthood/World Population estimates, three in ten girls nationwide who have had premarital intercourse have experienced premarital pregnancies and 75 percent of all first pregnancies of teen-agers were conceived before marriage.

• One out of every ten girls in the United States is a mother by the age of 17, according to statistics from the National Alliance Concerned with School-Age Parents (NACSAP).

But the news stories and statistics only give facts and figures. Across the nation, there are countless quiet tragedies daily as young lives are scarred by unplanned pregnancies.

The stories can be heartbreaking: dreams for education and careers abandoned, child abuse, premature marriages and divorces, grief over giving up a child for adoption or the emotional ordeal of abortion, or living with the painful mixture of love and frustration that seems inevitable when you're trying to be a parent and finish your own growing up at the same time.

These stories may be doubly tragic because they didn't have to happen.

Birth control is more available and advanced than ever before.

Birth rates are falling for every age group—except teen-agers.

Some, like Tracy's aunt, claim that sex education is to blame.

We disagree. If only *more* sexually active teens knew more about their bodies and were educated to use reliable methods of birth control.

An estimated 52 percent of teen-agers 13 to 19 years of age are sexually active, but less than 10 percent of these, in some surveys, use reliable contraceptives.

Why are teens taking such risks?

Among the reasons we have heard:

"Birth control just isn't romantic. Sex should be spontaneous."

"I didn't know I could get pregnant the first time . . . if I had sex standing up . . . etc."

"I didn't think it would happen to *me!*"

"He said he'd pull out . . ."

"I didn't think teens could get pills."

"Nobody ever told me about what really works."

Ignorance about their bodies, about how pregnancy occurs and how it can be prevented is taking a massive toll in the quality of young lives and in unmet potential.

An ounce of prevention—knowledge about the use of birth control—could save many young people from becoming such tragic statistics.

"CAN YOU GET PREGNANT IF . . ."

My boyfriend and I have decided we are mature enough to have sex. This may sound dumb, but we've made love once and I'm scared I'm pregnant. How long or how many experiences does it take to get pregnant? Is it possible your first time?

Anxious

Can a girl get pregnant from French kissing? I read in some article that you could. It sounds strange to me, but now I'm kind of worried.

Bonnie B.

Do you have to be on your menstrual period to get pregnant? Can pregnancy happen if a guy fondles a girl's sex organs?

L.K.

Can a girl become pregnant if the penis has touched or rubbed, but hasn't been placed into the vagina? Is it possible that the sperm cells could work their way up into the vagina and meet the egg cells?

Colleen

Can you get pregnant if the penis is removed before ejaculation?

Curious

Can you get pregnant if a guy ejaculates while lying on top of you—even if you're both wearing clothes?

Emily H.

This guy and I got into some heavy petting and one thing led to another. I didn't enjoy it. I just lay there. He got excited and had a discharge in my vagina. Could I get pregnant even if I didn't enjoy it? (I heard you had to "come" to get pregnant and nothing like that ever happened to me!)

Scared

I'm worried because I don't know what days I could get pregnant. Also, I'd like to know if I could get pregnant if both of us were naked and doing everything but going all the way?

Afraid

Can a girl get pregnant from a toilet seat after a male has ejaculated on it? Or if a male ejaculates near your genitals?

Worried

My friends told me that you can't get pregnant for the first few times that you have intercourse. Is this true or not?

S.Y.

These are only a few of the many "Can you get pregnant if . . . ?" questions we have received from young people. They reflect a lot of ignorance, confusion, and fear. Knowledge is the best defense against such fears.

Pregnancy occurs when the sperm of the male unites with the egg cell of the female.

As we saw in Chapter Two, a woman usually releases one egg per month in a process called ovulation, which occurs around the middle of her menstrual *cycle* (not period!). The exact time of ovulation is difficult to calculate, and it may be particularly impossible to pinpoint in a young teen-ager whose menstrual cycle is not well-established and regular.

For this reason, many teens who try to limit sex to "safe" days wind up pregnant.

It is best to go on the assumption that no time is safe. Women have been known to get pregnant at *all* times in their cycle, even during menstruation (although pregnancy may be less likely at this time).

Women usually get pregnant as a result of sexual intercourse, when the man ejaculates his sperm high up in the vagina near the cervix.

It doesn't matter which position you choose for intercourse. It's possible to get pregnant while standing up, lying down, sitting, or even hanging upside down.

Usually, a man must have an orgasm (ejaculate) to impregnate a woman, but there is evidence that sperm cells may also be present in the clear lubricating fluid that may ooze from his penis during sexual excitement. So, even if he "pulls out" before ejaculation, he may still leave some sperm behind in the vagina and pregnancy may result.

Contrary to a popular myth, it is not necessary for a woman to have an orgasm or to respond in any way in order to get pregnant.

You can't get pregnant from toilet seats.

You also can't get pregnant from French kissing or fondling unless such activities lead to sexual intercourse or, in the case of fondling, unless a male puts a finger that may have semen on it up the vagina.

Can you get pregnant in other ways that do not involve actual intercourse?

It is possible that if a boy ejaculates just outside the vagina that some of the semen may get inside. This is not the most common way to become pregnant, but it has happened.

In summary, you can get pregnant any time you have intercourse without birth control protection or from any kind of sex play that may enable sperm to get into the vagina.

COMMON MYTHS ABOUT BIRTH CONTROL

My boyfriend and I have talked about using birth control, but we agree it might destroy the naturalness of our sex life. We really enjoy being spontaneous and feel that it's wrong to plan in advance for sex. Yet I'm worried about getting pregnant. What should I do?

Leslie

Birth Control Is Not Romantic and Destroys the Spontaneity of Sex.

This is a particularly widespread and harmful myth that a great many teen-agers seem to believe.

But, if you're among the believers, consider this: How romantic is it to worry about pregnancy—before, during, and after sex? How romantic is it to sweat it out each month until your (or her) period comes?

The fact is, using a reliable method of birth control can free you to enjoy sex more.

It's true that seeking and using a reliable contraceptive may take some advance planning. But how terrible is planning—really? You plan other pleasurable things in your life: vacations, weekend trips, weddings, parties, and picnics. These occasions can be more fun when they are well-planned. Sex can be the same way.

Seeking birth control can mean admitting to yourself and possibly to others that you will have sex. However, if you really feel OK about having sex, this should not be a major problem.

When you can banish the constant fear of pregnancy, it may make a wonderful difference in your sexual relationships.

My boyfriend says he can feel when he is coming and can pull out. He says this is a good form of birth control. Could I still get pregnant if he pulls out in time and then puts his penis back in?

Merry B.

We've been hearing a lot about this new form of natural birth control and it sounds great! In fact, it's the only method my boyfriend and I would even consider using. All we want to know is how effective it is. The method is that a female drinks ice water right after sexual intercourse to freeze all her organs so she won't get pregnant. Would this work well?

Denise and David

I've heard that tampons make great contraceptives. True?

T. H.

A few months ago, me and my boyfriend had sex. He put a rubber band around the end of his penis and assured me that I wouldn't get pregnant, but I'm curious because I haven't had my period for about three months. Could I be pregnant? I'm only 14.

Kris

There Are Many Effective Methods of Birth Control That You Can Use on Your Own Without Going to a Doctor or Setting Foot in a Drugstore.

This myth has also caused a lot of harm, often in the form of unplanned pregnancies.

Rumors about what works and what doesn't work fly in adolescent circles. Most of these are half-truths or just plain fantasies. Some of these myth methods may be of minimal help in preventing a pregnancy. Others offer no protection at all.

Some famous last lines:

"Don't worry, honey! I'll pull out in time!"

The withdrawal method means that the man withdraws his penis, or attempts to do so, before ejaculating.

The problem is, many young men don't have such control. Ever-conscious of the need to pull out before ejaculation, the man may not enjoy sex as much. If he does start to enjoy himself, he may forget to pull out.

The biggest problem with the withdrawal method, however, is the fact that sperm may be in the lubricating fluid that is present before the man ever ejaculates. So the man may pull out in time for ejaculation, but may still leave several million sperm in the vagina.

"It's all right to have sex now. It's a safe day."

This type of guesswork is a form of roulette: If you're sexually active, it may be only a matter of time until pregnancy happens.

It's true that a form of the rhythm method (which recommends that the couple avoid sex during the woman's time of ovulation) is used by some couples. The problem is, rhythm, at best, is not a very effective method of birth control. "At best" means that the couple is highly motivated, that the woman has regular menstrual cycles, and that she has learned to keep accurate charts and graphs of changes in her body temperature, her menstrual cycle patterns and, possibly, changes in her cervical mucus as well.

Few teens trying to use the rhythm method take such elaborate precautions.

At worst, rhythm means guesswork and guessing means that you have a good chance of being wrong about your "safe" (nonfertile) days.

"It's OK. I'll just douche with the rest of this cola!"

Douching, which means washing or flushing the vagina with liquid, is never an effective method of birth control, although many people believe rumors that it is and try douching with anything handy—from water to colas.

The problem with this method is: before you even have a chance to sit up after intercourse, it's likely that sperm have already surged through the cervical os and into your uterus. Sperm travel faster than you possibly can! And douching with a soft drink or other liquid not meant for douching may cause a serious—even life-threatening—uterine infection.

"Don't worry about getting pregnant! I'll use plastic wrap . . . Baggies . . . balloons . . . a rubber band . . ." or, *"Oh, we're safe. I'll put in a tampon."*

Plastic wrap and Baggies are great for wrapping sandwiches. Balloons are fun to blow up and rubber bands are great for wrapping newspapers and zapping friends. Tampons catch the menstrual flow very well. But *none* of the above could be called effective contraceptives.

Drinking ice water, the method that Denise and David related to us, will neither freeze a woman's organs nor prevent pregnancy.

In short, any time you hear about a new, too-good-to-be-true, do-it-yourself birth control method . . . be wary.

I'd like to take the Pill, but people tell me that there's no way I could get birth control pills, since I'm only 15. Do I just take my chances until I'm 18?

Tammy

I hear it's against the law for people under 18 to get birth control and that clinics turn you away and drugstores won't sell you anything like that. So what do I do?

Liane K.

Effective Birth Control Methods Are Not Available to Teen-Agers.

The fact is, birth control services are available to young people at Free Clinics, Youth Clinics, and family planning clinics across the nation. These services may also be available from some physicians in private practice.

By 1976, 26 states and the District of Columbia upheld the right of those under 18 to receive contraceptive care. A number of court cases have been decided in favor of contraception for minors.

For example, the U.S. Supreme Court struck down a New York law stating that only pharmacists could sell contraceptives and then only to those over 16. The Court confirmed the right of citizens to make intimate decisions regarding contraception without government intervention. (New York was the only state that had a specific law about the sale of contraceptives to minors.)

In St. Louis, a 15-year-old girl, who wanted to receive birth control without parental consent, recently filed a class action suit in a U.S. District Court. Ul-

timately, the Eighth U.S. Circuit Court of Appeals ruled that "the girl's interest in privacy must outweigh any desire to accommodate parental concerns."

Contraceptive services are available to minors at clinics in all states. (See listing of Adolescent Clinics and Birth Control Facilities in the Appendix.) The legal question involved in such services usually does not deal with contraception directly, but with the issue of medical care of a minor without parental consent.

Some teens may have parental consent for contraceptive services. Most won't. Yet many receive such services.

A number of states have "emancipated minor" statutes declaring that emancipated minors (for example, those living away from home and/or supporting themselves and making their own decisions) and/or married minors may give their own consent for medical treatment.

A variation on this is the "mature minor" rule, which has been recognized by a number of states. Here, the rule states that "a minor can effectively consent to medical treatment for himself if he understands the nature of the treatment and it is for his benefit."

A number of other states have statutes that specifically authorize medical personnel to give birth control to minors without parental consent.

Even in states without such rulings, teens can get help. Although clinic personnel may ask a patient's age and whether or not that patient is emancipated, they will generally not ask for proof.

"Our program is designed to meet the health needs that may be met inadequately elsewhere," says one clinic official. "We do not ask for proof of age or residence. It may be that some of our patients are not emancipated. We do not wish to violate the law, but our first concern is for the adolescent who needs help."

Many would echo this sentiment. In fact, the American Medical Association, the American College of Obstetrics and Gynecology, and the American Academy of Pediatrics have all given public support to the issue of contraception for sexually active teen-agers.

So birth control information and help will probably be available to you—if you take the responsibility for seeking it.

WHAT METHODS WORK?

I love my boyfriend very much. We've been going together two years and now want to have sex. But I don't want to get pregnant. What kind of birth control is best and easiest to take and get?

Hilary H.

I'm tired of being a dummy. Please tell me some birth control methods that really work!

Judi

I'm 17 and want to know something. What is the best method of birth control? I can't take no more chances!

Rita Y.

There are a number of effective birth control methods.

But no method (except sexual abstinence and, possibly, sterilization) is 100 percent effective.

And there is no method that is right—or best—for everyone.

Some want a contraceptive that is, first and foremost, highly effective, even if it causes some side effects and possible health risks.

Others would rather use a method where the risk of pregnancy might be a bit higher, but the risk to health would be minimal.

Still others opt for methods that are easily obtained without a doctor's prescription.

Some people need continuous birth control protection. Others, who have sex only occasionally, may choose a method that needs to be used only at the time of sexual intercourse.

Still others put a high premium on spontaneity and prefer methods that require no special thought or preparation either just before or during sex.

Some women prefer to take sole responsibility for birth control, while others prefer to share this responsibility with the male partner.

As you can see, people have a variety of needs and there are a number of effective birth control methods that may fill these.

One or more of them may be right for you.

How do you find out which method may best suit your needs?

It's best to learn all the facts and possibilities, and then decide.

Think about your priorities.

If you want a highly effective method, read our information about the Pill and IUD with special care.

If you want an effective method with no side effects or health risks, pay special attention to what we have to say about the diaphragm and jelly, and condom-plus-spermicide methods.

If you need continuous protection, the Pill or the IUD may be the answer.

If you have only occasional sex, you might consider Encare Oval, the diaphragm, or condom-plus-spermicide combinations.

Before making up your mind which method you'll choose, it is a good idea to read about ALL the methods and then to discuss these with your sex partner and, if applicable, your physician or nurse practitioner. We can only give you information. The best method for YOU is a very personal decision.

The Pill (Oral Contraceptives)

What Is It?

Although people refer to "the Pill" when discussing oral contraception, there are a number of different brands of birth control pills.

Most pills are combinations of synthetic preparations of the hormones estrogen and progesterone. There is also a pill containing only progesterone, but the effectiveness of this "mini-pill" has been shown to be somewhat lower than that of the combination pills.

How Does It Work?

The synthetic hormones in birth control pills are similar to natural hormones and work to prevent pregnancy in several ways.

First, these hormones keep the ovaries from releasing an egg each month. If there is no egg, there can be no pregnancy.

These chemicals also affect the lining of the uterus so that if by chance ovulation and fertilization did occur, the egg would have difficulty attaching itself to the uterine lining.

Also, progesterone may cause cervical mucus to become thick and, essentially, hostile to sperm.

How Do You Use It?

Birth control pills are available in 21- and 28-day packets. If you take a 21-day packet, you will take pills every day for three weeks with seven days off, generally starting the new packet of pills on the fifth day after your menstrual period begins. Some family planning counselors are advocating starting a new cycle of pills on a certain *day* of the week (for example, a Sunday). Starting the new cycle of pills on the fifth day of your menstrual cycle will also give you continuous contraceptive protection.

If you have a 28-day pill packet, you will take a pill every day of your cycle. Seven of these pills, however, are non-functional sugar pills. They are included so that you can take a pill every day instead of trying to calculate when you should be starting and stopping your pills. Some people find this a much easier way to remember to take birth control pills.

Pills should be taken consistently at the same time

every day. (Some women prefer to take them first thing in the morning or before going to bed at night.)

Birth control pills should also be taken only as directed by a physician. In other words, do not borrow a friend's pills. You must have your own prescription, tailored to your needs.

It is also a good idea to know what brand of pill you are taking, so that if you should lose a pill packet or go to another health facility, you will be able to tell a physician which type of pill you have been taking.

How Effective Is It?

Most birth control pills are very effective with a less than 1 percent failure rate. Failures are most likely to happen if you forget to take a pill for one or two (or more) days during your cycle.

If this happens, take the forgotten pill (along with your regular one for that day) and, for the rest of the cycle, use a backup method of birth control—while continuing to take your pills!

Who Can Use This Method?

Generally, a woman who is menstruating regularly and has well-established cycles and who also has no condition that would preclude use of the Pill may use birth control pills.

However, most physicians and nurse practitioners will be very careful to discuss the Pill's disadvantages along with its advantages.

The Pill isn't for everyone.

Who Should Not Use This Method?

Women who have a history of abnormal vaginal bleeding, heart disease, blood clots, liver disease (for example, hepatitis), or cancer in the reproductive system should not take the Pill.

In addition, women who have high blood pressure, migraine headaches or diabetes may be advised to consider other forms of birth control. If a diabetic does take oral contraceptives, she should do so under the direction and supervision of the physician who treats her diabetes.

Also, if you tend to be rather forgetful, the Pill may not be for you. To be effective, birth control pills must be taken consistently, on a precise schedule.

What Are the Advantages?

Birth control pills are highly effective.

They are convenient to take and do not interfere with sex.

In addition, these pills may offer some relief from heavy and/or painful menstrual periods. The Pill may also regulate menstrual periods although this is not considered reason enough to prescribe it.

What Are the Disadvantages?

Birth control pills have a number of side effects, some relatively minor and some serious.

Among the (more or less) minor side effects may be nausea, weight gain, breast tenderness, migraine-like headaches, spotting between periods, and irritability.

Sometimes these side effects may be caused by a pill with a hormone balance that is not right for you and may be remedied by switching to another brand of pill with a different hormone concentration.

For example, if you experience nausea, you may be taking a pill that has too much estrogen for you. Switching to a lower estrogen pill may help. The same may be true for symptoms like headaches and breast tenderness. Weight gain may be due to too much progesterone and irritability may mean an estrogen deficiency. Spotting between periods may mean a progestin and/or estrogen deficiency.

There are some major health risks that may be connected with the Pill. These must not be overlooked.

Birth control pills can contribute to high blood pressure, changes in your blood sugar, migraine headaches, and skin changes. They have also been linked to blood clots, strokes, and liver tumors, among other complications.

Such major complications tend to be rare, but they *are* possibilities when you take the pill.

PLEASE NOTE: When sizing up the risks of the Pill, do consider this: The Pill is quite safe when compared to the risks involved in pregnancy and childbirth, especially if you're young. Medical studies attempting to find links between certain forms of cancer and oral contraceptives are in progress, but are inconclusive at this time.

How Do You Get It?

Birth control pills are available by prescription only and may be obtained from a physician in private practice or at a family planning facility, Youth Clinic, or Free Clinic.

Before prescribing the Pill, however, the physician and/or nurse practitioner will take a complete medical history and perform a physical examination that will include checking your blood pressure and your breasts as well as a gynecological exam, Pap smear, and urinalysis.

Annual health checkups are advised.

How Much Does It Cost?

The initial examination fee may vary widely depending on whether you go to a physician in private practice or to a clinic. Many clinics will examine you for a low fee or for no cost.

The pills themselves range in price from $2.00 to $3.50 for a month's supply.

The Intrauterine Device (IUD)

What Is It?

The IUD is a small, flexible plastic device, which may be coated with copper or hormones, that is placed into the uterus by a physician using a small tamponlike inserter.

IUDs come in all shapes and sizes, but the most common types, perhaps, are the Copper 7 (Cu-7), Copper T, Lippes Loop, and the Coil.

Whatever its shape, the IUD will have a tiny string that will protrude through the cervical os. This enables you to check periodically to make sure that the IUD is still in place.

How Does It Work?

There are a number of differing opinions regarding how the IUD works.

Probably the most widely held opinion is that the IUD causes a slight inflammatory reaction within the

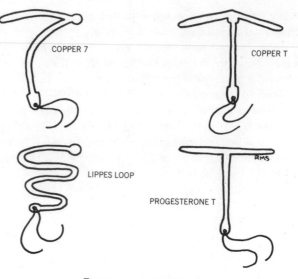

Four types of IUDs

uterus. This may be detrimental to sperm and to a fertilized egg as well, preventing it from attaching to the wall of the uterus.

The copper element of some of the IUDs may, as it reacts with various enzymes, work to immobilize sperm.

How Do You Use It?

After it is inserted into the uterus, the IUD requires no further care beyond checking the string from time to time to make sure that the IUD is still there. (Some women may expel the devices without realizing it.)

Many IUDs may be left in place indefinitely, al-

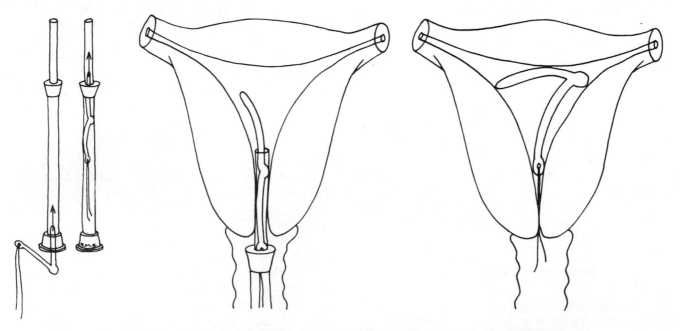

The IUD is inserted into the uterus. Once in place, it springs back to its original shape.

though those with copper should be changed every two to three years.

How Effective Is It?

Once in place, the IUD is a highly effective method of birth control with a 1 to 3 percent failure rate.

To minimize the risk of failure, make sure that the physician inserting the device has considerable experience with IUDs. Studies have found that the competence of the physician and his/her familiarity with the particular IUD is important to its proper placement and effectiveness.

Also, some physicians suggest using a backup method of birth control (for example, foam or condom) for the first month or so after the insertion of the IUD. This seems to be the time when most of the relatively rare IUD pregnancies occur.

An IUD can fail, too, if it is expelled from the uterus without your knowledge. So check the string, especially after your menstrual period. The IUD explusion rate tends to be higher among young women who have not had a baby.

Who Can Use This Method?

Any woman who does not have a condition that would preclude use of an IUD may be able to use one.

If you tend to be quite sexually active and/or forgetful, an IUD could be an excellent birth control choice—if you don't suffer side effects.

Some clinics, however, may restrict use of IUDs to women who have had a pregnancy.

Who Should Not Use This Method?

The IUD should not be used by women who have active or recurrent pelvic infection, inflammation of the cervix, valvular heart disease, uterine fibroid tumors, endometriosis, severe menstrual cramps and/or heavy periods, abnormal uterine bleeding, or anemia.

This device also should not be used by a woman who may be pregnant. This is one reason why the IUD is usually inserted during a woman's menstrual period. Another reason for insertion at this time is that, during menstruation, the cervical os is a bit dilated, making insertion easier and less painful.

What Are the Advantages?

The IUD is highly effective.

It is always there when you need it with no special thought or effort required on the part of the user.

It does not interfere with the sex act and usually

cannot be felt by either partner. Lengths of IUD strings may vary, however. If the male partner complains that he can feel the string during sex, a physician may simply shorten the string.

What Are the Disadvantages?

Especially in the early months after insertion, the IUD may cause heavy menstrual periods, cramps, and bleeding between periods.

In some instances, which are, fortunately, not too common, an IUD may cause pelvic inflammatory disease or perforation of the uterus. If you have severe pain or tenderness in the abdominal area, check with your physician immediately!

Another disadvantage: Insertion of the IUD may be painful. Some physicians, however, may use a local anesthetic to minimize this pain.

If, after the first few months, you continue to have pain and bleeding, the IUD may have to be removed.

How Do You Get It?

An IUD must be inserted by a physician either at his/her office or at a clinic.

How Much Does It Cost?

The cost of an IUD may vary from $3 to $25 depending on what kind you get *plus* the doctor's or clinic's fee, if applicable.

The Diaphragm

What Is It?

The diaphragm is a shallow, dome-shaped cup made of soft rubber. It is placed securely over the cervix and is used with spermicidal (sperm-killing) cream or jelly.

How Does It Work?

The diaphragm is a barrier between the sperm and the uterus. The contraceptive jelly or cream used with it offers added protection by immobilizing and killing the sperm cells.

How Do You Use It?

Contraceptive cream or jelly is applied to the rim and both sides of the diaphragm. Then the rim (which is reinforced by a metal spring) is squeezed and the device is placed high in the vagina, covering the cervix. You can tell if the diaphragm is properly placed by feeling for the cervix through the dome of the diaphragm.

This device may be inserted some time before intercourse. However, if it has been several hours since insertion, it is a good idea to add some more spermicidal jelly or cream with an applicator before having sex.

If intercourse is repeated within the next few hours, another application of jelly or cream should be inserted. *But do not remove the diaphragm!*

The diaphragm must remain in place for at least eight hours after intercourse. After this, it may be removed, washed, dried, and stored in its container.

How Effective Is It?

If fitted correctly and used every time, the diaphragm is a highly effective method of birth control.

Recent figures show that, if used properly, this method has only a 3 percent failure rate.

To minimize the risk of failure, follow directions for use exactly and check the diaphragm before insertion (by filling it with water or holding it up to a bright light) to make sure that there are no holes or tears in it.

Who Can Use This Method?

This method is safe for just about everyone, but works best with people who are emotionally mature, responsible, and highly motivated to practice birth control.

It also helps to have a certain amount of privacy and, ideally, access to a bathroom, since some cream

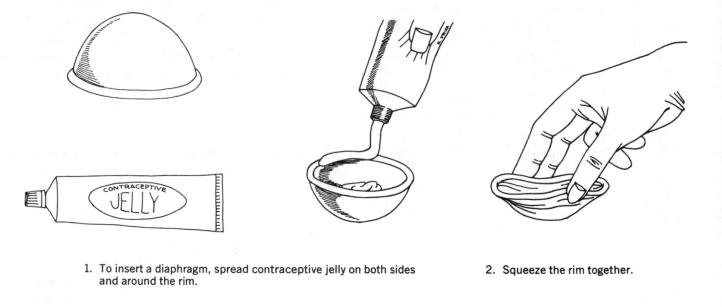

1. To insert a diaphragm, spread contraceptive jelly on both sides and around the rim.

2. Squeeze the rim together.

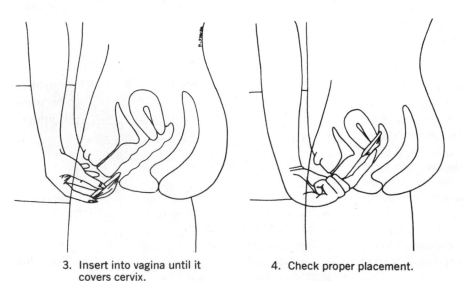

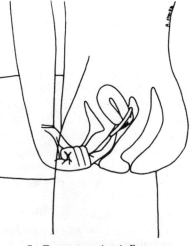

3. Insert into vagina until it covers cervix.

4. Check proper placement.

5. To remove, hook finger on rim and pull gently.

and jelly preparations can be a bit messy. Although some complain that this method is a hassle, many couples find that this is not so if the diaphragm is inserted well before love-making begins or if its insertion (often by the male) is incorporated into the couple's foreplay.

It can be an especially good method of birth control for someone who does not have sex regularly, since it is used only when one has sex.

Who Should Not Use This Method?

People who might be tempted to see this method as bothersome and be tempted to say "Let's not hassle with it, just this once . . ." should not try to use the diaphragm.

Also, people who do not have the maturity or the motivation to use this method properly would be advised against it.

What Are the Advantages?

The diaphragm is completely safe and has no adverse side effects. Physicians have reported widespread new interest in this older method of birth control as more women become disenchanted with the various side effects of the Pill and IUD.

The diaphragm is used only when you need it.

It can also catch the menstrual flow, making intercourse during menstruation a more acceptable option for some.

What Are the Disadvantages?

Some may see the diaphragm method as messy and inconvenient and as an interruption of lovemaking. Many people are not highly motivated enough to work around such disadvantages. Others, however, may minimize such problems by inserting the diaphragm some time before intercourse and by incorporating the insertion of more cream or jelly as part of foreplay.

In order to work at all, a diaphragm must be properly fitted by a physician and must be replaced if you lose or gain more than ten pounds, or if you have a baby, an abortion, or pelvic surgery. Also, it does not last indefinitely and, for best results, should be replaced about once a year.

Another disadvantage: the diaphragm may become dislodged during intercourse. With sexual excitement, the vagina may expand and even a properly fitted diaphragm may loosen. This possibility is increased if the couple is using the female superior (woman on top) position. In such a case, the woman may become pregnant even if her diaphragm usually fits well.

How Do You Get It?

You must be fitted for a diaphragm by a physician in his/her office or in a clinic.

While a diaphragm is available by prescription only, the spermicidal jelly or cream used with it may be purchased without prescription in any drugstore.

How Much Does It Cost?

The diaphragm itself (minus doctor's fees—if any) costs from $3 to $7.50. A typical month's supply of spermicidal cream or jelly will cost about $3 to $5.

The Condom

What Is It?

The condom (or "rubber") is a thin sheath of rubber or animal tissue that is slipped over the erect penis before intercourse. For best results, it is used in combination with spermicidal foam, jelly, or cream.

How Does It Work?

The condom prevents pregnancy by keeping sperm from entering the vagina. Instead, the semen is deposited in the reservoir tip of the condom or in a space left by the man at the end of the condom. It works best when used in conjunction with spermicides.

How Effective Is It?

Condom-user failure rates range from 10 to 20 percent. This percentage may be cut drastically if the man follows manufacturer's instructions carefully and uses foam or other spermicides as well.

Who Can Use This Method?

In this instance, responsibility for birth control is placed on the male partner. This method can be used by any male who is highly motivated and who understands how to use the condom correctly.

Who Should Not Use This Method?

Men who would see the condom as an inconvenience and be tempted to skip using it at times should not consider this method.

Men who don't have the motivation to follow package instructions are also bad candidates for this method.

What Are the Advantages?

The condom is safe, with no adverse side effects. It is available everywhere without prescription.

Particularly when used with vaginal spermicides, it can be a very effective method of birth control.

The condom may also help to prevent the transmission of venereal diseases and other infections.

What Are the Disadvantages?

Many couples complain that the condom interferes with lovemaking. It must be placed on the *erect* penis before any insertion into the vagina has taken place. (Some couples, however, simply make rolling the condom on part of foreplay.)

Some men also complain that condoms may detract somewhat from their physical sensations and enjoyment.

The condom can break, spilling semen into the vagina. This may be most likely to happen if the man forgets to leave a space at the tip for semen and/or if the condom is old or not of good quality.

The condom can slip off and spill semen in the vagina. To minimize this possibility, the man should withdraw his penis from the vagina before he loses his erection and should hold on to the condom as he withdraws.

How Do You Get It?

You can buy condoms anywhere—from many men's rest rooms to drugstores. Drugstore condoms may be fresher and of better quality.

How Much Does It Cost?

A package of three plain condoms is about one dollar. Special reservoir-tip and other high-quality condoms tend to be more expensive.

If spermicides are used, add on an extra $3 to $5 per month if you are having sex regularly.

The Encare Oval

What Is It?

The Encare Oval is a new spermicidal chemical barrier contraceptive that is bullet-shaped and not much larger than a thumbnail. It has been available in this country for less than a year, but has been widely used and tested in Europe for the past five years with excellent results.

How Does It Work?

The Oval is inserted with the finger high up in the vagina. Once there, it will melt at body temperature within ten minutes and will form a dense barrier over the cervix while its spermicidal ingredient Nonoxynol-9 destroys sperm. It is this double action that seems to make Oval as effective as it is.

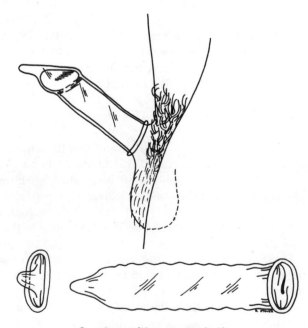

Condom with receptacle tip

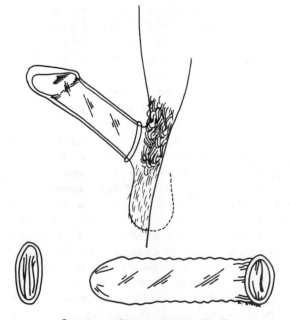

Condom without receptacle tip

The Oval offers protection against pregnancy from ten minutes to two hours after insertion. However, if intercourse is repeated within that time, another Oval should be inserted.

How Effective Is It?

Until extensive testing is done on the Oval in this country, family planning officials tend to take a rather conservative stand on the product, rating the Oval's effectiveness in the range of other chemical contraceptives like foam.

However, the news from Europe sounds promising. In a four-year study involving 10,000 West German women, the Encare Oval proved to be 99.14 percent effective. Studies made in the United States have yet to substantiate this effectiveness claim.

Who Can Use This Method?

As far as we know at this time, anyone can use this method, since it does not affect the body systems in any way.

Who Should Not Use This Method?

People who are not strongly motivated to use birth control and to follow instructions precisely should not use this method.

Also, people who tend to be forgetful, who might risk either forgetting to insert the Oval or forgetting to wait ten minutes before having intercourse, or those who may forget to insert a second Oval if intercourse is repeated might want to try another method.

This method may also not be ideal for a woman who objects to touching her own genitalia, although, in such instances, a cooperative sex partner might insert the Oval for her.

What Are the Advantages?

The Encare Oval, at least in preliminary studies, seems to be quite effective as a contraceptive.

It is safe. No side effects have been noted.

It is a nonprescription, over-the-counter birth control method and may be obtained easily in most drugstores.

It is easy to use and to carry. One Oval is only slightly larger than a thumbnail. A whole packet of 12 is about *half* the size of a paperback book!

What Are the Disadvantages?

The Oval, which is designed to melt at body tem-

perature, may soften prematurely if you carry it in your purse or pocket on a hot summer day.

Some may object to the fact that inserting the Oval and waiting ten minutes may interfere with the sex act. However, since it is effective for up to two hours after insertion, one might solve this problem by inserting it well before sexual activity starts. However, some may be bothered, too, by the fact that a new Oval must be inserted for each act of intercourse.

A minority of women may experience a feeling of warmth in the vagina as the Oval melts and foams, but a number of these women say that they rather enjoy this feeling.

How Do You Get It?

Encare Oval may be bought over the counter in most drugstores. It is also available at most family planning clinics.

How Much Does It Cost?

For a package of 12 individually sealed Encare Ovals, you can expect to pay about $3.75.

Foams and Other Chemical Contraceptives

What Is It?

Spermicidal foam, creams, and jellies are chemical contraceptives that, when inserted into the vagina via tamponlike applicators before intercourse, kill sperm. Foam will also block sperm trying to enter the cervix.

Foam, which comes in a container under pressure (like shaving cream) is generally considered to be the most effective of these chemical contraceptives.

For best results, it is a good idea to use a double dose of foam about 20 minutes or less before intercourse, repeating the double application as sex is repeated.

How Does It Work?

Contraceptive foam is stored in a container under pressure and transferred to a plastic inserter just before use and then placed—via the inserter—high into the vagina shortly before intercourse. Once in the vagina, foam quickly forms a barrier over the cervix, blocking the sperm. It also contains potent spermicides which immobilize and kill sperm.

How Effective Is It?

Statistics on the effectiveness of foam vary a great

deal, but it is generally considered to be less effective than the diaphragm or condom methods.

Vaginal jellies and creams, used without these barrier devices, are less effective than foam.

Foam can be a good backup method and can be very effective if used with a condom or diaphragm.

What Are the Advantages?

The advantages of foam are that it is readily available in most drugstores, it has no side effects, and it is used only when you have sex.

What Are the Disadvantages?

Some couples feel that this method interferes with sex, although some incorporate inserting the foam as part of foreplay.

Others object to foam and other chemical contraceptives because they can be messy and some may be allergic to the chemicals.

The greatest disadvantage, however, may be that, in general, chemical contraceptives are not as effective as the methods discussed earlier.

How Do You Get It?

Chemical contraceptives are readily available at drugstores. No prescription is necessary to purchase them.

How Much Does It Cost?

The cost of chemical contraceptives used on a regular basis may range from $3 to $5 a month.

Rhythm

What Is It?

There are several variations of the rhythm method, but all have one goal: helping the woman to estimate the days in her monthly cycle when risk of pregnancy may be lowest.

How Does It Work?

Rhythm may be practiced using a calendar system where the woman must document her menstrual periods for six months to a year, carefully calculating, from the cycle patterns, when ovulation may be taking place.

Changes in vaginal mucus and in basal body temperature may also be observed in an attempt to determine the time of ovulation.

Some couples use all three of these variations together.

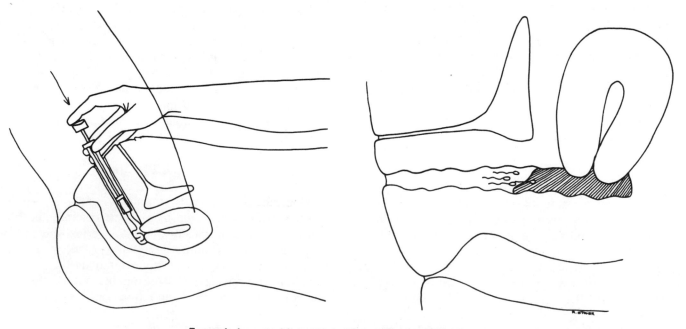

Foam is inserted into the vagina with an applicator.

How Effective Is It?

Unfortunately, despite the effort and careful calculations, rhythm is not a very effective method of birth control. It has about a 30 percent failure rate under optimum conditions and, due to the high motivation and long-range planning involved, this method is not recommended for most teen-agers.

What Are the Advantages?

Rhythm has no method-caused side effects.

It will reduce chances of getting pregnant—a 30 percent possibility versus an 80 percent chance if no contraceptive measures at all are taken.

It is also the only birth control method that is officially accepted by the Catholic church.

What Are the Disadvantages?

Rhythm is an unreliable form of birth control, no matter how careful one's calculations, because time of ovulation does not always follow a regular pattern. Thus, it may be very difficult to determine every month.

Also, this method requires a great deal of abstinence from sex during "unsafe" days. Patterns of desire do not always coincide with "safe" and "unsafe" days.

Sterilization

What Is It?

Sterilization is an increasingly popular method of birth control, especially for married people over 30 who have had all the children they want and for people married or single who have decided that they will never have children.

This permanent form of birth control is practically 100 percent effective. Sterilization operations may be performed on the male or female.

How Does It Work?

When the male is sterilized, the procedure is called *vasectomy* and means cutting and tying of the vas deferens (to effectively block the passage of sperm) via a simple operation that may be performed in a doctor's office.

This operation is not the same as castration. The male will be able to function just as well sexually and will ejaculate seminal fluid with no sperm in it. However, it may take 10 to 15 ejaculations after the surgery

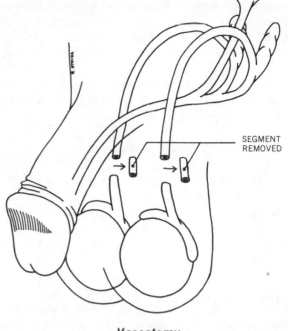

SEGMENT
REMOVED

Vasectomy

is performed before the ejaculate will be entirely sperm-free.

Sterilization for women is a bit more complicated, involving a brief hospital stay.

This procedure, called *tubal ligation,* means that the Fallopian tubes are severed to prevent the passage of the egg from the ovary to the uterus. The operation may be done through a tiny abdominal incision or through the vagina. The tubes may be severed by cutting, by blocking them with special clips, or by sealing them off with electric currents.

Who Can Use This Method?

Only people looking for a permanent method of birth control should opt for sterilization.

There is some research being done on reversing sterilization and some operations are actually being

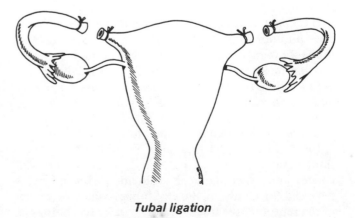

Tubal ligation

performed on men to reverse vasectomies. However, such reversals are only sometimes successful in terms of fertility and are always quite expensive. So, at this time sterilization must still be considered permanent and irreversible.

Because of its permanent nature and the expense involved, this form of birth control is not a common choice among young adults.

In an Emergency

I heard about a birth control pill you can take the morning after you have sex that will keep you from getting pregnant. That sounds great to me. I don't have sex all that much and I hate to take pills constantly. Could you tell me more about this "morning after" pill?

Kim C.

I'm 19 and have a boyfriend I plan to marry in two years after we finish school. I use the diaphragm as a form of birth control and I like it a lot because it doesn't mess up my body in any way. But lately I've been worried. There have been quite a few rapes in this area and I was wondering if you are raped, how you can keep from getting pregnant. I'd hate to take pills or something just in case I got raped, but I do worry about it.

Jean P.

In most cases, of course, sex is not an emergency. There is always time for the responsible couple to take adequate birth control precautions.

However, there are cases, particularly in the event of rape, when such safeguards are not possible.

In such an instance, what can you do to prevent pregnancy?

There is the so-called morning after pill, which is ten 25-mg tablets of diethylstilbestrol (DES), a synthetic estrogen that is taken over a five-day period. This hormone may also be given in the form of an injection.

If taken within 72—and preferably within 24—hours after an unprotected intercourse, this DES will often prevent pregnancy, causing changes in the uterine lining that make it inhospitable to the fertilized egg.

PLEASE NOTE: *This is an emergency procedure only and should not be considered as a regular form of birth control.*

There are two major reasons for this.

First, the safety of this pill is currently being questioned, since DES may be linked to certain forms of cancer and other medical problems. Women with a personal (or family) history of breast cancer or cancer of the reproductive tract should not take this hormone.

Women who have had hepatitis, heart disease, blood clots, or migraine headaches might also be advised against taking pills containing DES.

The second reason why the morning after pill is not a suitable form of ongoing birth control is this: It makes you sick, causing nausea and vomiting, dizziness and headaches during the days of treatment. While such symptoms may be preferable to an unwanted pregnancy, they would certainly be undesirable on a continuous basis.

For women who can't take DES or choose not to, the physician may insert an IUD (often a Copper 7) within a short time after intercourse. This would be, preferably, within 24 to 72 hours after unprotected intercourse. The IUD, which sets up an inflammatory reaction within the uterus, may also make the uterine lining inhospitable to the fertilized egg.

In studies involving women who had a Copper 7 inserted shortly after unprotected intercourse, the effectiveness of this method has been high and has not had the dangers and temporarily incapacitating side effects of DES. However, the IUD may cause some cramping and is not well-tolerated by some women.

The advantage of this method, though, is that the IUD may be left in place to offer continual contraceptive protection. But, of course, if you are thinking about getting an IUD, it's better to do so before having intercourse and a pregnancy scare.

Some women, after they have an unprotected intercourse, allow time to pass, waiting to see if they menstruate. When they don't and pregnancy is confirmed, they may opt for abortion. We will be discussing abortion at greater length in the next chapter. However, we would like to add here that, although an early legal abortion carries fewer health risks than pregnancy and childbirth, abortion does have its risks and may be relatively costly, both monetarily (when compared with common birth control methods) and emotionally. If abortion is an option you would consider, this, too, should be seen as an emergency procedure *only*—not as an ongoing form of birth control.

BIRTH CONTROL OF THE FUTURE

I'm 20 years old and have been using birth control for three years. I've gone from the Pill to the IUD and am now thinking about getting a diaphragm because I have some cramping and heavier periods with the IUD. The diaphragm won't be as convenient, but at least it won't hurt me. I hate to think of hassling with that for a lifetime though. Are there any new birth control discoveries coming up in the near or even the distant future that might be good?

Cindy S.

There are currently about 20 new contraceptives being researched and tested. Some or all of these may be available within the next ten years.

The following are only a few of the methods now being researched.

May Be Available Within the Next Two Years

The Collagen Sponge. Now being tested at the University of Arizona, this is much like a diaphragm, but scientists hope that it will be able to be used without cream or jelly and that it will be available over-the-counter. This small sponge, which can be inserted with a tamponlike device or by hand, is held in place by vaginal folds and may be left in for a number of days if desired. It is hoped that the sponge will prevent pregnancy not only by covering the cervix, but also, because of its acidity, by quickly deactivating sperm. The sponge may be available to the public late this year.

Once-a-Month Injections. These shots of synthetic hormones would do what birth control pills do now and may be more convenient for some. But safety and effect on future fertility are still being researched.

Contraceptive Implants. These are tiny rods containing contraceptive hormones that will be released constantly for one to five years. They will be put just beneath the skin in a woman's groin, arm, or buttock. This may be an effective long-term method of birth control, but the necessity of surgical implantation may make some shy away from this method.

New Breakthroughs in Rhythm. There are two small devices that may help to determine more accurately when ovulation occurs for couples who opt for the rhythm method of birth control. One of these devices notes changes in cervical mucus. The other, a small electrical device, measures electrical changes that may be linked to ovulation. Neither of these devices, however, can eliminate one of the major problems of the rhythm method: the necessity of sexual abstinence for a major portion of every month.

Reversible Sterilization. This is being researched particularly with men who have had vasectomies, using microsurgery to reconnect the severed vas. However, at this time, not all men achieve full fertility, even after such surgery.

May Be Available Within Ten Years

Birth Control Pill for Men. This pill, which contains male hormones, would block sperm production. Preliminary tests show mixed results in reducing fertility entirely and the male pill has some undesirable side effects. Since much more research is needed, it may be ten years before this is available.

Contraceptive Vaccine. Given to women, a single injection would block production of HCG, the substance that nourishes the fertilized egg. However, researchers are not sure yet whether this method may be reversible.

Vaginal Rings. A small plastic ring containing a synthetic preparation of the hormone progesterone would be placed in the vagina near the cervix and would gradually release the hormone, preventing ovulation. There are still a number of side effects that researchers are studying and the rings may not be available for some time.

These and other future advances in birth control methods may be exciting to contemplate.

However, there is a great deal you can do right now to prevent the tragedy of an unplanned, unwanted pregnancy. The birth control devices we have now are, in many instances, quite effective. But the crucial element for the success or failure of any birth control method is your own motivation to use a contraceptive and your determination to make it work. Personal responsibility is the most important ingredient in any method of birth control.

CHAPTER THIRTEEN

Pregnancy and Parenthood

CONSIDERING PARENTHOOD

I'm 14 years old and I want to have a baby. I try to be very sensible and think of the unfairness it would bring to a child to be without a father and to my family, but I still want to get pregnant. If I do have a baby, do you think it might be abnormal because I'm so young? Do you think I could take care of it? I'm pretty mature for my age and I've got a way with children. I love kids a lot and I'd be willing to get a job and support my child. I don't know what to do. I want a child very badly, but I want the best for it and don't want to live to regret it later on. What do you think I should do?

Anonymous

My husband and I are both 22 and graduating from college this year. We've been married for eight months. We don't know whether to have a baby within the next year or wait for a while. We're trying to see parenting in a realistic light and to decide whether it's for us at this point in our lives. We want children very much. It's just a question of . . . when?

Melody K.

I'm engaged to a wonderful guy and we plan to be married in August. We've been making a lot of plans for our life together and are not really sure children will fit into these plans. We are both very ambitious and plan to get graduate degrees and have lifelong careers. We'd also like to travel a lot. But Gene and I feel guilty. Especially when our parents go on about how nice it will be to be grandparents and how selfish childless people are. How can we make a decision we can live with?

Cynthia M.

Parenthood—or nonparenthood—is one of the most important choices you'll ever make. Because this choice can affect your life tremendously and, possibly, the life of a child as well, it is a decision that must be made with care, NOT left to chance!

Whether you're single or married, in early adolescence or in your twenties, there are some vitally important points to consider if you are thinking about having a baby.

1. *What are my plans for my own future?*

Do you have specific educational, career, or life-style goals?

How close are you to meeting these goals?

What do/will these goals require in terms of time, money, concentration, and personal flexibility?

If you *don't* have clear-cut goals, have you thought about your future in terms of how you will support yourself—and, possibly, a child?

If you have very hazy ideas about this and are thinking of having a baby, think twice.

This is especially important if you are single and a teen-ager. It has been found in various studies that teen-agers who get pregnant do not realize, in most cases, the power they possess to guide their own destinies. They tend to feel that life just happens to them.

Taking such a passive view of life, they may shrug off concerns about support, passing the responsibility on to others.

Some may say "Oh, my parents will help me to support and care for my baby."

This may be so—for a while. But such an arrangement cannot go on indefinitely. You may find yourself locked in a power struggle with your own mother over your baby's care and affections. You may find, too, that your parents may not be eager or able to assume the time commitment and expense of raising another child for the next 18 to 20 years.

A number of young women may say "Oh, I'll get married . . ."

However, many marriages today are ending in divorce, especially when both parents are under the age of 20 and there is a pregnancy involved in the decision to marry. Even in a stable marriage, many young couples need two incomes, for a time at least, just to make ends meet.

Many young people will say "Oh, well, I'll get a job . . ."

Good jobs do not abound, however. And if you're underage, undereducated, and lack a marketable skill, getting a job may be almost impossible.

So whatever your life situation at the moment, a marketable skill and *at least* a high school diploma are vital survival tools.

These will give you more choices and alternatives in life and will help to make parenthood, when it comes, an active, positive choice, not something that just happens because you have nothing else to do with your life.

2. *Why do I want a baby?*

There are many reasons that people voice for having children:

"To carry on the family name."

"It's the normal thing to do!"

"We wanted to share our love with another, to nurture another human being."

"We have so much to give."

"Our parents expected grandchildren."

"Because a woman is not complete until she has a child."

"Having kids means you're a man!"

"I wanted to show everyone I was grown up!"

"To have someone to love me."

These are a few reasons people have given us. There are many others. Reasons for having a baby are very personal and we are not saying that one reason is necessarily right or wrong. Most people have a number of reasons for deciding to become parents. Some of these reasons mirror expectations, however, that may bring inevitable disappointment.

For example, if your heart isn't in parenthood, if you're thinking of having a baby because you feel it's expected of you or to validate yourself as a man or woman or full-fledged adult, you may find yourself belatedly disappointed.

If you expect a baby to give you all the love you feel you lack, it may be a rude shock when you have this little stranger who makes enormous demands on *you* and on your time, energy, and patience!

3. *What do I expect of my baby?*

Some want a baby as a companion, as someone who will love them no matter what, or as security for old age.

Others see a baby as an instant fix-it for a faltering marriage or love relationship.

Some want miniature images of themselves—or of the selves they might have been.

Others want a flesh-and-blood version of the Ultimate Fantasy Child: the beautiful, cuddly, cooing, sweet-smelling baby who has an exotic name, precocious talents, and a high IQ. This child is also of a certain sex. (Statistics show that most first-time parents or would-be parents tend to prefer boys.)

Reality is often somewhat different.

A baby, especially for the first months of life, is by necessity self-centered and demanding. Only with time will the child possibly come to see and appreciate your needs, and even so, your needs may always come second. And the child may not be able to fill them—ever.

Babies cannot even help themselves, let alone your marriage or relationship. In fact, the changes that a baby may bring into your life may intensify any relationship problems that exist.

Babies are also separate people who may or may not resemble their parents. They cannot always achieve what we couldn't, nor do they always choose to try.

So, if the image of the Ultimate Fantasy Child has been haunting you, consider the following questions:

Would you love your child not as a mirror image of you, but as a separate person?

If your heart is set on a son, could you love and welcome a daughter? Or will only the desired sex do? If you have an inflexible sex preference for your baby, you have about a 50 percent chance of being disappointed. But it may be the child who suffers most.

Could you love your child as an average person?

Most kids will not be beauties or prize-winning scholars. But average children need just as much or more loving affirmation and care.

Real-life babies can be delightful and distressing. They can be charming and cuddly. They also have a penchant for screaming in the night, going through piles of diapers daily, and spitting up, quite systematically, on every piece of clothing you own. This is normal for a baby.

It's important to know that a baby is very helpless and dependent, especially at first. What you give this little person is much more important than what you'll get.

4. *What can I give my baby?*

Most of us want the very best for our children.

Can you offer your baby the best right now?

Unconditional love, a fair amount of economic security and freedom from hunger, and the emotional support of two parents is the ideal.

The ideal, of course, is not always possible.

Divorce, for example, has created a number of single-parent homes. While it may be preferable for a child to grow up in a loving single-parent home rather than a strife-torn two-parent home, the best possible situation is a two-parent situation where the couple's relationship is reasonably stable and loving, where *both* parents actively participate in the child's care and nurturing, and where there is a certain amount of economic security.

Single-parent families, especially when the parent is a woman under 25, do not fare as well. The suicide rate among teen mothers is seven times higher than the rate for teens without children. Young single mothers, struggling to cope, may be more likely to emotionally neglect or physically abuse their children. And, in a recent Rand Corporation survey in California, it was found that 90 percent of single-parent families, in which the household head was under 25, were on welfare. It was found that these parents—usually mothers—"are substantially underschooled, under-trained, and underskilled. . . ."

"It is difficult and time-consuming for *two* people to raise a child successfully and it can be even more difficult for a single parent," says noted child psychologist Dr. Lee Salk, whose book *Preparing for Parenthood: Understanding Your Feelings About Pregnancy, Childbirth and Your Baby* is an excellent guide for those contemplating parenthood. "Any single person planning to have a baby and raise it alone should be aware of the tremendous commitment this involves. It's easy to have a child, but difficult to be a parent."

While single parenthood does happen—through divorce, death of the other parent, or through unplanned pregnancies—Dr. Salk and others concerned with child welfare tend to discourage young people from the fourth cause of single parenthood: conscious and deliberate choice to conceive, give birth, and raise a child alone.

"It always raises a question in my mind whether these people who deliberately decide to be single parents are doing so in the best interests of the child or for the satisfaction of some unknown or hidden self-interest," says Dr. Salk.

Parenthood can be tough for a man or woman of any age. Although a baby may bring you very special joy, the emphasis will be on what you can give. In many instances, the child's needs will have to come before yours. The hardships and sacrifices involved are not always easy for anyone, but may be especially hard to take if you're still in the process of growing up and are feeling really needy, too.

Some young mothers cope beautifully with the demands of parenthood. Others can't face the responsibility at all. It may be helpful for you to know something about what is expected of you and the awesome responsibilities of parenthood before you're in the position of having to cope with such realities.

5. *Am I ready for the responsibilities of parenthood?*

Parenthood is a 24-hour-a-day, 18-year commitment *at the very least!*

It may involve giving up a certain amount of personal freedom and privacy, curtailing your social life, and being constantly concerned with your child's needs.

Many young people become parents before they realize how real and ever-present these responsibilities will be.

"Before Jennifer was born, I couldn't quite grasp the fact that she was a *person*," says Vicki, 17, who is married and the mother of a seven-month-old daughter. "I figured she'd cry and I'd feed her and that would be it. But that wasn't it! I was almost overwhelmed at first by her constant, unrelenting dependence on me. . . ."

Joy, 18, married and the mother of two children, says that "you do miss being free. . . . Tim and I used to go to the movies whenever we wanted to, but with two babies, I have to feed them, get bottles ready, and try to find a sitter. We stay home a lot. When I had my first baby, I was 16 and had a difficult time at first. I thought I could play with her and have fun right from the start. But all she did at first was cry, sleep, and eat. That was rough."

To give her "Adult Living" students an idea of what parental responsibility is like, a resourceful young Des Moines, Iowa, teacher named Jacqueline Schlemmer gives each of her students custody of a fresh, uncooked egg for a week. For the entire week, the student must carry the egg with him or her. If he/she will be pursuing an activity where it would be dangerous or highly inconvenient to carry the egg, the student must find someone else to care for it temporarily. Her students report that the exercise makes a strong impression. "It seemed like I was planning *everything* around that egg!" sighed one female student.

This situation is quite similar to parenthood, especially when a baby is involved.

Are you ready to plan much of your current life around a baby?

Are you ready to give up freedom to come and go as you please?

There are important points to consider honestly before you become a parent.

6. *Should I be a parent at all?*

How do you really feel about kids?

Do you enjoy them or barely tolerate them?

Do you like to spend a lot of time with them or does the idea turn you off?

Do you have a lot of patience?

Do you view parenthood as an exciting challenge or a grim duty?

Do you view parenthood as something to be anticipated?

When you dream of the future—as you really want it to be—are children in the picture at all?

These are some things you should consider before becoming a parent.

Of course, not all parents enjoy their kids and not all childless couples dislike children. And many people have very normal ambivalent feelings about parenthood. Maybe you're one of them. At times, you really feel you want a child. Then you see a toddler tantrum at the market or think of how you want to build a career, and you wonder if parenthood is for you. You may need time to be with your feelings, both positive and negative, before making a commitment one way or another. In time, you may discover that you feel predominantly that you do—or don't—want to have children.

You may opt for responsible parenthood, making sure before pregnancy occurs that you are in a position to meet your baby's needs without expecting him or her to meet yours.

You may opt for responsible nonparenthood, either temporary or permanent.

If you feel that you're not ready for a baby right now, waiting until you do feel better equipped to handle the unique demands of parenthood is a perfectly reasonable option, despite peer or family pressure to have a baby now. (This may be especially likely if you are married and in your twenties.)

You may feel, however, that parenthood is simply not for you—now or ever. This, too, is a viable life option.

Being childless (or "childfree") by choice is an often misunderstood life-style. In an attempt to educate the public about nonparenthood, the National Organization for Non-Parents (N.O.N.) came to be. Members of N.O.N. are single and married, parents and nonparents who believe that the childfree life-style is acceptable and should be respected, with no social or economic discrimination against couples who have no children.

What members of N.O.N. and many other nonparents try to point out is that being childfree does not mean that you hate children or want nothing to do with nurturing the next generation. Many nonparents, in fact, have more time and energy to devote to social causes, many of these for the benefit of children. They may be in a number of occupations, including teaching, social work, medicine, counseling, the arts, and any number of other professions that may help the younger generation.

Nonparents are often called selfish, but, in many cases, this is an unfair accusation. If you do not want to be a parent or feel unsuited to parenthood, it would be extremely selfish to bring a child into the world—just to avoid social criticism. (It may also be selfish to have a baby just to validate your femininity or masculinity or in an attempt to strengthen a faltering love or marriage relationship.)

Many parents have children for very unselfish and loving reasons. These same reasons may enter into another person's decision not to have a child. So labeling is unfair.

Actually, fewer people these days are likely to label you as selfish or abnormal if you choose not to have children. In the past few years, the question "Should I be a parent?" has been asked more and more. And the childfree life option is becoming more common and more widely accepted.

Whatever your decision about parenthood may be, it's important to give yourself a lot of time to think about it.

Parenthood can certainly be rewarding. It will also affect your life for years to come.

In choosing parenthood at a very early age, you may lose other life options—like further education, fulfilling employment, financial security, or a chance to come first for a while longer as you grow toward adulthood.

While researching and writing their new book *The Parent Test: How to Measure and Develop Your Talent for Parenthood,* Dr. William Granzig and Ellen Peck noted that parents who had the most positive feelings about parenthood tended to be those who had started their families after the age of 25.

"Time to do what you want before becoming a parent is very important," says Dr. Granzig. "So is maturity. Those who have babies at an early age may tend to live vicariously through their children or blame them for any misfortunes. On the other hand, those we surveyed who had babies while in their mid-twenties or later tended to accept the choice as their own and did not shift blame to their children. The old myth we used to hear was 'Have your children while you're young!' A more fitting motto these days might be 'Grow up first!' "

It's up to you which options you choose. But it is important to be aware of what you might gain and what you might give up before you become a parent.

It is also important to realize that, whatever your choice may be, it is *your* choice. You may choose actively, making a conscious decision to get pregnant. Or you may choose passively, letting pregnancy "just happen" to you. Whether planned or allegedly unplanned, pregnancy and parenthood are your responsibilities. It isn't fair to blame a baby who didn't ask to be born for holding you back from your dreams or causing you hardship.

Part of being a good parent means being responsible for yourself and responsive to your child's needs. It also means being prepared for the challenge of raising another human being from infancy to adulthood.

"I THINK I MAY BE PREGNANT . . ."

I'm scared I may be pregnant even though I haven't had sexual intercourse. My boyfriend and I have done everything but and I'm late with my period. Is it possible I could get pregnant without intercourse? What does it take for pregnancy to happen?

Lisa

What are the symptoms of pregnancy? Before it shows, I mean? Please tell me quick!!!

Scared

My mom and I were talking about pregnancy the other day and we both wonder if there's a way you can find out if you're pregnant without going to the doctor?

Curious

How pregnancy occurs is a mystery to many young people. Most know, of course, that pregnancy usually occurs as a result of sexual intercourse, but many wonder exactly what time of the month it is most likely to happen and whether it can occur as a result of heavy petting as well as intercourse.

Many factors are involved in the process of conception.

The female's egg, or ovum, must be fertilized by the male's sperm. While a man releases sperm whenever he ejaculates, a woman usually releases only one egg each month during ovulation. Although this is most likely to occur in mid-cycle between menstrual periods, the exact time of ovulation is very difficult to determine and has been known to occur at all times in the cycle. So it's almost impossible to know for sure whether or not you can get pregnant on a particular day.

Pregnancy may not occur at the exact time or day you have intercourse. The egg—once released—will live about two days. Sperm can survive in the uterus and Fallopian tubes for about the same amount of time. Fertilization could occur, then, at any time during these crucial days.

Pregnancy is usually the result of sexual intercourse, but it can happen as a result of heavy petting if the man ejaculates close to the vagina or if he secretes a clear, lubricating fluid (which may contain sperm) close to the vaginal opening. These sperm may travel into the vagina and then on to the uterus, and pregnancy may occur. This is not the most common way to get pregnant, but it has happened.

What if you think you may be pregnant?

What are the symptoms of pregnancy?

Usually, a missed menstrual period may be your first clue to pregnancy, but this is not invariably the case.

You may skip a period if you're not eating properly, if you are under a great deal of stress, or if you're afraid of getting pregnant. This fear may cause you to display other signs of pregnancy, too. Such false pregnancy symptoms are called *pseudocyesis*.

Other symptoms of pregnancy may be: feeling tired *all* the time—even when you've had adequate rest; tenderness and swelling of the breasts, similar to what may happen before your period, but this persists rather than going away after a few days; more frequent than usual urination; a more copious vaginal discharge; and morning sickness. This feeling of queasiness and possible vomiting can happen at any time of the day (especially when you smell food cooking), but it is often most likely to strike just as you're getting out of bed in the morning. This sickness is triggered by high levels of HCG (human chorionic gonadotrophin) which the fetus produces at an especially high level during the first three months. This is why morning sickness is most likely to occur in early pregnancy.

These symptoms are a signal to check with a physician. Only he/she can confirm an early pregnancy via urine and/or blood tests and a physical examination.

In the physical exam, the physician may note changes in the size and firmness of the uterus as well as a bluish hue to the cervix. All of these may be signs of pregnancy.

Tests can confirm this. A urine test to measure HCG levels in the urine will diagnose pregnancy 42 days after conception—or when you've missed two periods. However, a blood test, measuring HCG in your bloodstream, can diagnose pregnancy with greater accuracy as early as seven days after conception.

The Food and Drug Administration recently approved a new test called Biocept G (from Wampole Laboratories). This test can measure HCG levels in blood or urine as early as one day after the first missed menstrual period or approximately ten days after conception. The results of this test can be available within an hour.

Early, accurate pregnancy testing is vital. It can be obtained from your physician, from an adolescent clinic, or from Planned Parenthood (see Appendix) at no or low cost.

Why is early diagnosis of pregnancy important?

The first three months of fetal development are crucial and the sooner you know you are pregnant, the sooner you can take precautions, like avoiding drugs, alcohol, and other habits that may endanger your baby's health. (More on this later.)

Second, if this is a "problem pregnancy"—either a health risk, unplanned, unwanted, or premature (in a young adolescent mother)—you may need to review your options and make a decision about what you will do early in the pregnancy.

While such a problem pregnancy may make you feel scared and alone, making you wish it would just go away, it's important to find out for sure if you are pregnant. If you aren't, you can stop worrying (and start taking reliable birth control precautions to avoid such scares in the future). If you are pregnant, you will have more time to decide which option you will choose.

WHEN CAN PREGNANCY BE A PROBLEM?

I'm 16 and have a very serious problem. I'm pregnant. I don't know whether to have an abortion or to have the baby. I'd kind of like to have the baby because I know I could raise it by myself and I love to play with little kids. What should I do?

Helpless

I'm pregnant (three months along) and am 15 years old. This could ruin my whole life. I don't want to have a baby! I can't have a baby!! There's no one to talk to. I can't talk to my parents. This baby would ruin all the plans I've made for the future. What can I do about the mess I've made of my life?

Sorry

I'm 12 years old and have an extremely big problem. I'm slightly pregnant. I don't know who the father is. I'm about five months along (I think) and so far I've been able to hide it from my parents, but I don't know how much longer I can. If they find out, I'll be in deep trouble, since I'm only 12. What can I do?

Katie

Many people equate a "problem pregnancy" with an unplanned, unwanted one. This is often, but not always, the case. An unplanned and unwanted pregnancy can certainly cause emotional anguish, possible health risks and, in some cases, limited life options.

But not all problem pregnancies are really unplanned—or unwanted.

Some may be in the problem category because of parental medical problems or disease possibilities. Some mothers (for example, diabetic mothers) may need special care during pregnancy. Some young couples who may be carriers of hereditary disorders like sickle-cell anemia or Tay-Sachs disease may be at risk of producing an afflicted child and need some genetic counseling. (Some of these couples may opt for a test

called *amniocentesis* in which a needle is inserted into the uterus fairly early in pregnancy and a sample of the amniotic fluid drawn out for examination. If the fluid cells show that the child is afflicted, the couple may opt for abortion or may prepare for the birth of a child with special needs.)

Other pregnancies may constitute a problem because they are *premature*. That is, they are occurring in mothers who may be too young and/or immature to care for a child adequately. In some cases, the mother may be so young that her health may be endangered significantly by the pregnancy.

Some recent statistics:

• More than one million teen-age girls get pregnant every year, one third of them intentionally.

• While birth rates have started to decline in all age groups including older teens, the birth rate is increasing rapidly in the *10- to 14-year-old* age group! These are the mothers who have the highest risk of a myriad of complications.

• The death risk for mothers under the age of 15 is 60 percent higher than for mothers over 20.

• Babies born to young teen-age mothers are two to three times more likely to die in their first year of life.

• Babies born to teen mothers are twice as likely to have low birth weight (implicated in many infant deaths and physical and mental defects).

• Health risks for teen-age mothers may be increased due to a number of factors. Lack of prenatal care is one of these. It is estimated that 70 percent of these teen-age mothers get no medical care at all during the critical first three months of pregnancy and 25 percent get none at all until their babies are born. This lack of medical care is especially dangerous for teens. A very young body may be able to conceive a baby, but carrying a baby to term may be extremely stressful. Teen mothers are more likely to have high blood pressure, toxemia, prolonged and difficult labor, more vaginal lacerations during childbirth, and more after-delivery complications and infections. To minimize these medical risks, good medical care is vital!

A premature pregnancy can be a problem from a nonmedical standpoint, too.

Young teen mothers are likely to drop out of school and face a high risk of unemployment, poverty, and welfare dependence. If they marry due to the pregnancy, their risk of divorce is high. The young mother is also, statistically speaking, more likely to be angered and disillusioned by her baby's demands and may become an abusive parent.

Each mother is a distinct individual, of course. Some young women make wonderful mothers and manage to build satisfying lives for themselves as well. Unfortunately, however, these tend to be in the minority.

Chances are, then, if you are a pregnant teen-ager, your pregnancy is a problem for you and/or your family.

WHAT ALTERNATIVES DO YOU HAVE?

Basically, you have four options if you are pregnant: have the baby and keep it, have the baby and give it up for adoption, marry the father and have the baby, or have an abortion.

No one of these options is right for everybody. Not all will be available or acceptable to everyone. Not one of these is an *easy* option. But there may be one that is best for you, given your unique circumstances.

You may find that those around you have a lot of opinions about what you should do. For example, some teens have told us that they would have preferred to give their babies up for adoption, but they were afraid that their peers would put them down for "copping out" and not keeping the baby. Others have complained that their parents just assumed that they would end the pregnancy through abortion. These are only two examples of pressures you may encounter. Pressures exist, but you have to live with your decision.

To make a responsible decision, listen to what your parents, physician, or counselor may be saying, but also listen to your own feelings. Consider the direction you want your life to go, what you could or could not offer as a parent and talk about this with those close to you. Together, you may work toward making a decision you can live with.

We are not advocating one option above another. We will simply review the four choices that you may be facing, giving you brief information about each choice and opinions from young people who have been there.

Have the Baby and Keep It.

This is an option that many teens are choosing.

We've already talked about some of the pitfalls of single motherhood for a teen: the risk of being under-educated, unemployed, impoverished, and disillusioned by the demands of parenthood.

Obviously, this is not the story for everyone. Some young mothers cope well with the parenting challenge, sometimes with the loving support of their families.

The Children's Home Society in California runs rap groups for teen mothers to help them to cope with

parenthood, and some of the mothers one sees in these rap groups are, indeed, coping well.

Johanna, 17 and the mother of an infant daughter, has just graduated from high school. She plans to study for a career as a nurse at a local junior college. Her mother takes care of her baby when Johanna is at school, but once she gets home, the baby is entirely Johanna's responsibility. While Johanna enjoys her daughter and looks forward to combining a satisfying career with motherhood, she is quick to add that, even in a situation as promising as hers, there are sacrifices to be made. "I don't go out at all between going to school and taking care of the baby," she says. "Being a mother means a lot of responsibility and loss of freedom to come and go. This rap group is my big night out each week!"

Robin, who became a mother at 17, is another resourceful and determined young woman who has managed to finish high school, take college classes toward a degree in social work, and support herself and her daughter with her wages from an office job. Robin and her daughter, Sashya, live in a modest apartment. An aunt looks after Sashya while Robin works. "Life is not without problems," says Robin. "But things seem to be working out. Having a baby is a huge responsibility, but it shouldn't mean giving up your whole life. I get so upset with some girls I know who give up and don't try to grow or become persons in their own right. I've experienced a lot of pain and a lot of changes since Sashya was born, but I've grown because of these."

A young woman named Ogie is an outstanding example of a mother who is coping beautifully with single parenthood. Her son, Patrick, is a beautiful, charming, intelligent, and happy toddler. Ogie is patient, mature, and enthusiastic. She also had a high school diploma and job skills before she became pregnant. Patrick attends nursery school while Ogie works in the office of a local hospital. Ogie admits, however, that there are some times when even a child as delightful as Patrick can try her patience. "But I'm careful of his feelings," she says. "He's little, but he *is* a separate person with feelings of his own. I'm learning to be careful with them."

Others do not fare as well.

Laurie, whose baby nearly died at birth (she was 16, had not received early prenatal care, and her baby was premature) is now trying to cope with the demands of an active, independent little boy who is visually handicapped. Sometimes it gets to be too much for her. "It would be OK if he'd mind," she sighs. "But he's learned the word *no*. When he throws a tantrum, I make him stand against the wall with his nose touching it and if he cries, I make fun of him, calling him a big crybaby!"

Sandra, 15, has two children already—the elder 18 months old. She neglects both babies, not because she doesn't love them, but because she finds it hard at her age to take on the awesome responsibility of two children consistently. As she watches her daughter grow and learn to speak, Sandra looks wistful. "She knows the names for lots of things and people now," she says sadly. "But she almost never says 'Mama.' Almost never." In her eyes, there is a flash of longing for a myriad of emotional needs unmet.

"When children get older and more independent, many single teen mothers realize they can't cope and give their babies up for foster care or adoption," says Charlotte De Armand of the Children's Home Society in Los Angeles. "This can be an emotional trauma for mother and child. And older children are much harder to place for adoption."

CHS social worker Claudia Chase laments the fact that often those single mothers most in need of special help are the least inclined to seek or accept such help. "Not long ago, I visited a girl who had turned 13 only two weeks before her baby was born," says Claudia. "She sat there in her room surrounded by dolls, with her own live doll in her arms, insisting that she didn't need our help, that she could cope alone."

Most single teen mothers cannot cope alone. Unless you have an extremely supportive family, special services like the Children's Home Society or the National Alliance Concerned with School-Age Parents (NACSAP) (see Special Needs Resources in Appendix), an adequate education and marketable skills, the going can be rough.

At best, single motherhood means a lot of hard work, resourcefulness, and sacrifices. Some people handle this challenge very well. Others can't handle it at all and all too often it is the child who suffers most.

If you're thinking of keeping your baby, consider your situation and your feelings honestly and share your thoughts with people who may be able to help you to decide how ready and able you may be to assume the challenge of single motherhood.

Have the Baby and Give It Up for Adoption.

This alternative, which used to be the one most often chosen by unmarried mothers, is less frequently the *first* option chosen these days, but some young mothers who find they cannot cope with their babies put them up for adoption at a later date.

Since later relinquishments and adoptions can be a trauma for both mother and child and since a child's chances to be adopted decrease as he or she grows out of the infancy stage, health professionals strongly encourage young mothers considering this choice to make the choice either before the baby is born or as soon as possible after the birth of the child.

This choice can, in many cases, be best for the baby. Extensive studies of some 17,000 children, which were revealed at the International Planned Parenthood Congress in Sydney, Australia, pointed up the fact that children conceived and born out of wedlock fare better when placed for adoption. Adopted children in this study were more confident and better adjusted socially than those who had remained with the natural mother.

These days there are many more would-be adoptive parents than available babies and adoption agencies can be highly selective in screening and choosing prospective parents. Particularly if your child is a healthy infant, his/her chances of placement in a fine, loving adoptive home are excellent.

While adoption may, in many cases, be the best alternative for the baby, making such a decision may be very difficult for the mother.

"When you're pregnant, it's very easy to say you're going to give your baby up," says 17-year-old Julie. "But when my baby boy was born and I saw him for the first time after nine months, it was very hard. It hurt very, very much to give him up. But you have to think of the child, not yourself. I am told that my baby is happy with two wonderful adoptive parents who love him dearly. I will always miss him, wonder about him, and hurt a little about this. But I won't let it get me down because I know I did the best thing for him and for myself."

Sandi, 17, just graduated from high school, a year after giving her baby boy up for adoption. "I felt a mixture of grief and relief when I gave my baby up," she says. "But I feel I gave *both* of us a chance at life. I'll always wonder about him, but I know the agency found a good home for him. I know that two parents who want a baby enough to go through the screening of an adoption will give him more than I could right now. I'm glad to have the chance to pick up my life—to graduate and go to college. If I had kept the baby, this wouldn't be possible and I might come to resent the baby for that."

"I've grown up on welfare and it's a bad way to live," says 15-year-old Deb. "So when I got pregnant and had a baby at 13, I gave her up for adoption. I wanted the best for her. I don't want to live my whole life in poverty. A good education will help me to get a good job and live a good life, so that when I have kids I can give them the best. I'm not trying to say that my decision or my life since I gave up the baby is peaches and cream. It was hard, really hard to give up my baby. But I couldn't have made it. It was the best decision for both of us. But that doesn't mean a peachy happy ending to the story. You know, a nice ending where everything turns out for the best and nobody gets hurt. That's not true. You *do* get hurt—no matter what choice you make and however sensible or right it is for you.''

Making the decision to give up your baby for adoption is not an easy one, but there are many excellent services that can help you to weigh the pros and cons to see if this may be the right option for you. There are a number of excellent agencies. Crittenton Services and BirthRite, which operate nationwide, and the Children's Home Society in California are among the best known and most established of the nonjudgmental services.

Marry the Father and Have the Baby.

While the statistics on teen marriages, especially those prompted by pregnancy, may be grim, showing a divorce rate twice that of other couples, there *are* teen couples who are coping with both early marriage and parenthood.

''While I wouldn't always encourage people to try it and while I realize that my husband and I are the exceptions to the rule, I just wanted to say that early marriage and parenthood don't always mean unhappiness,'' says Peggy, 19, who has been married for two years and has an 18-month-old daughter.

There are many variables: the age, education, and maturity levels of the couple, how supportive their families are, and whether or not the couple would have married anyway—minus the pregnancy crisis. Those couples who planned to marry eventually—pregnancy or not—may adapt best to the sudden new responsibilities and demands. It can be quite an adjustment, however.

Vicki, 17, married for a year and the mother of a seven-month-old daughter, says that she and her husband have always loved each other very much. ''But right after the baby came, our relationship was very shaky,'' she says. ''Greg felt left out and jealous of the time I spent with the baby. He's over that now, but for a time it was very trying. Jennifer is very attached to Greg now and that helps a lot. Also, at first, both of us felt trapped, Greg as the family breadwinner and me at home with the baby. Finally, my mother agreed to watch the baby several hours a day so I could work part-time as a typist. So now Greg and I both work, take college courses at night, and share caring for the baby. We're lucky to have parents who help us, good educations and job skills, a healthy baby, and a wonderful doctor who has helped me over some real rough spots. But life isn't easy. I'm very young to be a wife, let alone a mother. My school friends have kind of drifted away. My life is so very different from theirs. So it's really just the three of us:

me, Greg, and the baby. Sometimes I get very lonely.''

''My high school friends don't come around much either,'' says Joy, 18, the married mother of two children. ''They've got different lives. All they worry about is clothes. I have a husband and family. But I feel I have a good life really. Money is our main problem. And since we have no car, we spend a lot of time at home. Marriage and motherhood is what I wanted, though.''

''I'd like Joy to have some career training and develop interests of her own,'' says her husband, Tim, 20. ''I think she should have pursuits and interests all her own. Joy has so much to offer as a person. I want her to make the most of herself.''

Not all teen marriages have two partners willing to work and sacrifice to cope with their new responsibilities, however.

''I married Chris when I was 16 and pregnant,'' says Linda, 18. ''He was 17 and the best student in the senior class. He was really looking forward to college. But I was afraid he'd meet someone else there, so I got pregnant so that he would marry me. I cried and begged and convinced him to forget about college and take a job in a shoe store and marry me. Our marriage, which lasted ten months, was a nightmare. He hated the job, hated not going to college, hated me, and resented the baby. He spent most of his time out with his friends. I never saw him. Finally he told me that he hated me, that I was ruining his life and he wanted a divorce. So now I'm 18, divorced, a high school dropout, a mother of one baby who has just hit the 'Terrible Two's.' I feel like my life is pretty much over—at only 18!''

''My husband was a nice person, but he was so restless and just too young to be married,'' says 19-year-old Jan, whose pregnancy at 16 prompted her marriage. The marriage ended in divorce when Jan was 18.

''I had stars in my eyes when I was 16,'' she says. ''I was happy to drop out of school and say good-bye to my ambition to become a fashion designer. I thought Joe and I would be happy forever. Instead, I found out how much you can grow and change in just a few short years. Now I'm trying to take up where I left off: finish school, get some training, get off welfare, and get a job. It isn't easy. And there's several years of my youth gone forever. I can never get those years back.''

Teen couples who do make it as marriage partners and parents seem to have a lot of love, a mutual commitment to struggle, and supportive others: families, counselors, physicians, and NACSAP affiliates (see Appendix) to help when the going is rough.

In making the decision whether or not to try marriage and parenthood simultaneously at a young age, it's important to determine if you are both willing to try—and if the two of you have outside help available for those rough times.

Have an Abortion.

This is a controversial option, but one chosen by many teens. It is estimated that about one in three abortions in the United States is performed on a teenager.

Although abortions have been legal in this country since the 1973 Supreme Court decision, antiabortion sentiment runs strong, especially in some areas. Some people have strong moral/religious objections to abortion, feeling that to end life at *any* time after conception is wrong. Without commenting on the political and moral issues, we simply want to point out that an abortion is fairly easy to obtain in most states, but may be difficult in states like Arkansas, Idaho, Louisiana, North Dakota, South Dakota, Utah, and West Virginia. Women who live in some of these states often choose to go to an adjacent state for an abortion, although legal abortions can be obtained within these states, too.

In general, legalizing abortion has not necessarily meant more abortions per se, simply more legal, *safe* abortions. In the days before abortion was legalized, great numbers of women died as a result of illegal abortions performed by incompetent practitioners or under unsanitary conditions with no proper medical follow-up. Many more died trying to induce their own abortion via a grim array of methods. The fact is, women have always had abortions and probably always will. The difference that legalization has made seems to be primarily in the area of greater safety for women.

Medically speaking, legal abortions—most of which are done in the first trimester (three months) of pregnancy—are usually very safe. Most of these early abortions are, statistically, nine times safer than carrying a pregnancy to term, according to a study by the Center for Disease Control in Atlanta. This difference may be intensified for teen-agers. While teens have a 60 percent higher death rate for pregnancy and childbirth than older mothers, they have the *lowest* abortion mortality rate!

What do abortions cost?

Generally, a first-trimester abortion done in a clinic may cost between $100 and $200. The more complicated second-trimester abortion can cost around $500 to $1,000.

How is an abortion performed?

First, pregnancy is confirmed and necessary lab tests are performed. Then the abortion may be done in one of several ways—often with a local anesthetic.

The *vacuum aspiration* method is used in 75 percent of first-trimester abortions. Here a small tube connected to a suction device is inserted through the cervix and the contents of the uterus are, in effect, vacuumed out.

In some cases, a spoon-shaped instrument called a *curette* may be used to scrape out the uterine contents. The procedure (which can also be done as a diagnostic test in nonpregnant women) is called a *dilation and curettage,* or D and C.

Both of these procedures are, with local anesthesia, essentially painless. Some women, however, may choose to have a general anesthetic. Having a general anesthesia may mean somewhat greater health risk and a few hours longer stay at the clinic. Usually, however, if you have a clinic abortion, you can be home the same day. Some women experience menstrual-like cramps for a while, but few have serious medical aftereffects.

It is more difficult—legally and medically—to perform an abortion during the second three months of pregnancy. The maternal health risks are greater, doctors willing to perform these are fewer, and the expense and pain considerably more.

Here, a saline or prostaglandin solution is injected into the uterus, replacing the amniotic fluid. This causes the death of the fetus, which is then expelled within 24 hours. This can be a painful procedure—both physically and emotionally—since it involves going into labor and giving birth to a dead fetus. In some areas, such an abortion is done only in case of dire need, and many states have laws setting time limits—often 20 or 24 weeks gestation—after which an abortion may not be performed at all.

Some medical facilities are now doing a combination of suction and D and C techniques for second-trimester pregnancies with, reportedly, safe results.

Those working in the abortion, family, and sexuality counseling services, however, emphasize that an early abortion is preferable and that abortion is no substitute for reliable birth control measures.

"The decision to have an abortion may be a painful one," says sex educator and counselor Elizabeth Canfield. "What most of us are advocating is *not* abortion per se, but freedom of choice to have a safe, legal abortion. No woman should ever be compelled to have an abortion against her will. No woman should have to continue a pregnancy she doesn't want either."

What emotional aftereffects can abortion have?

According to a Harvard study, 91 percent of postabortion patients studied felt relieved and at peace with their choice. Much depends, of course, on how the woman felt about having an abortion and how those around her reacted.

"If a girl feels forced into an abortion by her parents or her boyfriend, or if she has strong convictions against abortion, she may have emotional problems afterward," says Rev. Hugh Anwyl of the Clergy Counseling Service in Los Angeles. "Some of these girls may become pregnant again right away to replace the fetus that was lost."

Recent studies have indicated that about 25 percent of women who have aborted a pregnancy may have postabortion depression. Some health professionals feel that this may be due only in part to emotional responses; others point out that such depression may be due largely to hormonal reactions, the same that may occur after childbirth, when such feelings are called postpartum depression or postpartum blues. The end of pregnancy by abortion or by childbirth brings a number of hormonal changes in the body and this may trigger a feeling of depression as well in some women.

Other women many feel depressed because they feel guilty and that they have done something that many people would see as a crime. It is significant, perhaps, that studies in Japan, where abortion has been legal and socially sanctioned for years, show no feelings of guilt at all among women having abortions.

Reactions to abortion in this country may vary a great deal, however.

"I was relieved, just relieved afterward," says 18-year-old Ellen. "The doctor and nurses at the clinic were great. I talked to the counselor there for a long time and felt that I was really making the right decision. I hope I'm never in the position of having an unwanted pregnancy and abortion again, but I don't feel guilty or like my life has been scarred by the abortion."

"It wasn't really physically painful and everyone was real nice," says Betty, 17. "But I cried afterward. I wondered what the baby might have been and wondered if I had made the right decision. One of my girl friends has refused to speak to me since, except for calling me a 'murderer' when she found out about the abortion. I felt terrible about that. But my parents have helped me a lot and so did the counselor at the clinic. I felt depressed for a time. It still hurts when I think about it. Maybe it always will. I feel like I probably did make the right decision for me, but who can say—really?"

Only you can decide whether abortion may be the right decision for you. Counselors at Planned Parenthood clinics across the country can help you to review your options in a clear, unbiased way. The Planned Parenthood-Clergy Counseling Service affiliates (listed in the Appendix) can offer you a wide range of services from pregnancy testing to nonjudgmental counseling to abortion referrals if abortion is the option you choose.

HEALTHY PREGNANCY/HEALTHY BABY

My husband and I (both 22) are planning to have only one or two children and are thinking about having our first baby within the next year. I want the baby to be as healthy as possible. What steps can I take during pregnancy or even before pregnancy to insure that our baby will be normal and healthy?

Marlene B.

I'm 17 and three months pregnant. This isn't a planned baby. I plan either to keep it or to give it up for adoption. I got a pregnancy test at a clinic and the nurse there was talking about getting prenatal care and how important this is. How soon should I get it?

Val

Planning for a healthy baby should start long before conception and continue through pregnancy.

Before You Become Pregnant

• Have a complete physical examination, including blood tests to determine whether you are immune to rubella (German measles) and to discover, if you don't know already, what blood type you have.

If you are Rh negative and have had a previous pregnancy (even one that ended in miscarriage or abortion), some medical precautions may have to be taken during your future pregnancy to safeguard your future baby's health against the Rh antibodies that may have built up in your bloodstream.

While some states require a blood test to determine a woman's immunity to rubella (as well as to make sure that neither she nor the man has syphilis) before a couple can get a marriage license, if you are planning to conceive soon, be sure to have this blood test if you are not married or if you live in a state where the premarital rubella titer test is not required.

If the test shows that you are susceptible to rubella, you should get a vaccination, which is usually effective for a lifetime, *at least four months before you stop taking contraceptives*. Waiting four months and having a follow-up blood test to make sure that the vaccination took will help you to be certain that you have no live virus in your system and that you are, indeed, immune.

Why is immunity to rubella so important?

While German measles is a rather mild disease in adults and many children, it can be a disaster for a fetus, especially one in its first three months of development in the womb. Rubella can cause miscarriages and numerous birth defects, including mental retardation, eye and heart disorders, and deafness—among others. If the fetus is infected during its first month of development, chances are about 50 percent that it will have significant abnormalities.

(If you are already pregnant and are not immune to rubella, do not take the vaccine. Simply try to avoid exposure to the disease during your first trimester.)

A pre-pregnancy physical examination will also pinpoint any health problems that may need to be treated with medication *before* conception occurs. It will also give you a chance to talk with your doctor if you have a chronic condition that may require special care and medication during pregnancy. It's important to discuss with your doctor what effect, if any, such medication would have on the baby.

• Minimize the obvious risks. Statistics show that if you have a baby before you're 20 years old or less than two years after a previous pregnancy, the risks that the infant will die can be 50 to 100 percent greater. While some young mothers have healthy babies in closely spaced intervals, they tend to be the lucky ones. We get no guarantees about a baby's health, but waiting until your body is fully mature and better able to nurture the growing fetus and spacing pregnancies in at least two-year intervals can put the odds in your favor.

• If you have a family history of genetic disorders, like hemophilia, sickle-cell anemia, Tay-Sachs disease, or muscular dystrophy, for example, do get genetic counseling. Your physician may be able to refer you to someone who can counsel you, or your local March of Dimes office will be able to give you more information about this. Many couples who are carriers of genetic disorders may elect to conceive and then, once pregnancy is under way, the woman will have a test called amniocentesis. As we discussed previously, an analysis of the cells in a sample of the amniotic fluid withdrawn may reveal if the child is afflicted with one of a number of genetic disorders that can be spotted in this way. The test also reveals the sex of the child, which may be significant in cases where there is a family history of hemophilia, which tends to afflict males only. This test can also reveal if the baby will be a victim of Down's syndrome (mongolism). If the fetus will be seriously afflicted with a crippling or even potentially fatal disorder (like Tay-Sachs disease), the couple may decide to terminate the pregnancy. If the pregnancy is continued, at least the parents and the physician will know that the baby may have special medical needs before, during, and after birth, and special preparations can be made.

• Begin eating a balanced diet—if you're not already! Also, get your weight as close to ideal as possible. Mothers who are notably overweight *or* underweight tend to run a higher risk of complications during pregnancy and childbirth. Also, stringent dieting is definitely not a good idea during pregnancy.

• If you're taking oral contraceptives, stop taking these well before you plan to conceive. For three to four months before you plan to get pregnant, use another reliable form of contraception (condom and foam, Encare Oval, diaphragm and jelly). There is some evidence that babies conceived while their mothers were intermittently taking the Pill or whose mothers had just stopped taking oral contraceptives may run a higher risk of having birth defects.

When You're Pregnant

• Check with your doctor as soon as possible for confirmation of the pregnancy. Once it is confirmed, prenatal ("before birth") care is vital. The doctor can monitor your health and your baby's health and growth during the months ahead, anticipating and dealing with any possible problems. If you're a teenage mother-to-be, you're in a higher risk category, so prenatal care is especially important.

• Don't take any drugs—even aspirin—without checking with your physician. A number of drugs can reach the baby and cause detrimental effects. This may be particularly true during the first three months when the baby's internal organs, arms and legs, teeth, eyes, and ears are forming.

It goes without saying that hard drugs can be harmful to the fetus, but even tetracycline (which can cause staining of the baby's teeth) and aspirin (which, taken in large doses, may cause increased risk of bleeding in both mother and child) should only be taken under a doctor's supervision, if at all.

Some physicians even caution against drinking large amounts of coffee, tea, and other beverages containing caffeine during pregnancy. Although caffeine has not been linked to birth defects in humans, it is a drug and a central nervous system stimulant that may affect the baby in ways we don't yet know. So it is a good idea to cut down on or cut out coffee and tea consumption, perhaps making a switch to decaffeinated or herbal varieties.

• Stop smoking—or cut down drastically. As we saw in Chapter Seven, smoking can have harmful—even lethal—effects on a fetus. Women who smoke during pregnancy are twice as likely to lose their babies or have a stillborn child or a low birth-weight infant. Low birth-weight infants tend to have twice as many physical and mental handicaps as other new-borns and account for half this nation's infant deaths.

A recent study also found a possible link between smoking and the tragic Sudden Infant Death Syndrome, or "crib death," in which a seemingly healthy baby dies for no apparent reason. This study found that a higher proportion of mothers who smoked before, during, and after pregnancy were in the SIDS group. (For more information on smoking and your baby's health, please refer to Chapter Seven.)

• Don't drink alcohol. Abstaining from alcoholic beverages during pregnancy—or restricting yourself to an occasional glass of wine or beer—can help to protect your baby against the threat of Fetal Alcohol Syndrome, a tragic disorder that has been linked in the past to heavy maternal drinking. Now researchers are finding that even moderate drinking may cause this in some infants.

Scientists in Seattle found that in a group of 164 women who drank only two ounces of hard liquor (like whiskey) a day during pregnancy, nine had infants with FAS. A baby afflicted with fetal alcohol syndrome may have heart, face, and body defects as well as being mentally retarded. Because of the seriousness of this affliction and the risks that even moderate drinking may involve, the National Council on Alcoholism recommends that pregnant women stay away from liquor completely during pregnancy.

• Eat a balanced diet, take iron and other vitamins as your physician may direct, and *exercise*. A well-nourished, well-toned body can help make pregnancy and childbirth easier. Check with your physician first for his/her recommendations. Many women jog, play tennis, and swim during pregnancy. There is, in fact, a new book out on fitness and exercise for pregnant women—*Your Baby, Your Body: Fitness During Pregnancy*, by Carol Stahmann Dilfer—that has some excellent suggestions.

• Prenatal care is important. So is vigilance on your part. If you notice any symptoms like bleeding (even spotting), swelling or puffiness of your face or limbs, sudden weight gain, blurred vision, or a severe, unrelenting headache, call your doctor immediately! He/she may be able to help prevent these symptoms from growing into serious complications.

• Read as much as you can about the care of your body before, during, and after pregnancy. An excellent start for your new library would be the book *Prenatal Care* published by the Department of Health, Education, and Welfare. This publication gives excellent information about maintaining health during pregnancy, what to look for between visits to your doctor, and how to handle common complaints like morning sickness and fatigue. (To get your copy, send $1.05 to: Consumer Information Center, Dept. 121E, Pueblo, Colo. 81009.)

Your Baby Is Born

I'm 16 years old, 7 months pregnant, and live with my boyfriend. We both believe in natural childbirth. In fact, my boyfriend wants to deliver the the baby himself in our own home. I was all for that a few months ago, but now I'm a little nervous. He said he read a book about childbirth once and he knows what he's doing. He won't let me go to a doctor at all. Do you think I have anything to worry about?

Nervous

I'm 21 and expecting my first baby in about five months. My husband and I are interested in natural childbirth and having him with me the whole time. Is this possible in a hospital setting?

Gayle

My husband and I are having an argument about where I'll have my baby—even though I'm only three months along! I'd like to give birth at home. I hate impersonal hospitals. He wants to be with me and have our baby born as naturally as possible, but says he'd feel better if I could be in a hospital with help available if something went wrong. What do you think? We're both 18, if that matters.

Barb C.

I'm scared. I'm due to deliver in a few weeks and my husband and I have taken Lamaze training. One friend of mine, who also had the training, recently had her baby and is going through a real crisis because she feels guilty that she had a lot of pain and had to have pain-killers and finally a spinal anesthetic. She feels like such a failure for having had pain. I feel sorry for her and scared for me. Is it possible to have bad pain, even if you have studied prepared childbirth? Is it a sign of failure, or something that would happen regardless? I'd really like to have my baby without a lot of pain-killing drugs as I hear it's better for the baby.

Shari Y.

We read the letter from "Nervous" with considerable alarm. Here is a young, high-risk parent who has had no prenatal care and whose boyfriend (who read a book once) intends to deliver the baby at home. (We hastened to inform her that natural childbirth does not have to mean taking needless risks and told her to run, not walk, to the nearest clinic!)

Most parents are not as misinformed as "Nervous"

and her boyfriend. However, more and more people are interested in natural childbirth these days. In fact, there has been a revolution of sorts among parents during the last decade.

• About 60 percent of fathers now see their babies born and some even deliver the infants under a doctor's supervision.

• There has been a move away from general anesthesia during childbirth to local or spinal anesthetics that reduce the pain of birth without making the mother unconscious. The woman can now fully experience her child's moment of birth, often sharing this with the father. Many women have no anesthetic at all if they have taken training in prepared childbirth.

• Many couples are taking prepared childbirth training. One of the most popular of these is the Lamaze method, developed by a French obstetrician. The prospective parents take a six-week course to learn about how labor and delivery progress and how muscle control and breathing techniques can help minimize discomfort and help the process of the child's birth.

This natural childbirth may make childbirth less frightening and painful. Many women say that the better prepared you are, the less frightened you will be. Some women find that muscle control and breathing make pain seem bearable, too.

But pain thresholds differ widely. Some women, despite correct use of breathing and relaxation exercises, will have pain. It's important not to put yourself down for feeling such pain or to feel that accepting pain-relievers or a local or spinal anesthetic makes you an inferior person or bad mother. If you are having an extremely painful labor, taking some pain medication so that you can relax a bit may actually help the baby. If you are under the stress of severe pain, this may also take its toll on the uterine blood/oxygen supply that goes to the baby. So you and your baby can both benefit from pain reduction via any method that works for you.

• There is a heightened interest in home or homelike deliveries. Many couples are turned off by the traditional hospital system, which they may see as impersonal and insensitive, and are becoming interested in the possibility of home delivery.

The practice of home delivery with a doctor and/or nurse-midwife in attendance has its advantages and its disadvantages. It may provide a supportive home setting with family and friends all around. It means that the child is not whisked away from its parents and into a nursery right after birth. Instead, they are a complete family right away!

There are some disadvantages, however. Medical personnel who will attend a home delivery are still a minority. Many physicians, while admitting that, in an uneventful birth of a healthy baby, a home delivery may be quite safe, stress the fact that if there have been any complications in pregnancy or any signs of fetal distress, home delivery should not be attempted. Some are even more skeptical, pointing out that, even in the most uneventful pregnancies, complications can occur during the birth itself. When these complications happen, seconds count, and the time it may take to get mother and child to a hospital can spell the difference between life and death.

As a compromise, a number of hospitals are remodeling delivery rooms, creating special homelike birth rooms or suites in Alternative Birth Centers where family and friends, in some instances, are welcome.

For example, birthing rooms at Manchester Memorial Hospital in Connecticut are cheery and personal, with colorful wallpaper, drapes, and a gold-framed mirror that enables the mother to watch the birth. The father is encouraged to take pictures if he wishes, and after the birth, there is a general champagne toast.

At the Alternative Birth Center at Santa Ana Tustin (Calif.) Community Hospital, the birth room is lovely, equipped with an old-fashioned rocking chair, a big quilt-covered bed, TV, stereo, and a crib for the baby right by the bed. The father is not only encouraged to be present for the birth, but also urged to stay overnight before the family leaves the hospital the next day. Friends and family may also be present to celebrate the birth.

At San Francisco General Hospital, a woman can choose between a conventional or family-style delivery. If she opts for the latter, she will have her child in the homelike surroundings of the Alternative Birth Center there.

At Phoenix (Ariz.) Memorial Hospital, the home-style delivery room is a suite with a big living room and a bedroom. Family and friends are encouraged to share the joyous event—either waiting in the living room or actually watching the delivery in the bedroom.

Many hospitals, too, whose delivery rooms still look quite conventional are giving much more personalized service these days.

Combining the warm personal feeling of a home delivery with the extensive services of a hospital may, in many cases, be the ideal approach to childbirth at this time. Natural childbirth in homelike surroundings can be a wonderful experience for all concerned, but it's also good to know that, should anything go wrong, help is available within seconds. And seconds do count in a crisis.

"I was disappointed when my doctor wanted me to have my baby at a large hospital," says Sharon, 20.

"I just hated the thought of an impersonal hospital. But it wasn't that way at all. The nurses were super and very supportive. I had a private labor room and could choose whether or not to have pain medication. I felt like *I* had control. People weren't bossing me around. My husband was with me the whole time. It was beautiful. What made me really glad I had followed my doctor's suggestion was when my daughter was born with the umbilical cord twisted around her neck. She wasn't breathing. A pediatrician was right there to give her special care and when she finally cried, it was such a relief that we all cried, too! She was in intensive care for a brief time and since then has been just fine. We had no idea, until she was born, that there might be a problem. A lot of birth problems can't be predicted in advance. I was really glad Shawna got help immediately. If I had been at home and help had been delayed, she might have had brain damage from lack of oxygen. She might even have died."

Sharon's story points up the fact that, in considering what birth style you want, the baby's health and safety should be very high on your list of considerations.

Alternatives abound these days. Talk with your physician. He/she will know your individual situation and, together, you may be able to find a birth style that is not only right for you, but safe for your baby.

PARENT SHOCK

I'm about to have a baby and have been planning to breast-feed it. Is breast-feeding best for the baby? I'm not sure I'll be able to on account of inverted nipples. I have a friend with the same problem. She couldn't breast-feed and she feels like a real failure.

Raelene

I don't know what to do. I have one one-month-old baby and one 25-year-old baby (my husband). And then there's depressed me. My husband is jealous of the time I spend with the baby, but he never offers to help so that I can get a rest or get finished sooner so that we can have some time to ourselves. He is depressed because he feels stuck in his job. I feel stuck here. I was a super student, a class officer, and a cheerleader. Now I drag and nag. We were so happy when Cindy was born, but the novelty wore off quickly. I find myself resenting both of them and feeling bad about it. What should I do? I can't go on like this!

Susan L.

I think I need help. I love my daughter, who is only two weeks old, but I hate her sometimes. Is this nor-

mal? Does anyone else ever feel that way? I feel like it's almost too terrible to mention! I'm 22 and pretty mature, but maybe I'm not mature enough to be a good mother. I haven't slept—practically—since Robin was born. She keeps waking up in the night. The pediatrician says this isn't so unusual for a newborn and that it will get better. I don't know how it could get any worse! I don't have a minute to myself. I feel like crying half the time. Robin cries, throws up, dirties diapers, and that's it, folks! I was really looking forward to being a mother. I wonder now if I'm suited to it or if I'm doing something wrong. I sometimes get the urge to hit Robin when she starts screaming and won't stop. But I never do hit her. I can understand, though, how child abuse can happen. Please help me!

Desperate

Parenthood—especially at first—can be extremely stressful. Some studies have shown that birth of a first child can be almost as stressful as the death of a family member. We have already talked a bit about how hormonal changes after childbirth can trigger an attack of the postpartum blues.

Feelings of stress and depression can stem from other causes, too.

You may be exhausted.   Few newborns are known to sleep through an entire night. Some seem to scream most at night. Lack of sleep can get to anyone. All new parents get tired, even those who seem to be coping well.

Cammie has always been very bright, efficient, and on top of things, a natural leader. But the first month of her daughter's life nearly unhinged her.

"I never got any sleep!" she remembers. "Sometimes I was so tired, angry, and frustrated, I'd just cry along with the baby! About the third week, my mom took the baby for the night and I got a good nights rest. It made a lot of difference. I had been trying to be supermother and do everything. After that, I learned to ask for help when I needed it, especially from my husband. Particularly on weekends, he gets up with the baby. Sharing responsibilities has helped both of us. I feel less burdened. He feels less shut out by my constant attention to the baby."

You may be anxious.   First-time mothers, especially, are often very concerned about measuring up. You may feel secretly that you fall far short of the madonna ideal: the serene, in-charge person who breast-feeds with ease and grace, and who can soothe her child out of any crying fit.

Some mothers become upset if they can't do what many other mothers do for their children. At this time, this may be especially true of breast-feeding, a trend that has become quite popular again.

Breast-feeding can be beneficial to your baby, not only providing him/her with vital nutrients, but also with antibodies against infection. For this reason, many mothers *are* nursing their infants these days. Even if you have inverted nipples, you may still be able to nurse your baby by wearing special nipple shields.

There can be certain disadvantages to breast-feeding if you work outside the home, if you are ill and/or are taking certain medications, or if you tend to drink. The effects from the alcohol or medications may be passed on to the baby via the breast milk.

There are some women who, for various reasons, cannot breast-feed their babies at all. If you're one of these, there is no reason to feel guilty or like a failure. Your baby will be fine. Although commercial formulas cannot duplicate the antibodies of human breast milk, these formulas can duplicate the nutritional components quite closely.

If you are feeling anxious because you can't always soothe your child when he/she is crying . . . relax! You can love a newborn dearly, but you can't reason with it. When you relax a bit, your child may, too.

If you're anxious about your baby's health, find a pediatrician you like, someone with whom you can communicate. Your doctor may be able to alleviate some of your fears and lend support as you learn to care for your child.

You may be feeling emotionally unsettled, like your whole life has turned around. In a way, it has. You are now a parent. The new responsibilities may weigh heavily on you. You may feel the new restrictions on your freedom acutely. If you're married, you and your husband are no longer simply a couple, but a family. Jealousies can arise. You can both feel trapped by the parental role and its responsibilities. You may miss the privacy you used to have and the luxury of sleeping through the night or making love without interruption or being free to go out whenever you felt like it. Such changes in your life-style are undeniably stressful, even if you were prepared for them. It may help if you and your partner can communicate your feelings to one another, share responsibilities, and understand that some stress now is quite normal. If your problems are compounded by poor communication, a Family Service counselor (see Appendix) may be able to help you to start communicating. In some communities, too, there are parent hotlines where empathetic volunteers can help you to cope with the stress that such a major change in your life may bring.

You may have mixed feelings about parenthood. You love your baby, but . . . well, it's hard to admit, but sometimes you don't like him/her very much. What seemed like a little miracle yesterday looks like a red, wrinkled, testy little tyrant today.

When the baby has been screaming half the night, thrown up twice before 9 A.M., gone through half a dozen diapers and two complete sets of sheets, and is still fussing and fixing you with an accusatory stare, you may get a sudden urge to forget the whole thing and get a one-way ticket to anyplace that is peaceful— and far away. You may even feel, for a moment, like hurting your baby. Then, guilt almost overwhelming you, you hug the baby and tell him/her how much she/he is loved.

"It is not uncommon for a mother to get feelings of rejection toward her child shortly after birth," says Dr. Lee Salk. "Ambivalent feelings about parenthood and toward the child are really very common. Fortunately, your feelings of love will usually predominate. But this love does not preclude periodic feelings of anger, hostility, and rejection. You can be emotionally healthy and still have these feelings. Recognizing these feelings is the first step toward coming to terms with them. Having a child *is* a burden at times and there may be moments when you get an impulse to hurt your baby. Even good parents have these feelings at times. However, if you find yourself unable to control these impulses, seek professional help right away. There is nothing unusual about occasionally wanting to wring your child's neck, but you mustn't *do* it!"

LIVING WITH YOUR CHOICE

I think I'd like to have kids, but the idea scares me a little. What if I have a baby and then hate the whole parenthood scene? I think I could be a good parent, but when I think of the bad things about parenthood, I get nervous.

Ginny

My husband and I were recently married and have been talking about not having any kids ever, although we haven't made a final decision. I find myself worrying a little. I feel fine about no kids now, but is it something I'll regret when I'm older and it's too late to have a baby?

Karen W.

The important life choice of parenthood or nonparenthood is not one that can necessarily be made quickly, easily, or without some mental reservations.

If you look at both options realistically, you will see that neither is all joy or all pain.

If you choose not to be a parent, you will have more personal freedom, more time to pursue careers and causes, time to travel and experience many new things, and time, of course, to yourself, time just to *be.*

There may be moments of longing, however, when you see a particularly charming child and catch yourself wishing you had one, too.

There may be moments of quiet sadness when you're feeling especially close and loving with your partner and, for a moment, have a flash of regret that no child will grow from—or be nourished by—your love.

There may be times, too, when you wonder what might have been, times when wistful visions of the Ultimate Fantasy Child cross your mind.

However, as one young nonparent explains, "I'd rather live with an hour or so of regret every few weeks over *not* having a child than live with regret every day for having had one! Most of the time, I feel I made the right decision for me. (Even if I *am* prone to cry over old Shirley Temple movies!)"

Parenthood, too, can be a mixed blessing.

It can be exhilarating and exhausting. Watching a child experience a holiday, a new discovery, or a new sensation (like catching snowflakes on his/her face) can be a special thrill. Watching your child fall down, make mistakes, be sick, or get hurt can be excruciating. It can be exciting to watch a child grow, but painful to see him or her grow away.

"It seems that the highs are higher and the lows are lower since I became a parent," says one young mother. "When things are good, I'm on top of the world. When things are bad, it's really the pits. But most of the time, I find parenthood to be a challenge and a joy."

Parenthood can be one of the most challenging, taxing, painful, and joyous roles you'll ever fill. It's far too important to be left to chance.

CHAPTER FOURTEEN

Help! When You Need It / How to Ask

Please tell me what to do. I am 14 years old and have symptoms that I think might mean diabetes. (I'm thirsty all the time, keep losing weight no matter how much I eat, and urinate a lot!) I know I ought to go to a doctor, but I'm scared. I'm scared of finding out that I might have diabetes or something else seriously wrong. I'm also just plain scared of doctors! Should I go get help anyway or just wait to see if my symptoms get worse?

Scared

I've been feeling real tired for the past few weeks and my mom thinks I ought to have a physical checkup, but I'd feel stupid going in and saying "Uh, well, Doc, my problem is that I'm tired a lot!" Doctors must get really sick of stuff like that. I hate to be a bother. What do you think I ought to do?

Doug

Please don't take this personally, but . . . I don't like doctors! It's not that I hate them. It's just that I'm afraid of them. I've never had a physical exam that I can recall. What can I do not to be afraid of doctors?

Petrified

"Do I really *have* to go to a doctor?" is what all of these letters seem to be asking, albeit in different ways.

Going to a doctor may be scary, especially if you have never been in the habit of seeking medical care on a regular basis. However, asking for help when you need it is an excellent health safeguard.

When do you need help? In a variety of situations.

In an Emergency

An emergency doesn't mean just a serious injury or unmistakable signs of an appendicitis attack. Severe depression and suicidal feelings can constitute an emergency. So do symptoms of a serious, or potentially serious, medical condition. If, for example, on reading Chapters Eight and Nine, you noted similarities between your symptoms and those of the medical problems discussed, it is a very good idea to consult a physician.

Don't hope that such symptoms will just go away. Don't adopt an "I'll wait and see!" attitude. In the long run, you'll be far less scared if you seek medical testing, help, and advice.

You may find that you do have a special medical need. In that case, you will benefit a great deal from early diagnosis and treatment.

On the other hand, you may find that your condition is not as serious as you had feared. The sooner you find this out, the less time you will spend agonizing over the possibilities.

Many teens, however, are afraid of what the doctor might think of them if they do turn out to be healthy after all. "The doctor will think I'm dumb . . . hysterical . . . a hypochondriac . . . a nuisance . . ." are often-voiced fears.

While we can't speak for all doctors, we have found that most doctors won't feel this way at all.

Your doctor will think that you're wise for being concerned about your body and for seeking help promptly when it seemed that something might be wrong. Your doctor will also be just about as relieved as you are that nothing serious is wrong.

If You Are Sexually Active

Both males and females who are sexually active should be aware of the availability of confidential venereal disease testing and treatment, and birth control services.

Certainly, if you note any symptoms that might mean venereal disease, do get tested and treated immediately. (VD doesn't just go away!)

If you are extremely sexually active with multiple sex partners, it is a good idea to get routine tests for syphilis and gonorrhea every two to three months.

Birth control, as we have seen in previous chapters, is another concern that must not be neglected.

Also, sexually active females should have pelvic examinations and Pap tests once a year. If you are on the Pill or have an IUD, your physician may want to see you every six months.

Many teens fear seeking such medical help because they are afraid that a doctor will be judgmental about their sexual activity.

Some doctors may be judgmental, but, especially if you seek help at a youth-oriented facility like a Free Clinic, Youth Clinic, or hospital-based Adolescent Clinic or at a family planning service like Planned Parenthood, chances are excellent that you will receive competent and nonjudgmental help. These health-care professionals who care primarily for adolescents are likely to be sensitive to your needs and difficult, if not impossible, to shock.

If you go to such a facility for a sexuality related reason, you will have lots of company. "I would say that about 90 percent of the caseload I see on my day at the Los Angeles Free Clinic is sexuality related," says Dr. Tony Greenberg, a Free Clinic volunteer doctor who is also chief of the adolescent clinic and assistant professor of pediatrics at UCLA. "Sexuality related services would include birth control, VD testing and treatment, pregnancy testing and counseling, and gynecological problems. The other 10 percent of patients come in with general medical complaints."

Adolescent medicine specialists (called *ephebiatricians*) are often physicians with basic training in pediatrics or internal medicine who have done special training in the subspecialty of adolescent medicine. They may be found in a number of clinics or in private practice where they may combine practice of adolescent medicine with pediatrics, internal medicine or another specialty, or, in some cases, may see adolescents exclusively. These physicians may be particularly in tune with your feelings and needs.

Of course, there are nonjudgmental doctors in all specialties and settings—from clinics to private practice. If you have bad luck with one doctor, don't give up on finding no-hassle health care. There will be someone else who is better able to help you, if you continue to seek such help.

As Part of Your Regular Health Maintenance

Preventive medicine is a growing concept in health care these days, but it isn't really such a new idea.

Seeking competent medical advice for relatively minor complaints like colds or flu may help keep these from becoming major problems and may enable you to care for yourself more effectively.

Routine physical examinations are vitally important, too.

If you are under 18, you should have routine physical examinations.

After the age of 18 and through the twenties, you should have a physical once every two years.

However, a woman 18 or over—or a younger woman who is sexually active—should have a gynecological (pelvic) examination and a Pap test once a year or every six months if you take the Pill or have an IUD.

These routine checkups are important. They may enable you and your doctor to spot any possible problems before you experience a major health crisis. These examinations can also make you more aware of your body and how it works. These may also offer you an opportunity to ask questions and share ideas with your physician about what you can do to maintain your health and fitness.

If You Have Questions About Your Body

A health professional—a doctor, nurse, or nurse practitioner—is an excellent person to consult if you have any questions at all about your growth, development, or body in general.

"But I'd feel dumb!" you may be saying. "I'd hate to bother a person like that with questions. They might put me down for being stupid and silly. They might say 'I don't have time for you.' "

It could happen that you encounter a health professional who has neither the time nor the inclination to answer your questions. If so, he/she is obviously not the person for you.

Many of those who treat adolescents—primarily or exclusively—tend to be extremely sensitive to the special needs you may wish to talk over.

"When you're treating a teen-ager, you *have* to be sensitive to the whole person, not just a particular symptom or disease," says Dr. Dick Brown, director of the Adolescent Unit at Children's Hospital in San Francisco.

This special kind of caring is evident every day in a myriad of settings.

During a visit to the Los Angeles Free Clinic not long ago, for example, we noticed an overflow of patients, with the line spilling out of the door and onto the sidewalk. One of those waiting was a 14-year-old girl named Debbie who wanted to talk with a doctor about her body changes to find out if she was developing at a normal rate.

Despite the heavy patient load that day, Dr. Tony Greenberg was delighted to see her and happy to answer her questions. He gave her some reading materials and they made plans for her to come back the next week and talk some more.

"She's the kind of teen-ager I'm delighted to see and talk with," says Dr. Greenberg. "She's really concerned about her health and her body. I think it's wonderful when a teen-ager asks questions. I only wish more would. Sure, I spent a lot of time with her and the clinic is busy, but she *needed* that time. When you're treating teen-agers, it's important to be there when they need you.''

There are many other physicians who care, in clinics and in private practice, across the nation.

CLINIC OR PRIVATE PHYSICIAN?

I've been going to our family doctor since I was little and I'm tired of it! He's a good friend of my parents and he sees himself as a kind of father-type to me and treats me like a kid, even though I'm nearly 16! I'd never ask him about birth control (and I have some questions about that). Would a Free Clinic be a better place for me to go?

Suzanne

How good are clinics like teen clinics and Free Clinics? Are they really free? Are the doctors really qualified? Do they spend time with you or are you just a number? What are the advantages of a clinic like this?

John H.

I'm 17 and want medical care, not for a specific problem right now, but for physicals and questions about my body and things like that. My parents say I should go to a pediatrician until I'm 21, but I feel silly going and sitting in a waiting room with two-year-olds! But then my parents' doctor isn't so hot either. He's always so busy and doesn't seem too interested in how you feel emotionally. I guess what I'd like is a doctor who is good and can listen and try to understand me. I'm afraid if I went to a clinic, the doctor wouldn't have time to talk to me. What kind of doctor should I go to? If I went to a doctor or to a clinic, would I have to have my parents' permission to be treated? Usually that wouldn't be a problem, but if I wanted to get birth control some time in the future, could I by myself?

Joanne L.

There are a number of health-care alternatives for young people. Which type of care you choose may depend on your particular needs.

If you want low- or no-cost care, generally nonjudgmental doctors and nurses who are particularly interested in treating young people, a youth-oriented clinic may be for you.

There are several different kinds of these clinics with special services for teen-agers.

Free Clinics

These clinics really are free—but, if you are able and so inclined, most would not mind a donation.

Free Clinics vary a great deal in their services, but many do offer a full range of services, not only sexually related ones (like VD testing and treatment, pregnancy testing, birth control, and gynecological exams), but also general medical services, psychological counseling, and sometimes legal counseling as well.

Because Free Clinics do depend on donations—often from the community at large—their longevity varies. This is why we do not have listings for Free Clinics in the Appendix. It's impossible to keep a current, up-to-date list of existing clinics. (Check your current phone directory to see if there is a Free Clinic in your city.)

Some Free Clinics—like the Los Angeles Free Clinic—thrive for years and enjoy volunteer services from a number of competent health-care professionals, including physicians from the community who are happy to spend one day or evening (or more) a week to meet the needs of people who might otherwise be unable to receive medical care.

A drawback of some of these clinics—besides the possible lack of longevity—is the fact that there may be many patients during peak treatment hours and you may have a long wait to see a doctor, nurse practitioner, nurse, or counselor. Also, you may not see the same doctor each time you go to the clinic, since certain physicians work only at certain times and the turnover can be high in some of these facilities. If you find that you relate to a particular doctor very well, you may plan visits to coincide with his or her availability and ask for that person. Many clinics may be cooperative and try to accommodate your request.

Youth Clinics

These may be tied in with county health departments and can offer many of the services that Free Clinics do as well as many others such as nutritional counseling.

Since these clinics are often county-funded, they usually have excellent facilities and less staff turnover with some staff members working full time and others—especially doctors from the community—who are paid to work part time in the evenings. These clinics—and *most* teen-oriented facilities—tend to be open in late afternoons after school as well as evenings.

Some county youth clinics are highly organized, accepting only a certain number of patients each day, to guarantee that each patient will get the maximum amount of time with the doctor.

"We usually take only 40 patients an evening," says nurse Eunice Skelton of the Van Nuys (Calif.) Youth Clinic, which is part of the excellent Youth Clinic system sponsored by the Los Angeles County Health

Department. "Our services are free, except for the premarital blood–rubella test, which costs three dollars. Our patients range in age from 13 to 20. Some are accompanied by their parents, but most come in on their own."

At the Van Nuys Youth Clinic, patients register at 3 o'clock in the afternoon for evening clinic hours, which run from 5 to 10 P.M. Prospective patients then return at 5 o'clock to settle into the large, cheery waiting room (where movies are sometimes shown to alleviate boredom) to await medical help.

This help may take many forms. Many come for pregnancy or VD tests. Others come for birth control. Still others seek premarital blood tests or nutritional counseling from staff nutritionist Betty Waldner, who has counseled overweight and underweight teens as well as aspiring vegetarians or those concerned with building and maintaining good health via good nutrition.

There are generally two doctors on duty every night to see patients with sexuality related needs, general medical problems, and any psychological problems that may be involved. (So many times we've seen a young person come in with a physical problem, yet end up talking more about an emotional crisis. This is not at all unusual.) Physicians who work for the Youth Clinics (as well as other teen-oriented clinics) usually have a special interest in and empathy for young people. Usually, they are people you can talk with, people who are concerned about your feelings as well as any physical symptoms you may have.

To see if there are any Youth Clinics in your area, check with your local county health department or look in your telephone directory.

College Health Services

Many of these clinics—especially ones in major, nonsectarian universities—have come a long way in the past decade.

In the not-so-distant past, the typical college health service had a staff of older, often semiretired doctors and limited, if any, sexuality related services. This may still be so in some schools, but in many major, nonsectarian institutions, there are many such services, and more and more younger doctors—often with a special interest in adolescent medicine—are staffing the clinics.

The college health service, which is usually financed by a flat fee charged each student every semester, quarter, or on an annual basis, can be an excellent source of low-cost medical care if you happen to be a college student.

Some students, however, fear that if they have certain kinds of treatment—like psychological counseling

or sexuality related services—records of such treatment may be available on demand to any prospective employer or admissions committee for professional schools (like medicine or law) or other graduate programs, and prove to be a handicap. This is not likely to happen, however.

"You are protected legally from this happening," says Dr. Tony Greenberg. "Your medical records are confidential by law. So you shouldn't be afraid to seek whatever help you need."

Specialized Clinics

These would include clinics such as Planned Parenthood that specialize in sexuality related services at low cost. Many Planned Parenthood affiliates offer special youth rap groups and sex education seminars, parent-teen classes, gynecological services, pregnancy testing and counseling, as well as referral and birth control services.

"Many Planned Parenthood centers have special hours and/or programs for teen-agers," says Gene Vadies, director of Youth and Student Affairs for Planned Parenthood Federation of America, Inc. "Under no circumstances will a teen-ager in need of information or services ever be turned away from any of our affiliates. And all young people will be afforded the same confidentiality as any other patient."

See the Appendix for a complete listing of Planned Parenthood clinics and other specialized services nationwide.

Adolescent Clinics

There are about 100 of these comprehensive care, hospital-based clinics in the United States and Canada. (See listings in the Appendix.) These special clinics, staffed by physicians and other medical personnel who have special training in the physiology and psychology of adolescents, offer a variety of services at low cost, usually based on ability to pay.

The Adolescent Unit at Children's Hospital of Los Angeles, for example, is a facility serving teens with a whole range of needs and concerns—from cancer to diabetes, weight control, gynecological problems, or psychological counseling needs.

The unit is also a famous training facility for doctors specializing in adolescent medicine and is active in the community as well, acting as a health advocate for the young and extending care to adolescents in youth homes and facilities and participating in school health-education programs. There is also a crisis hotline, a special obesity clinic, and rap groups for teens who have cancer or other serious illnesses, those with weight problems or emotional concerns. There are even parent-teen rap groups to improve at-home communication as well as family counseling available.

Sensitivity to a teen's needs—whether that teen has a major illness or a relatively minor problem—is at the heart of this successful program, which combines the advantages of a clinic (low cost and a variety of services) with the personal concern that your very own physician can offer. Each patient at the clinic has his or her own primary physician.

"We attempt to treat the whole person, being sensitive to his or her medical and psycho-social needs," says Dr. Richard MacKenzie, director of the unit. "We have a strong emphasis on preventive medicine and health education. We feel it's important to have a primary physician who will be most concerned with your care. But we don't promote dependency, the doctor-as-father-figure idea. We don't say 'You bring me a problem and I'll give you an answer!' We say, instead, 'I have special knowledge that may help you, but you're only sharing your life and problems with me. YOU have the choice to follow the advice or not.' We try to emphasize taking responsibility for your own health."

A Private Physician

For their health care, some teens prefer to seek a physician who is in private practice.

The advantages of this are that, with the right doctor, you may develop a more personal, long-lasting one-to-one relationship. You have someone you can contact quickly in a crisis.

However, on the negative side, going to a private physician is more expensive than seeking services at a clinic and the doctor may or may not offer you nonjudgmental sexuality services like birth control or see you without a parent—if that is a need that you have.

How do you choose a doctor?

You might begin by asking for recommendations from another doctor—your parents' physician or your pediatrician (if that physician is primarily interested in treating children rather than adolescents)—or other health-care professionals like your school nurse, nurses, counselors, or social workers in clinics or hospitals. They might know of a number of competent doctors who may be able to meet your needs. Your local medical society can give you doctors' names, too, although they cannot recommend one over another.

You might also check with the Society for Adolescent Medicine (see Appendix) to get the names of doctors in your area who belong to the society. These may be pediatricians or internists or other specialists who have special training and interest in treating adolescents. In some cases, a physician may treat adolescents *only*. Society members, because they have worked extensively with young people, are likely to be nonjudgmental and sensitive to your needs, although, as in any profession, there may be some exceptions.

After you have the names of some recommended doctors, you might go to the library and look them up in the *American Medical Association Directory* to find out how old the doctors are, where they received their training, when they were licensed, and whether they are board-certified (which means that they have trained additional years after medical school and passed stringent examinations in certain specialties).

After checking their on-paper credentials, think about some of your own preferences. Do you want a young doctor or an older one? You might prefer a doctor closer to your age. You can get excellent medical care, however, from a number of doctors, no matter how old they are. You may prefer a female physician. Many young teen girls do. Although more women than ever are now entering medical schools, female doctors still are a minority and may be difficult to find in some areas and/or specialties. (There are quite a number of female physicians in adolescent medicine, however.)

If a female physician is not available and you find yourself—feeling shy and self-conscious—faced with the prospect of a male physician, it may help to examine your feelings. Why do you feel that a male doctor may not be acceptable to you? If you feel this way because you're self-conscious about your developing body, this is very understandable. Many teens become very modest at this time and may be upset at the thought of a doctor of the opposite sex examining them. Many, too, may wonder if he will see them with any spark of sexual interest. In a sense, it can be a no-win situation: You would feel mortified and insulted if the doctor regarded you as an object of sexual interest or commented on your shape or appearance, and you might have the same feelings if he saw you as just another body on his examining table, not looking at you as attractive one way or another, or as a person instead of a number. These feelings—conflicting at times—are very normal and understandable. It may help for you to know how the typical physician may see you.

We can't speak for all physicians, but the majority of male doctors will not feel any sexual interest while examining you. The doctor is, in a sense, a medical scientist and is seeing your body in a scientific way, checking for signs of normal and abnormal body development and function. This does not mean that he doesn't care about you as a person or about your feelings. The doctor, if he is a good one, will be very concerned about your feelings, including your feelings of being embarrassed or threatened by a man examining your body.

It is likely that he will do everything possible to help you to feel more at ease. Most physicians, for example, have their patients undress in private and drape themselves in a gown. While examining you, the doctor will pull back only a small part of the gown at a time so that you are never totally undressed in front of him.

He may also assume a whole new attitude as he does the physical exam. Many doctors, particularly young males, are aware of how embarrassed you may be and most will try very hard—almost to the point of seeming aloof—not to embarrass you further. Your doctor may be a man of few words during the exam, confining his conversation to simple directives like "Relax . . . cough . . . take a deep breath . . . sit up, please . . ." and observations to the nurse or assistant (who is present to help as well as to chaperone for his legal safety and your emotional reassurance) to be entered on your medical chart. If he senses that you are really uptight, the doctor may engage you in a conversation that has nothing to do with the exam, encouraging you to talk as he continues to examine you. This can have a calming effect on some young people, although others (and some physicians, too) may find it distracting.

A doctor who is truly professional will not make any sexual overtures or suggestive remarks as he examines you.

You may find his professional attitude and the presence of the nurse immensely reassuring.

Some doctors and clinics, too, have nurse practitioners (usually female) who can do physical examinations and many routine health-care procedures under a physician's supervision. For example, Diane Stafanson, who is assistant coordinator of Family Planning for the University of California, San Francisco, Nurse Practitioner Program and who works in the local Planned Parenthood affiliate as well, interviews and counsels patients, taking medical histories and doing pelvic examinations.

There are more and more nurse practitioners, who have received special postgraduate training, working with doctors these days. Often they care for well patients with an emphasis on preventive health measures. So if you feel strongly that you would prefer to be examined by a woman and cannot find a female doctor, a nurse practitioner working with a male physician or in a clinic may be a good alternative to consider.

We all want competent medical care. We may prefer one sex of examiner over another, or one age group over another. Beyond that, there are many variations in individual requirements. You may like a doctor who is friendly and outgoing, or you may prefer one who is more reserved.

The personality of your ideal doctor may be very much a matter of personal taste, but it's important to have a doctor who will examine you thoroughly, take a careful medical history, and listen to you, not putting you down. If you can't ask him or her questions about your health or your treatment or any tests that he or she may perform, if your doctor is not *askable,* you might want to look for another doctor.

Speaking of asking, it's OK to ask the doctor (or his/her secretary) what the costs will be for an examination and/or for particular tests.

LEGAL ASPECTS OF YOUR MEDICAL CARE

One question that many teen-agers have (and are almost afraid to ask) is, "Can I be treated without my parents' knowledge or consent?" or "Will everything I say here get back to my parents?"

As we discussed in Chapters Eleven and Twelve, there are instances where you can get medical treatment without parental consent. Briefly, once again, if you have or feel you might have a venereal disease or any other reportable communicable disease, you can get medical testing and treatment on your own and on a confidential basis if you are 12 or over.

Many states allow minors who are "emancipated" (living away from home, supporting themselves, and so forth) or "partially emancipated" (their parents have lost control over them in a certain area) to receive birth control help without parental knowledge or consent.

In many places, too, there is recognition of the "mature minor" concept. That means that you are capable of understanding medical treatment and are thus able to give your own consent to it.

In practice, some doctors and/or clinics will take your word for it—without asking for proof—that you are emancipated. Others will be more cautious and ask that you get parental consent or have a parent accompany you. If parental consent would be a problem for you, it's a good idea to find out immediately what the policies of a particular doctor or clinic are while you are considering your health-care alternatives.

A number of parents do know and give consent for their teens' care in clinics and with physicians, and feel that it's all fine. But some of these teens—sensitive about their individual privacy—may be concerned that everything they say will get back to their parents. Some teens, for example, are afraid to tell a doctor that they are sexually active, fearing that the news will travel back home.

Again, we can't speak for all doctors, but most will respect your privacy and keep such information confidential.

"Most of our patients have parental consent for treatment, but we do insist on doctor-patient confidentiality," says Dr. Richard MacKenzie of the Adolescent Unit at Children's Hospital of Los Angeles. "Parents generally agree with this stipulation. We will not allow parents to call and ask what a young person has told us. I will say 'Ask your child . . .' If the patient is diagnosed as having a certain disease—like ulcerative colitis, for example—we will *ask* the patient if we can talk with his or her parents. Almost invariably, the young person will say it's OK.''

COMMUNICATING WITH A DOCTOR

I have a problem with doctors: No matter how nice they are, I freeze when I try to ask questions! Half the time, I forget and the other half I'm afraid the doctor will think I'm dumb. But there are some things I really need to ask. My doctor asks me if I have any questions and I go "Ummm . . . no . . . ummm . . ." while trying to get my nerve up, you know? By that time, I'm halfway home! How can I get over this?
Sally

How much are you supposed to tell a doctor? This doctor I went to when I had a problem with my period asked if I'd ever been pregnant. He also wanted to know if I was sexually active. What's it to him?
Marianna

I'm upset with both me and my doctor. I want birth control pills, but don't have the nerve to ask for them. So I went to my doctor complaining of cramps and wanting a pelvic exam. See, I thought if he did the exam, he could tell I wasn't a virgin and would suggest birth control pills for cramps and birth control. But he didn't seem to notice. He just suggested some relaxation exercises and prescribed a mild pain-reliever. How can I get the pill I really want?
Upset

What do you do when you want to see your doctor about something really private and embarrassing, but his secretary asks you over the phone or, even worse, while you're waiting, what you want to see him about?
Worried

Good communication with your doctor is vital.

There are several ways you can help your doctor—and help yourself at the same time.

Be Honest. Don't lie to your doctor about symptoms, sexual activity, or anything else he/she may ask you. Don't be afraid. Your confidential relationship should be respected. And doctors are notoriously difficult to shock. A doctor is there to help you, not to pass judgment.

If a doctor asks you a specific question, it may be important to his/her diagnosis. Your lie might make a correct diagnosis more difficult. So it is to your benefit to be honest.

Don't Expect Your Doctor to Be a Mind Reader. Some doctors are very perceptive and can sense sometimes that you really want to talk about something. Some others, who are still sensitive to your needs, may not know you well enough to discern this or may get confusing signals from you.

The doctor may be in a tough spot. He/she may realize that you have unexpressed areas of need, but may also be aware of the fact that if he/she seems overly inquisitive, you may be offended. So you can both help each other a bit here. If you want to talk about something, but find it difficult, say so and your doctor may be able to help you discuss your concern.

Don't Be Afraid to Ask Questions. Asking questions can help you to learn and to better understand your body and whatever treatment you may be getting.

Most doctors would *prefer* that you ask questions. He/she will probably think that you're intelligent and concerned to ask, not dumb or troublesome.

Ask about specific treatments, medications, or tests you're getting. Why are these being given? Are there any side effects? How can you help increase the effectiveness of the treatment? How long should you take medications? Will the tests hurt? Will they be expensive?

Ask about any bodily function or aspect of development that you don't understand. Most doctors will be happy to explain this to you. If you understand your body, it will help the two of you to communicate better and will also help you to take better care of yourself.

If you don't understand a direction or suggestion your doctor has given you, *ask* him/her to clarify the point. Don't pretend to understand if you really don't. That's not fair to you. All medical conditions can be explained in plain English, so if your doctor gets carried away with long Latin phrases and other medical jargon, call a halt and ask for an instant replay—in *English!*

And again, if your doctor is not askable, maybe you need a new doctor.

Give a Good Medical History. This is one of the most important ways you can help your doctor to help you.

Some of the questions the doctor might ask will seem dumb, like ones about your family's medical history, but these can be important, since certain medical conditions can run in families.

If your doctor asks about your sexuality, he/she isn't trying to be nosy or to embarrass you. Your sexual activity, birth control method, possible pregnancy, VD risk, and so forth may all impinge on your health.

Some questions asked may take a little research on your part. You may have to check which immunizations you have had, for example, or look at a calendar and do some counting to recall the first day of your last menstrual period.

What are some of the questions a doctor is likely to ask you?

The following are just a general selection of questions that might be asked.

- What brings you here today?
- (If it is a problem or symptom) How long have you had this?
- How old are you?
- Has anyone in your family had cancer? Diabetes? Heart disease? High blood pressure? Allergies? TB? Kidney disease? Asthma? Any other serious health problems?
- Do you have (or have you had) any of the following diseases? If so, when? German measles (rubella), red measles, mumps, chicken pox, allergies, pneumonia, bronchitis, tonsillitis, diabetes, epilepsy? Other health problems or diseases?
- Do you ever have any of the following (answer "never," "sometimes," or "frequently")? Sore throat, colds, headaches, dizziness, ear infections, constipation, diarrhea, excessive weight loss or gain, excessive thirst, difficulty in concentrating, feelings that trouble you, suicidal thoughts? Any other troublesome feelings or physical symptoms?
- Have you ever been hospitalized? If so, when? Why?
- How much sleep do you get each night?
- Do you eat a balanced diet? Do you eat breakfast?
- Do you smoke? Drink alcohol? Drink coffee, tea, or colas? In what amounts?
- Have you experimented with drugs or taken drugs on a regular basis? If so, which ones?
- Are you taking any medications now? (Either prescription or over-the-counter drugs.) If so, what are you taking and for what reason?
- Are you sensitive to any particular drug?
- Have you had immunizations for polio? Measles? Rubella? Mumps? Tetanus-diphtheria? When did you have your last tetanus-diphtheria booster? (NOTE: This is recommended between the ages of 14 and 16 and every ten years thereafter).
- When did you first begin to develop physically?
- At what age did you begin to menstruate?
- Are your periods regular?
- What date did your last period begin?
- How many days does your period last?
- Is the flow light, medium, or heavy?
- Do you have cramps? If so, how long have you had them? How severe are they? Do you have nausea with these cramps?
- Do you have premenstrual symptoms? (Tension and irritability, weight gain, tender breasts, a bloated feeling, headaches?) How long do these symptoms last?
- Do you ever spot or bleed between periods?
- Are you sexually active?
- If so, what method of birth control do you use? Have you ever had any problems or symptoms stemming from this method?
- Have you ever been pregnant? If so, how long did the pregnancy last and how did it end? (Abortion, miscarriage, stillbirth, live birth of a premature baby, live birth of a full-term baby?)
- Have you ever had a problem with vaginal discharges or infections?
- Have you had any operations or surgical procedures (like a D and C)? If so, why and when?
- Do you have any pain when you urinate?
- Have you had any discharge from your penis?

THE PHYSICAL EXAMINATION

I'm scared to have a physical exam. Could you tell me (in detail) what the doctor does and why?

Ray

My friend told me that doctors examine your insides when you're a mature woman. Please tell me how doctors do this and why.

Carol

Before I go to a doctor, I want to know what the doctor will do. I want to prepare myself. Otherwise, I'll be too scared to go!

L.S.

I would like more information about a complete medical checkup. Most people say that your heart and pulse are checked in addition to a blood and urine test. Is that all there is or is there more? Is there a difference between a woman's checkup and a man's? This may all sound really dumb to you, but I've never had a physical before and so I have no way of knowing.

Wondering

The physical examination is, with the medical history, one of the best ways for a physician to assess your health. It is important that the examination be thorough, covering the body quite literally from head to toe.

Every physician has his or her own way of performing a complete physical, but there are many similarities. The following rundown will give you a general idea of what to expect.

After you finish talking to the doctor, you will go to an examining room (after stopping off at the bathroom to leave a sample for a urinalysis).

As we said before, you will usually be able to undress and put on an examining gown before the doctor knocks on the door, asks if you're ready, and enters the room.

First, he/she will usually measure your height, weight, blood pressure, pulse, and perhaps even take your temperature.

Then the top-to-toe examination will begin. The thoughtful physician will, as a courtesy to you, only uncover one area of your body at a time, keeping the rest covered. If your doctor doesn't do this and/or makes you feel like "Exhibit A: Nonperson," tell him/her that you are feeling uncomfortable and embarrassed. This is important for you and for the doctor, who may not mean to be thoughtless. Your gentle reminder may help the examiner to be more considerate now and in the future.

First, the doctor will examine your skin for any abnormalities—like any moles that may have increased in size, any rashes, or any signs of bleeding under the skin.

Next, he/she will examine your head, starting with your hair. (Some diseases may cause changes in the texture of the hair or significant hair loss.)

Your ears will probably be examined with an ear speculum, which enables the doctor to see into the ear canal. A hearing test may also be included.

The physician will check your eyes by shining a light into them to check pupil reaction and then will ask you to follow his/her moving finger with your eyes. This enables the physician to see if you have any weakness in the eye muscles. The doctor may also examine your retina with a special instrument. This test is extremely important, since disorders such as diabetes, high blood pressure, and brain tumors may be, in many cases, diagnosed by examining the retina in this way. The physician may also check your vision, by asking you to read a special chart on the wall.

In examining your nose, the doctor will look to see if there are any abnormalities of the nasal bones or if there are any abnormalities of the nasal cavity itself.

When examining your mouth, the doctor will look carefully at your teeth, gums, tongue, and throat. Although the doctor usually does not have dental training he/she can tell if the teeth are in fairly good condition or if you need immediate dental care. Also, some diseases have symptoms that can appear in the mouth.

Moving to your neck, the doctor will feel for an enlargement of the lymph glands or any enlargement or abnormality of the thyroid gland.

Examination of your breasts, lungs, and heart—the chest area—follows.

The breast examination for the female is extremely important. The doctor will gently feel the breasts (in the circular manner we have described in Chapter Two) in order to detect any lumps, dimples, or other abnormalities of the breast tissue. She/he will probably also gently squeeze the breasts to see if any fluid comes from the nipples. (If such fluid is present, it could be a sign of a breast disease.) The underarms will probably also be checked for any lymph gland enlargement, which can be a sign of a breast disease or tumor.

Then the doctor will listen to your lungs with a stethoscope, checking for any signs of lung disease, like asthma, which may manifest itself with a wheezing sound, or pneumonia or chronic lung disease, which may have a symptom like decreased air exchange.

The physician will also use the stethoscope to listen to different areas of your heart.

As your doctor begins to examine your abdominal area, it's important to relax, since tense abdominal muscles can make an accurate examination difficult.

If the doctor touches a ticklish spot, don't be ashamed to giggle. We all have such spots. You're normal. So giggle, then take a deep breath and try to relax.

In this part of the physical examination, the physician will check the size of the liver and spleen as well as look for any signs of tenderness of these organs. She/he will also gently examine this area for any evidence of abdominal masses, tumors, or tenderness.

She/he will also probably examine the lower back for any sign of kidney tenderness, which can be a sign of kidney disease.

Often, in doing the abdominal exam, the doctor may feel or press the area where your bladder is located. It is a good idea, then, to empty your bladder (perhaps giving a sample for a urinalysis) before the examination begins. This is especially true for women, since during the pelvic examination, direct pressure may be placed on the bladder.

Examination of the genitalia usually follows.

In the male, this includes examination of the penis to see if there are any abnormalities. If you are uncircumcised, the doctor will check to see if your foreskin retracts easily. She/he will also look for any signs of

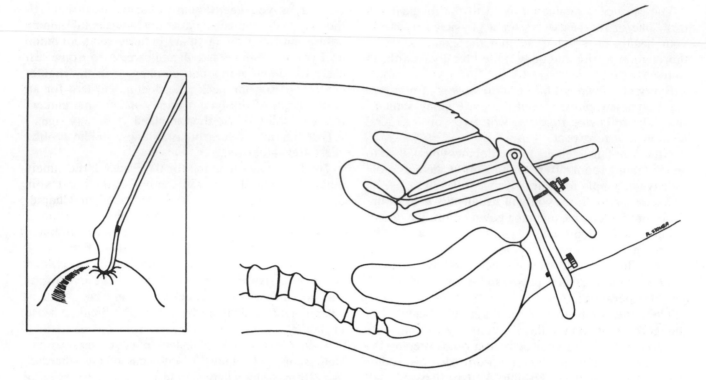

Pelvic examination with speculum enables the physician to see cervix.
Wooden stick is used to collect cells for Pap smear.

abnormal growths, such as small skin tumors or venereal warts on the penis.

The testicles will also be examined for any signs of tumors, unusual pain, or signs of hernia. Here the physician will ask you to cough or exert pressure (as if you were moving your bowels) to enable him or her to see if there is any evidence of a possible hernia.

In the female, a physician will do a pelvic examination after putting your feet in stirrups. Many women find this position to be embarrassing, but it seems to be the best way to do an adequate pelvic examination.

The physician will first examine the labia for any signs of growths, cysts, rashes, or other irritations.

Then she/he will put a gloved finger in your vagina to ascertain which size speculum may be needed. These instruments, which help the physician to see and examine your cervix, come in a variety of sizes, from infant to adult size. Before inserting the speculum, the physician may warm it with water and then gently insert it into the vagina, taking great care not to hurt or pinch you.

With the speculum in place, the doctor can see the cervix clearly and can note any abnormalities, like redness, erosion, cysts, polyps, or irritation. By looking at the cervical os the doctor can tell if you have ever been pregnant, and a bluish hue to the cervix may indicate pregnancy now.

A Pap test will be done with the speculum still in place. Here, the doctor will insert a very small, specially designed wooden applicator to obtain a small sample of the superficial lining around the mouth of the cervix. (Or, to get a better sampling, she/he will put a cotton-tipped applicator into the cervical os.) This procedure does *not* involve cutting, simply gentle scraping, and it is painless. After the sample is obtained, the spatula/applicator is placed on a slide and sent to a pathologist for examination.

The Pap test is very important, since it can detect changes in the superficial cells, which can reflect changes in the cervix itself. These changes may vary from inflammatory changes that happen with a vaginal infection like Trichomonas to abnormal cells that may be a sign of cervical cancer. This type of cancer is quite treatable if caught early and regular Pap tests can detect such cancer early.

This test is usually not done during menstruation, so if you are scheduled for a physical examination and get your period, let the physician know. She/he may want to reschedule your examination or your Pap test.

After this test, the speculum is gently removed from the vagina and the physician begins the bimanual examination of the uterus and ovaries. She/he will insert one or two fingers into the vagina until they touch the cervix while placing his or her other hand on the abdomen above the uterus.

In this way, she/he can examine the uterus for position, shape, size, and tenderness. The ovaries will be examined for enlargement, cysts, tumors, or tenderness in much the same way.

If a woman has a uterus that is tipped toward the back, the physician may need to insert a second finger into the rectum (with one remaining in the vagina) to adequately examine the uterus. If you're tense, this can be painful, so do try to relax.

Relaxation is important for the whole pelvic examination. If you're tense, it can be uncomfortable. If you breathe deeply, even closing your eyes, and try to relax, the procedure should not cause any real discomfort. Most doctors try to be as gentle and considerate of your feelings as possible during this examination.

A rectal examination is important for both males and females. Here, the examiner will check for hemorrhoids, rectal disease, or fissures (splits in the skin of the rectum). She/he may also examine the male's prostate gland through the rectal wall for an enlargement or tenderness.

To detect whether or not you may have any bleeding in the intestinal tract, the physician may get a small stool sample on his or her glove for further examina-

tion. This may seem unpleasant or embarrassing, but can be of critical importance, since intestinal bleeding can be an early sign of possible major health problems.

After a thorough check of your genital organs and rectum, the physician will look carefully at your extremities—your arms, legs, hands, and feet—for any signs of joint swelling or bone deformities and will often examine your back (spine), too, for any signs of abnormal curvature, since scoliosis can be a problem for a number of teen-agers.

A neurological examination, where the doctor checks your reflexes, coordination, sensory and motor functions as well as cranial nerves, may conclude the physical examination.

Certain lab tests—blood and urine—may follow, if they didn't precede, the examination.

The *urinalysis,* of course, is painless and can help to detect a number of problems like kidney disease, urinary infections, and diabetes.

The *blood test* may be a bit painful and scary for some, but it is very brief and is an important way of checking for anemia and other blood disorders.

The two tests above are done routinely when you have a physical examination. There may be other lab

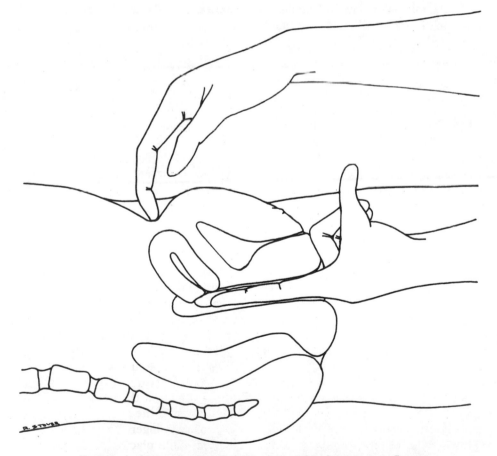

During a pelvic examination, the physician inserts two fingers into the vagina and feels the uterus through the abdomen.

tests that your doctor may suggest or that you may request.

For example, tests for syphilis (a blood test) or for gonorrhea (a culture taken with a cotton-tipped applicator from possible sites of infection like penis, cervix, rectum, mouth, or throat) may be done at your request and are a good idea if you are very sexually active with multiple partners.

The venereal diseases may not be detected in the physical exam or in a regular blood test. The blood test for syphilis is called the VDRL. Ask for it and for a gonorrhea culture as well if you want these, since these may not be done routinely.

And while pregnancy can be detected by urine or blood tests, these tests, too, are special ones that you must request. (See Chapter Thirteen for more details about pregnancy tests.)

GROWING TOWARD A HEALTHY FUTURE

You and your doctor are, ideally, a team working in unison to keep your body as healthy as possible.

You are the most important member of this health-care team.

Many people make the mistake of casting the doctor into the role of guardian of their health and well-being, giving him or her all of the responsibility.

This is a mistake.

A doctor can only diagnose, treat, and advise.

You live in your body and you are the person most responsible for its care. Your body is you. And do you really want anyone else trying to make the choices that are yours alone?

There are many choices you can make that will influence your health. We have examined many of them in this book. Some of the choices enabling you to safeguard your health include:

- Understanding your body's growth and functions
- Eating well and exercising regularly
- Cultivating healthy (rather than harmful) habits
- Learning to manage stress and deal with other troublesome feelings
- Accepting and caring for your special medical needs
- Exercising special responsibility in the area of sexuality
- Asking for help when you need it

Doctors may advise you about your health and your options.

This book may have given you some necessary information and new ideas about some of your health options.

We can—and do—wish you a full, healthy, and happy life.

But only YOU can make this wish reality!

Help! Where to Get It

Adolescent Clinics and Birth Control Facilities

The following is a special state-by-state guide to low- or no-cost youth services and birth control facilities, listed in alphabetical order by state and city. Listings for adolescent clinics are courtesy of the Society for Adolescent Medicine, P.O. Box 3462, Granada Hills, Calif. 91344. The Planned Parenthood Affiliates and Chapter entries are printed with permission of the Planned Parenthood Federation of America and list all major U.S. affiliates and chapters. All welcome teen-agers and some even have special teen clinics or hours. Many of these chapters provide medical services in a number of additional locations, so if you don't see a listing in your hometown, don't despair! Just call the closest Planned Parenthood clinic for information on services available to you.

ALABAMA

Planned Parenthood-Birmingham Area
2301 Arlington Avenue
Birmingham, Alabama 35205
(205) 933-8444

Department of Pediatrics
University of Alabama Medical Center
Birmingham, Alabama 35294

Planned Parenthood Association of Madison County
125 Earl Street
Huntsville, Alabama 35805
(205) 539-2746

ALASKA

Anchorage Planned Parenthood League
c/o Ms. Diane Newman
8601 Vigor Circle
Anchorage, Alaska 99504

ARIZONA

Planned Parenthood Association of Phoenix
1301 South Seventh Avenue
Phoenix, Arizona 85007
(602) 257-1515

Department of Pediatrics
University of Arizona
College of Medicine
Tucson, Arizona 85724
(602) 882-6173

Planned Parenthood Center of Tucson, Inc.
127 South Fifth Avenue
Tucson, Arizona 85701
(602) 624-7477

CALIFORNIA

Southern California-Permanente Kaiser Hospital
9400 East Rosecrans Avenue
Bellflower, California
(213) 920-4881

Adolescent Clinic
Naval Regional Medical Center
Camp Pendleton, California
(714) 725-5556

Planned Parenthood of Humboldt County
P.O. Box 6272
Eureka, California 95501
(707) 442-5709

Adolescent Clinic
Valley Medical Center
445 South Cedar
Fresno, California 93702
(209) 251-4833

Planned Parenthood of Fresno
416 West McKinley
Fresno, California 93728
(209) 486-2411

Planned Parenthood/World Population Los Angeles
3100 West Eighth Street
Los Angeles, California 90005
(213) 380-9300

Department of Pediatrics
Division of Adolescent Medicine
Children's Hospital of Los Angeles
4650 Sunset Boulevard
Los Angeles, California 90027
(213) 660-2450

Oakland Children's Hospital
Outpatient Department
Oakland, California

Planned Parenthood Association of Orange County
704 North Glassell
Orange, California 92667
(714) 639-3023

Planned Parenthood of Monterey County, Inc.
229 Seventeenth Street
Pacific Grove, California
(408) 373-1691

Planned Parenthood Committee, Inc.
1045 North Lake Avenue
Pasadena, California 91104
(213) 798-0708

Planned Parenthood Association of Sacramento
1507 Twenty-first Street, Suite 100
Sacramento, California 95814
(916) 446-5034

Department of Pediatrics, Adolescent Clinic
Naval Regional Medical Center
San Diego, California 92134
(714) 233-2722

Planned Parenthood of San Diego County
2100 Fifth Avenue
San Diego, California 92101
(714) 231-1282

Planned Parenthood Alameda-San Francisco
1660 Bush Street
San Francisco, California 94109
(415) 441-0555

University of California Medical Center
Adolescent Clinic
400 Parnassus Avenue
San Francisco, California 94143
(415) 524-1485

Children's Hospital of San Francisco
3700 California Street
Sant Francisco, California 94119
(415) 387-8700

Planned Parenthood Association of Santa Clara
   County
17 North San Pedro
San Jose, California 95110
(408) 287-7526

Planned Parenthood Association of San Mateo County
2211-2215 Palm Avenue
San Mateo, California 94403
(415) 574-2622

Planned Parenthood Association of Marin County
710 C Street, Suite 9
San Rafael, California 94901
(415) 454-0471

Planned Parenthood of Santa Barbara County, Inc.
322 Palm Avenue
Santa Barbara, California 93101
(805) 963-4417

Planned Parenthood of Santa Cruz County
421 Ocean Street
Santa Cruz, California 95060
(408) 426-5550

Planned Parenthood of San Joaquin County
116 West Willow
Stockton, California 95202
(209) 464-5809

Stanford University Medical Center
Stanford, California 94305
(415) 497-6891

Planned Parenthood of Contra Costa County, Inc.
1291 Oakland Boulevard
Walnut Creek, California 94596
(415) 935-3010

Planned Parenthood Association of Yolo County
327 College Street, Suite 102
Woodland, California 95695
(916) 662-4646

COLORADO

Boulder Planned Parenthood
4500 North Broadway
Boulder, Colorado 80302
(303) 447-1040

Colorado Springs Planned Parenthood
1619 West Colorado Avenue
Colorado Springs, Colorado 80904
(303) 475-7162

Denver Chapter, Planned Parenthood, Central
  Denver Clinic
2030 East Twentieth Avenue
Denver, Colorado 80205
(303) 388-4777

Adolescent Clinic
University of Colorado Medical Center
4200 East Ninth Avenue
Denver, Colorado 80220

Adolescent Medical Clinic
Fitzsimons Army Medical Center
Denver, Colorado 80232

Rocky Mountain Planned Parenthood
2030 East Twentieth Avenue
Denver, Colorado 80205
(303) 388-4215

Larimer County Planned Parenthood
149 West Oak Street, No. 8
Fort Collins, Colorado 80521
(303) 456-0517

Pueblo Planned Parenthood
151 Central Main
Pueblo, Colorado 81003
(303) 545-0246

CONNECTICUT

Bridgeport Planned Parenthood
1067 Park Avenue
Bridgeport, Connecticut 06604
(203) 366-0664

Danbury Planned Parenthood
240 Main Street

Danbury, Connecticut 06810
(203) 743-2446

Hartford Planned Parenthood
297 Farmington Avenue
Hartford, Connecticut 06105
(203) 522-6201

Division of Child and Adolescent Behavior
University of Connecticut, Department of Pediatrics
Mount Sinai Hospital
500 Blue Hills Avenue
Hartford, Connecticut 06107
(203) 242-4431

Meriden/Wallingford Planned Parenthood
Box 2119
Meriden, Connecticut 06450
(203) 235-3231

Middlesex Planned Parenthood
79-81 Crescent Street
Middletown, Connecticut 06457
(203) 347-5255

New Britain Planned Parenthood
Box 292
New Britain, Connecticut 06050
(203) 225-9811

Planned Parenthood League of Connecticut, Inc.
129 Whitney Avenue
New Haven, Connecticut 06511
(203) 865-4250

Medical Program for Adolescents
Yale University School of Medicine
333 Cedar Street
New Haven, Connecticut 06510

Southeast Chapter, Planned Parenthood
420 Williams Street
New London, Connecticut 06320
(203) 443-5820

South Fairfield Planned Parenthood
259 Main Street
Stamford, Connecticut 06901
(203) 327-2722

Northwest Chapter, Planned Parenthood
27 Pearl Street
Torrington, Connecticut 06790
(203) 489-5500

Waterbury Planned Parenthood
115 Prospect Street
Waterbury, Connecticut 06702
(203) 757-1955

Northeast Chapter, Planned Parenthood
791 Main Street
Willimantic, Connecticut 06226
(203) 423-1500

DELAWARE

Delaware League for Planned Parenthood
825 Washington Street
Wilmington, Delaware 19801
(302) 655-7293

DISTRICT OF COLUMBIA

Adolescent Medicine
Children's Hospital of D.C.
2125 Thirteenth Street, Northwest
Washington, D.C. 20009
(202) 835-4352

Planned Parenthood of Metropolitan Washington,
    D.C.
1109 M Street, Northwest
Washington, D.C. 20005
(202) 387-4711

Adolescent Medicine Clinic
Howard University Hospital
2041 Georgia Avenue, Northwest
Washington, D.C. 20060
(202) 745-1592

Division of Adolescent Medicine
Department of Pediatrics
Georgetown University Medical Center
3800 Reservoir Road
Washington, D.C. 20007
(202) 625-7383

Washington D.C. Chapter, Planned Parenthood
1120 M Street, Northwest
Washington, D.C. 20005

Adolescent Clinic
Walter Reed Army Medical Center
Washington, D.C. 20012
(202) 576-2051

FLORIDA

South County Center-Planned Parenthood
162 West Palmetto Park Road
Boca Raton, Florida 33432
(305) 368-1023

Planned Parenthood of North Central Florida
P.O. Box 12385
Gainesville, Florida 32604
(904) 377-0881

Planned Parenthood of Northeast Florida
305 East Church Street
Jacksonville, Florida 32202
(904) 354-7796

Planned Parenthood, Naples Center
482 Tamiami Trail North
Naples, Florida 33940
(305) 649-5484

Planned Parenthood Association of South Florida,
    Inc.
3400 N.W. 135th Street
Opa Locka, Florida 33054
(305) 685-7571

Planned Parenthood of Southwest Florida
Sarasota Memorial Hospital
P.O. Box 2532
1224 S. Tamiami Trail
Sarasota, Florida 33578
(813) 959-4648

Planned Parenthood-Palm Beach Area
800 N. Olive
West Palm Beach, Florida 33401
(305) 655-7984

GEORGIA

Planned Parenthood Association of the Atlanta Area
118 Marietta Street, Northwest
Atlanta, Georgia 30303
(404) 688-9302

Planned Parenthood of East Central Georgia
P.O. Box 3293, Hill Station
Augusta, Georgia 30904
(404) 724-5557

HAWAII

Hawaii Planned Parenthood, Inc.
1164 Bishop Street, 12th Floor
Honolulu, Hawaii 96813
(808) 521-6991

Adolescent Medicine Service
Tripler Army Medical Center
Honolulu, Hawaii APO SF 96438

Adolescent Unit
Straub Clinic and Hospital
888 South King Street
Honolulu, Hawaii 96813

Kauikeolani Children's Hospital
226 North Kaukini Street
Honolulu, Hawaii 96812

IDAHO

Planned Parenthood Association of Idaho, Inc.
P.O. Box 264
Boise, Idaho 83701
(208) 345-0760

ILLINOIS

Planned Parenthood of McLean County
McBarnes Memorial Building
201 East Grove Street, 2nd Floor
Bloomington, Illinois 61701
(309) 827-8025

Planned Parenthood of Champaign County
314 South Neil Street
Champaign, Illinois 61820
(217) 359-8022

Adolescent Clinic
Rush-Presbyterian Hospital
1753 West Congress Parkway
Chicago, Illinois 60612
(312) 942-5000

Planned Parenthood Association-Chicago Area
55 East Jackson Boulevard
Chicago, Illinois 60604
(312) 322-4200

Planned Parenthood of Decatur, Inc.
988-990 South Main Street
Decatur, Illinois 62521
(217) 429-9211

Planned Parenthood Association of Peoria Area
313 S.W. Jefferson
Peoria, Illinois 61602
(309) 673-6911

Planned Parenthood-Springfield Area
624 South Second
Springfield, Illinois 62704
(217) 544-2744

INDIANA

Planned Parenthood of South Central Indiana
421 South College Avenue
Bloomington, Indiana 47401
(812) 336-0219

Planned Parenthood-Elkhart County Health Unit
315 South Second Street
Elkhart, Indiana 46514
(219) 293-7715

Planned Parenthood of Evansville, Inc.
1610 South Weinback Avenue
Evansville, Indiana 47714
(812) 479-1466

Planned Parenthood of Northwest Indiana, Inc.
740 Washington Street
Gary, Indiana 46402
(219) 883-0411

Planned Parenthood of Indianapolis, Inc.
616 North Alabama Street
Indianapolis, Indiana 46204
(317) 634-8019

Planned Parenthood Association of Tippecanoe
County
P.O. Box 1114
Lafayette, Indiana 47902
(317) 742-9073

Planned Parenthood of East Central Indiana, Inc.
4020 Rosewood Avenue
Muncie, Indiana 47304
(317) 282-8011

Marshall County Planned Parenthood
218 LaPorte Street
Plymouth, Indiana 46563
(219) 936-8680

Planned Parenthood of North Central Indiana
201 South Chapin
South Bend, Indiana 46625
(219) 289-7027

Planned Parenthood Association of the Wabash
  Valley, Inc.
330 South Sixth Street
Terre Haute, Indiana 47807
(812) 232-3578

Kosciusko County Planned Parenthood
P.O. Box 555
Warsaw, Indiana 46580
(219) 267-3889

IOWA

Planned Parenthood of Des Moines County
521 North Fifth
Burlington, Iowa 52601
(319) 753-2281

Planned Parenthood of Iowa
P.O. Box 4557
Des Moines, Iowa 50306
(515) 280-7000

Planned Parenthood of North Lee County
631 Avenue H
Fort Madison, Iowa 52627
(319) 372-1130

Adolescent Medicine
Departments of Medicine/Pediatrics
University of Iowa Hospitals—E304
Iowa City, Iowa 52240
(319) 356-3447

Planned Parenthood of South Lee County
927 Exchange Street
Keokuk, Iowa 52632
(319) 524-2759

Planned Parenthood of Southeast Iowa
125½ West Monroe
Mt. Pleasant, Iowa 52641
(319) 385-8322 or 385-4310

Planned Parenthood of Sioux City
2825 Douglas Street
Sioux City, Iowa 51104
(712) 277-3330

Planned Parenthood of Louisa County
407 Washington
P.O. Box 182
Wapello, Iowa 52653
(319) 523-8297

Planned Parenthood of Washington County
Clara Barton and Fourth
P.O. Box 44
Washington, Iowa 52353
(319) 653-3525

Planned Parenthood of Northeast Iowa
1825 Logan Avenue
Waterloo, Iowa 50703
(319) 235-3731

KANSAS

Planned Parenthood of Kansas
158 North Grove Street
Wichita, Kansas 67214
(316) 686-3356

KENTUCKY

Mountain Maternal Health League
P.O. Box 429
Berea, Kentucky 40403
(606) 986-4677

Lexington Planned Parenthood Center, Inc.
331 West Second Street
Lexington, Kentucky 40507
(606) 252-0448

Division of Adolescent Medicine
Department of Pediatrics, Children's Hospital
University of Louisville
Louisville, Kentucky 40206
(502) 589-8750

Planned Parenthood Center, Inc.
843–845 Barrett Avenue
Louisville, Kentucky 40204
(502) 584-2471

MARYLAND

Planned Parenthood Association of Maryland, Inc.
610 North Howard Street
Baltimore, Maryland 21201
(301) 752-0131

Division of Child and Adolescent Psychiatry
University of Maryland, School of Medicine
Baltimore, Maryland 21201

Planned Parenthood of Prince George's County
Landover Mall
East Tower Building, No. 203
Landover, Maryland 20785
(301) 773-5601

Adolescent Clinic
Montgomery County Health Department
8500 Colesville Road
Silver Spring, Maryland 20910
(301) 587-4565

Planned Parenthood of Montgomery County
1141 Georgia Avenue
Wheaton, Maryland 20902
(301) 933-2300

MASSACHUSETTS

Boston City Hospital
Boston, Massachusetts 02118

Boston Floating Hospital
Boston, Massachusetts 02111

Adolescents' Unit
Children's Hospital Medical Center
300 Longwood Avenue
Boston, Massachusetts 02115

Adolescent Unit
Children's Hospital
Boston, Massachusetts 02115

Kennedy Memorial Hospital
Brighton, Massachusetts 02135

Planned Parenthood League of Massachusetts
99 Bishop Richard Allen Drive
Cambridge, Massachusetts 02139
(617) 492-0518

Teen Health Clinic
St. John's Hospital
Lowell, Massachusetts
(617) 458-1411

MICHIGAN

Planned Parenthood-Alpena County
2330 Sandy Lane
Alpena, Michigan 49707
(517) 356-1137

Adolescent Clinic
University Hospital
Ann Arbor, Michigan 48104

Washtensaw County League for Planned Parenthood
912 N. Main Street
Ann Arbor, Michigan 48104
(313) 769-8530

Planned Parenthood Association of Southwestern
  Michigan
785 Pipestone
Benton Harbor, Michigan 49022
(616) 925-1306

Mecosta County Family Planning
P.O. Box 1156
Big Rapids, Michigan 49307
(616) 796-8644

Cadillac Planned Parenthood
c/o Ms. Kathy Tunney
110 North Park Street
Cadillac, Michigan 49601
(616) 775-4956

Ambulatory Adolescent Service
Children's Hospital of Michigan
James Couzeun Clinic
Detroit Medical Center
Detroit, Michigan 48201
(313) 494-5050

Planned Parenthood League, Inc.
13100 Puritan
Detroit, Michigan 48227
(313) 861-6700

Adolescent Medical Program
Michigan State University
B-240 Life Sciences
East Lansing, Michigan 48824

Adolescent Clinic
Hurley Medical Center
Flint, Michigan 48502

Flint Community Planned Parenthood Association
YWCA
310 East Third Street
Flint, Michigan 48503
(313) 238-3631

Planned Parenthood of Ottawa County
Box 728
Grand Haven, Michigan 49417
(616) 842-4569

Planned Parenthood Association of Kent County,
   Inc.
425 Cherry, S.E.
Grand Rapids, Michigan 49503
(616) 774-7005

Planned Parenthood of Ionia County
111 Kidd
Ionia, Michigan 48846
(616) 527-3250

Planned Parenthood of Kalamazoo County
612 Douglas Avenue
Kalamazoo, Michigan 49007
(616) 349-8631

Marquette-Alger Family Planning Association
c/o Ms. Audrey Trautman
410 E. College
Marquette, Michigan 49855

Muskegon Area Planned Parenthood Association,
   Inc.
1095 Third Street
Muskegon, Michigan 49440
(616) 722-2928

Shiawassee County Planned Parenthood Association
P.O. Box 542
Owosso, Michigan 48867
(517) 723-6420

Northern Michigan Planned Parenthood Association
316½ North Mitchell
Petoskey, Michigan 49770
(616) 347-9692

Sault Ste. Marie Planned Parenthood
P.O. Box 246A
Route 1

Sault Ste. Marie, Michigan 49783
(906) 632-8103

MINNESOTA

Planned Parenthood of Bemidji Area
722 Fifteenth Street
Box 822
Bemidji, Minnesota 56601
(218) 751-8683

Central Minnesota Planned Parenthood
502 Front Street
Brainerd, Minnesota 56401
(218) 829-1469

Planned Parenthood of Northeast Minnesota
504 East Second Street
Duluth, Minnesota 55805
(218) 722-0833

South Central Planned Parenthood
Liberty Building, Room 203
Mankato, Minnesota 56001
(507) 378-5581

Teenage Medical Service
Adolescent Out-Patient
Department of Children's Health Center
2425 Chicago Avenue
Minneapolis, Minnesota 55404

Planned Parenthood of Metropolitan Minneapolis
230 Walker Building
803 Hennepin Avenue
Minneapolis, Minnesota 55403
(612) 336-8931

Planned Parenthood of Rochester Area
116½ South Broadway
Rochester, Minnesota 55901
(507) 288-5186

Planned Parenthood Chapter, St. Paul
   Metropolitan Area
408 Hamm Building
408 St. Peter Street
St. Paul, Minnesota 55102
(612) 224-1361

Planned Parenthood of Minnesota, Inc.
1965 Ford Parkway
St. Paul, Minnesota 55116
(612) 698-2401

MISSISSIPPI

Keesler AFB Medical Center
Department of Pediatrics
Adolescent Medicine
Biloxi, Mississippi 39531

MISSOURI

Planned Parenthood of Central Missouri
800 North Providence Road, Suite 5
Columbia, Missouri 65201
(314) 449-2475

Adolescent Clinic
Children's Mercy Hospital
240 Sillham Road
Kansas City, Missouri 64108
(816) 471-0626

Planned Parenthood of Western Missouri/Kansas
1001 East Forty-seventh Street
Kansas City, Missouri 64110
(816) 756-2277

Planned Parenthood of Northeast Missouri, Inc.
P.O. Box 763
Kirksville, Missouri 63501
(816) 665-5674

Planned Parenthood of the Central Ozarks
Box 359
1032B Kings Highway
Rolla, Missouri 65401
(314) 364-1509

Planned Parenthood of Southwest Missouri, Inc.
1918 East Meadowmere
Springfield, Missouri 65804
(417) 869-6471

Planned Parenthood Association of St. Louis
2202 South Hanlety Road
St. Louis, Missouri 63144
(314) 781-3800

MONTANA

Planned Parenthood of Billings
2718 Montana Avenue
Billings, Montana 59101
(406) 248-3636

Planned Parenthood of Missoula County
301 Alder
Missoula, Montana 59801
(406) 728-5490

NEBRASKA

Planned Parenthood of Lincoln
3830 Adams Street
Lincoln, Nebraska 68504
(402) 466-2387

2221 South Seventeenth Street
Lincoln, Nebraska 68502

Adolescent Clinic
Children's Memorial Hospital
3925 Dewey Avenue
Omaha, Nebraska 68131

Planned Parenthood of Omaha
2916 North Fifty-eighth Street
Omaha, Nebraska 68104
(402) 554-1045

NEVADA

Planned Parenthood of Southern Nevada, Inc.
601 South Thirteenth Street
Las Vegas, Nevada 89101
(702) 385-3451

Planned Parenthood of Northern Nevada
406 Elm Street
Reno, Nevada 89503
(702) 329-1781

NEW HAMPSHIRE

Planned Parenthood Association of the Upper
  Valley
1 Foundry Street
Lebanon, New Hampshire 03766
(603) 448-1214

NEW JERSEY

Planned Parenthood-Greater Camden Area
590 Benson Street
Camden, New Jersey 08103
(609) 365-3519

Planned Parenthood Center of Bergen County
485 Main Street
Hackensack, New Jersey 07601
(201) 489-1140

Planned Parenthood Association of Hudson County
777 Bergen Avenue, Room 218
Jersey City, New Jersey 07303
(201) 332-2565

Adolescent Services and Clinic
Morristown Memorial Hospital
Morristown, New Jersey
(201) 540-5199

Planned Parenthood of Northwest New Jersey, Inc.
197 Speedwell Avenue
Morristown, New Jersey 07960
(201) 539-1364

Planned Parenthood-Essex County
15 William Street
Newark, New Jersey 07102
(201) 622-3900

Department of Pediatrics
New Jersey Medical School
Martland Hospital
65 Bergen Street
Newark, New Jersey 07107
(201) 456-5481

Planned Parenthood League of Middlesex County
84 Carroll Place
New Brunswick, New Jersey 08901
(201) 246-2554

Passaic County Planned Parenthood Center
145 Presidential Boulevard
Riverview Terrace
Paterson, New Jersey 07522
(201) 274-3883

Planned Parenthood of Union County Area, Inc.
234 Park Avenue
Plainfield, New Jersey 07060
(201) 756-3736

Planned Parenthood of Monmouth County, Inc.
69 Newman Springs Road
Shrewsbury, New Jersey 07701
(201) 842-9300

Planned Parenthood Association of the Mercer Area
437 East State Street

Trenton, New Jersey 08608
(609) 599-3736

NEW MEXICO

Bernalillo County Planned Parenthood Association,
    Inc.
113 Montclaire, S.E.
Albuquerque, New Mexico 87108
(505) 265-3722, Ext. 21

Planned Parenthood of South Central New Mexico
302 West Griggs Avenue
Las Cruces, New Mexico 88001
(505) 524-8516

Planned Parenthood of Southwest New Mexico
524 Silver Heights Boulevard
Silver City, New Mexico 88061
(505) 388-1553

NEW YORK

Planned Parenthood Association of Albany
225 Lark Street
Albany, New York 12210
(518) 434-2182

Frankfurt Youth Health Center
APO New York 09710

Planned Parenthood of Broome County, Inc.
710 O'Neill Building
Binghamton, New York 13901
(607) 723-8306

Comprehensive Adolescent Medical Program
Brookdale Hospital Medical Center
Linden Boulevard-Rockaway Parkway at Brookdale
    Plaza
Brooklyn, New York 11212
(212) 240-5901

Division of Adolescent Medicine
Montefiore Hospital and Medical Center
111 East 210th Street
Bronx, New York 10467
(212) 920-4045

Adolescent Unit
Roswell Park Memorial Institute
Buffalo, New York 14263
(716) 845-4406

Planned Parenthood Center of Buffalo
210 Franklin Street
Buffalo, New York 14203
(716) 853-1771

St. Lawrence County Planned Parenthood
15 Main Street
Canton, New York 13617
(315) 386-2441

Planned Parenthood of Nassau County
1940 Hempstead Turnpike
East Meadow, New York 11554
(516) 794-8380

Planned Parenthood of the Southern Tier
200 East Market Street
Elmira, New York 14901
(607) 734-3313

Planned Parenthood of Ontario County
435 Exchange Street
Geneva, New York 14456
(315) 781-1092

Southern Adirondack Planned Parenthood
   Association
126 Warren Street
Glens Falls, New York 12801
(518) 792-0994

Planned Parenthood Center of North Suffolk
17 East Carver Street
Huntington, New York 11743
(516) 427-7154

Planned Parenthood of Tompkins County
512 East State Street
Ithaca, New York 14853
(607) 273-1513

Lockport Planned Parenthood
555 Pine Street
Lockport, New York 14094
(716) 433-4464

Lewis County Planned Parenthood
7552 State Street
Lowville, New York 13367
(315) 376-2741

Franklin County Planned Parenthood
109 East Main Street
Malone, New York 12953
(518) 483-7150

Planned Parenthood of Orange-Sullivan, Inc.
91 DuBois Street
Newburgh, New York 12550
(914) 562-5748

Adolescent Medicine
Long Island-Jewish Hillside Medical Center
New Hyde Park, New York 11040

Department of Pediatrics
New York University Medical Center
550 First Avenue
New York, New York 10016

Department of Pediatrics
New York Medical College
106th Street and Fifth Avenue
New York, New York 10029
(212) 860-8000

Mt. Sinai School of Medicine
Fifth Avenue at 100th Street
New York, New York 10029

Roosevelt Hospital
428 West 59th Street
New York, New York 10019

Planned Parenthood of New York City, Inc.
300 Park Avenue South
New York, New York 10010
(212) 777-2002

Division of Adolescent Medicine
Department of Pediatrics
New York Hospital
525 East 68th Street
New York, New York 10020

Planned Parenthood of Niagara County
906 Michigan Avenue
Niagara Falls, New York 14305
(716) 282-1223

Planned Parenthood Association of Delaware and
   Otsego Counties, Inc.
48 Market Street
Oneonta, New York 13820
(607) 432-2250

Planned Parenthood of East Suffolk, Inc.
127 South Ocean Avenue
Patchogue, New York 11772
(516) 475-5705

Planned Parenthood of Clinton County
94 Margaret Street
Plattsburgh, New York 12901
(518) 561-4430

Planned Parenthood of Dutchess-Ulster, Inc.
85 Market Street
Poughkeepsie, New York 12601
(914) 471-1540

Adolescent Clinic
601 Elmwood Avenue
Rochester, New York 14604

Threshold
115 South Clinton Avenue
Rochester, New York 14604

Planned Parenthood of Rochester and Monroe
    Counties, Inc.
24 Windsor Street
Rochester, New York 14605
(716) 546-2595

Planned Parenthood of Schenectady and Affiliated
    Counties, Inc.
414 Union Street
Schenectady, New York 12305
(518) 374-5353

Planned Parenthood Center of Syracuse, Inc.
1120 East Genesee Street
Syracuse, New York 13210
(315) 424-8260

Planned Parenthood Association of the Mohawk
    Valley, Inc.
1424 Genesee Street
Utica, New York 13502
(315) 724-6146

Planned Parenthood of Northern New York, Inc.
161 Stone Street
Watertown, New York 13601
(315) 782-0481 or 788-8065

Planned Parenthood of Rockland County
37 Village Square
West Nyack, New York 10994
(914) 358-1145

Planned Parenthood of Westchester, Inc.
149 Grand Street
White Plains, New York 10601
(914) 428-7876

NORTH CAROLINA

Planned Parenthood of Greater Charlotte
East Independence Plaza Building
951 South Independence Boulevard
Charlotte, North Carolina 28202
(704) 377-0841

NORTH DAKOTA

Fargo Clinic
737 Broadway
Fargo, North Dakota 58102

OHIO

Planned Parenthood Association of Summit County,
    Inc.
39 East Market Street
Akron, Ohio 44308
(216) 535-2671

Planned Parenthood of Southeast Ohio
306 Security Building
8 North Court Street
Athens, Ohio 45701
(614) 593-3375

Planned Parenthood of Stark County
626 Walnut Avenue, N.E.
Canton, Ohio 44702
(216) 456-7191

Adolescent Service
Cincinnati General Hospital
Cincinnati, Ohio 45229
(513) 559-4681

Planned Parenthood Association of Cincinnati
2406 Auburn Avenue
Cincinnati, Ohio 45219
(513) 721-7635

Pickaway Family Planning Association
Berger Hospital
600 North Pickaway
Circleville, Ohio 43113
(614) 374-5143

Department of Pediatrics, Adolescent Clinic
Cleveland Metropolitan General

3395 Scranton Road
Cleveland, Ohio 44109
(216) 398-6000

Cleveland Clinic Foundation
Adolescent Diagnostic Center
9500 Euclid Avenue
Cleveland, Ohio 44106
(216) 444-5516

Planned Parenthood of Cleveland, Inc.
2027 Cornell Road
Cleveland, Ohio 44106
(216) 721-4700

Planned Parenthood of Central Ohio, Inc.
206 East State Street
Columbus, Ohio 43215
(614) 224-8423

Planned Parenthood Association of Miami Valley
224 North Wilkinson Street
Dayton, Ohio 45402
(513) 226-0780

Maternal Health Association of Lorain County
266 Washington Avenue
Elyria, Ohio 44035
(216) 322-9874

Planned Parenthood Association of Crawford County
200 Harding Way East
Galion, Ohio 44833
(419) 468-9926

Planned Parenthood Association of Butler County,
    Inc.
305 South Front Street
Hamilton, Ohio 45011
(513) 894-3875

Planned Parenthood Association of Mansfield Area
35 North Park Street
Mansfield, Ohio 44902
(419) 525-3075

Planned Parenthood Association of East Central
    Ohio
17 North First Street
Newark, Ohio 43055
(614) 345-5450

Family Planning Association of Lake and Geauga
    Counties
1499 Mentor Avenue

Painsville, Ohio 44077
(216) 352-0608

Planned Parenthood of West Central Ohio
401 North Plum Street
Springfield, Ohio 45504
(513) 325-7349

Teen Health Center
St. Vincent Hospital and Medical Center
2213 Cherry Street
Toledo, Ohio 43608
(419) 259-4795

Planned Parenthood League of Toledo
Hillcrest Hotel, Sixteenth and Madison
P.O. Box 10003
Toledo, Ohio 43699
(419) 246-3651

Planned Parenthood of Wayne County
111 South Buckeye
Wooster, Ohio 44691
(419) 262-4866

Planned Parenthood of Mahoning Valley
105 East Boardman Street
Youngstown, Ohio 44503
(216) 746-5662

OKLAHOMA

Pediatric Adolescent Medicine Program
Department of Pediatrics
Oklahoma Health Sciences Center
P.O. Box 26901
Oklahoma City, Oklahoma 73190
(405) 751-9065

Adolescent Unit
University of Oklahoma Medical Center
800 Northeast Thirteenth
Oklahoma City, Oklahoma 73103

Planned Parenthood of Oklahoma City
10 N.E. Twenty-third Street
Oklahoma City, Oklahoma 73105
(405) 528-2157

Planned Parenthood of Northeastern Oklahoma
808 South Peoria Avenue
Tulsa, Oklahoma 74120
(918) 587-8419

OREGON

Planned Parenthood of Benton County, Inc.
2750 N.W. Harrison
Corvallis, Oregon 97330
(503) 753-3348

Planned Parenthood Association of Lane County
134 East Thirteenth Avenue
Eugene, Oregon 97401
(503) 344-9411

Planned Parenthood of Jackson County
650 Royal Avenue, Suite 18
Medford, Oregon 97501
(503) 773-8285

Planned Parenthood Association, Inc.
1200 S.E. Morrison
Portland, Oregon 97214
(503) 234-5411

PENNSYLVANIA

Planned Parenthood Association of Lehigh County
806 Hamilton Street, 2nd Floor
Allentown, Pennsylvania 18102
(215) 439-1033

Planned Parenthood Association of Bucks County
721 New Rodgers Road
Bristol, Pennsylvania 19007
(215) 785-4591

Planned Parenthood of Northampton County, Inc.
275 South Twenty-first Street
Easton, Pennsylvania 18042
(215) 253-7195

Monroe County Planned Parenthood Association
162 East Brown Street
East Stroudsburg, Pennsylvania 18301
(717) 421-4000, Ext. 630

Adolescent and Youth Center
801 Old York Road, Suite 222
Jenkintown, Pennsylvania 19046

Cambria/Somerset Planned Parenthood
502 Main Street
Johnstown, Pennsylvania 15901
(814) 535-5545

Planned Parenthood of Lancaster
37 South Lime Street
Lancaster, Pennsylvania 17602
(717) 394-3575

Children's Hospital of Philadelphia
Adolescent Clinic
Thirty-fourth and Civic Center Boulevard
Philadelphia, Pennsylvania 19102
(215) 387-6311

Planned Parenthood Association of Southeastern
 Pennsylvania
1220 Sanson Street
Philadelphia, Pennsylvania 19107
(215) 574-9200

Planned Parenthood Center of Pittsburgh
102 Ninth Street
Pittsburgh, Pennsylvania 15222
(412) 434-8950

Planned Parenthood Center of Berks County
48 South Fourth Street
Reading, Pennsylvania 19602
(215) 376-8061

Planned Parenthood Organization of Lackawanna
 County
207 Wyoming Avenue, Suite 322
Scranton, Pennsylvania 18503
(717) 344-2626

Planned Parenthood of Chester County
113 West Chestnut Street
West Chester, Pennsylvania 19380
(215) 692-1770

Planned Parenthood Association of Luzerne County
63 North Franklin Street
Wilkes-Barre, Pennsylvania 18701
(717) 824-8921

Planned Parenthood of Central Pennsylvania
710 South George Street
York, Pennsylvania 17403
(717) 845-9681

RHODE ISLAND

Planned Parenthood of Rhode Island
187 Westminster
Providence, Rhode Island 02903
(401) 421-9620

SOUTH CAROLINA

Planned Parenthood of Aiken County
P.O. Box 277
Clearwater, South Carolina 29822
(803) 593-9283

Planned Parenthood of Central South Carolina, Inc.
2719 Middleburg Drive, Suite 202
Columbia, South Carolina 29204
(803) 256-4908

Medical Park Pediatric and Adolescent P.A.
3321 Medical Park Road, Suite 501
Columbia, South Carolina 29203

Greenville Hospital Systems
Adolescent Clinic
Department of Pediatric Education
Greenville General Hospital
Greenville, South Carolina 29601
(803) 242-7000

TENNESSEE

Planned Parenthood Association of Knox County
Lincoln American Insurance Building
2611 Magnolia Avenue
Knoxville, Tennessee 37914
(615) 522-0191

Memphis Planned Parenthood Association, Inc.
Suite 1700, Exchange Building
9 North Second Street
Memphis, Tennessee 38103
(901) 525-0591

Planned Parenthood Association of Nashville
University Plaza
112 Twenty-first Avenue South
Nashville, Tennessee 37203
(615) 327-1066

Planned Parenthood Association of the Southern
   Mountains, Inc.
162 Ridgeway Center
Oak Ridge, Tennessee 37830
(615) 482-3406

TEXAS

Panhandle Planned Parenthood Association
604 West Eighth Street
Amarillo, Texas 79101
(806) 372-8731 or 372-8732

Planned Parenthood Center of Austin
1823 East Seventh Street
Austin, Texas 78702
(512) 477-5846

Planned Parenthood of Cameron County
15 East Levee Street
Brownsville, Texas 78520
(512) 546-4571

South Texas Planned Parenthood Center
801 Elizabeth
Corpus Christi, Texas 78404
(512) 884-4352

University of Texas
Southwestern Medical School
Department of Pediatrics
Dallas, Texas 75207
(214) 688-2925

Planned Parenthood of Northeast Texas
2727 Oak Lawn, Suite 228
Dallas, Texas 75219
(214) 522-0290

Adolescent Clinic
El Paso, Texas 79920

Planned Parenthood Center of El Paso
214 West Franklin Street
El Paso, Texas 79901
(915) 542-1919

Planned Parenthood Center of Fort Worth
301 South Henderson
Fort Worth, Texas 76104
(817) 332-9101

Adolescent Division
University of Texas Medical Branch
Galveston, Texas 77550
(713) 765-2355

Baylor College of Medicine
c/o Texas Children's Hospital

6621 Fannin Street
Houston, Texas 77030

Planned Parenthood of Houston
3601 Fannin Street
Houston, Texas 77004
(713) 522-3976

Planned Parenthood Association of Chaparral
    County
117 South Fifth Street
P.O. Box 1134
Kingsville, Texas 78363
(512) 592-2649

Planned Parenthood of Webb County, Inc.
2000 San Jorge
Laredo, Texas 78040
(512) 723-4606

Planned Parenthood Center of Lubbock
3821 Twenty-second Street
Lubbock, Texas 79410
(806) 795-7123

Planned Parenthood Association of Hidalgo County
P.O. Box 1069
Mission, Texas 78572
(512) 585-4575

Permian Basin Planned Parenthood, Inc.
American Bank Commerce Building, Suite 401
Odessa, Texas 79761
(915) 563-2530

Planned Parenthood Center of San Angelo
122 West Second Street
San Angelo, Texas 76901
(915) 655-9141

University of Texas
Health Science Center at San Antonio
Robert B. Green Hospital
San Antonio, Texas 78219

Planned Parenthood Center of San Antonio
106 Warren Street
San Antonio, Texas 78212
(512) 227-2227

Adolescent Medicine Service
Department of Pediatrics
Brooke Army Medical Center
San Antonio, Texas 78234
(512) 221-4407 or 221-6735

The Central Texas Planned Parenthood Association
P.O. Box 6308
Waco, Texas 76706
(817) 754-2392

UTAH

Planned Parenthood Association of Utah
Chapman Building
28 East 2100 South
Salt Lake City, Utah 84115
(801) 487-8914

VERMONT

Planned Parenthood Association of Vermont
158 Bank Street
Burlington, Vermont 05401
(802) 862-9637

VIRGINIA

Planned Parenthood of Northern Virginia
5622 Columbia Pike
Falls Church, Virginia 22041
(804) 820-3335

Peninsula Planned Parenthood
1520 Aberdeen Road, Room 314
Hampton, Virginia 23666
(804) 826-2079

Planned Parenthood of Norfolk and Chesapeake,
    Inc.
222 West Nineteenth Street
Norfolk, Virginia 23517
(804) 625-5591

Adolescent Medicine
Department of Pediatrics
Children's Hospital of the Kings Daughters
609 Colley Avenue
Norfolk, Virginia 23507
(804) 622-1381

Adolescent Clinic
Department of Pediatrics
Naval Regional Medical Center
Portsmouth, Virginia 23708
(804) 397-6541

MCV Adolescent Clinic
Medical College of Virginia
Box 151
Richmond, Virginia 23298
(804) 770-6506

Virginia League for Planned Parenthood
1218 West Franklin Street
Richmond, Virginia 23220
(804) 353-5516

Planned Parenthood of Roanoke Valley, Inc.
920 South Jefferson Street
Roanoke, Virginia 24016
(703) 342-6741

Tri-County Area Planned Parenthood
P.O. Box 1400
Suffolk, Virginia 23434
(804) 539-3456

WASHINGTON

Planned Parenthood of Whatcom County
P.O. Box 4
Bellingham, Washington 98225
(206) 734-9095

Planned Parenthood of Snohomish County
2730 Hoyt Avenue
Everett, Washington 98201
(206) 259-0096

Planned Parenthood of Benton-Franklin Counties
P.O. Box 6842
Kennewick, Washington 99336
(509) 586-2164

Group Health Cooperative
10200 First Northeast
Seattle, Washington 98125
(206) 545-7138

Planned Parenthood of Seattle-King County
2211 East Madison
Seattle, Washington 98112
(206) 447-2350

University of Washington
Division of Adolescent Medicine
University of Washington (WJ-10)
Seattle, Washington 98195

Planned Parenthood of Spokane
North 507 Howard Street
Spokane, Washington 99201
(509) 624-3271

Planned Parenthood of Pierce County
312 Broadway Terrace Building
Tacoma, Washington 98402
(206) 572-6955

Planned Parenthood of Walla Walla
329 South Second Street
Walla Walla, Washington 99362
(509) 529-3570

Planned Parenthood of Yakima County
208 North Third Avenue
Yakima, Washington 98902
(509) 248-3625

WEST VIRGINIA

Planned Parenthood Association of Parkersburg
210 Fifth Street
Parkersburg, West Virginia 26101
(304) 485-1144

WISCONSIN

Planned Parenthood Association of Fox Valley
128 Durkee Street
Appleton, Wisconsin 54911
(414) 731-6304

Beaumont Clinic Ltd.
Pediatric and Adolescent Department
1821 South Webster Avenue
Green Bay, Wisconsin 54301
(414) 437-9051

Planned Parenthood of Green Bay
Bellin Building
130 East Walnut Street
Green Bay, Wisconsin 54301
(414) 432-0031

Planned Parenthood of Dodge-Jefferson Counties
159 West Garland Street
Jefferson, Wisconsin 53549
(414) 674-2233

Planned Parenthood of Kenosha
5621 Eighteenth Avenue
Kenosha, Wisconsin 53140
(414) 654-0491

Teenage Clinic
University of Wisconsin Hospitals
1552 University Avenue
Madison, Wisconsin 53705
(608) 262-1170

Planned Parenthood of Madison-Dane County
Regent Mills Professional Building
1051 Regent Street
Madison, Wisconsin 53715
(608) 256-7257

Planned Parenthood of Manitowoc-Two Rivers
910A South Eighth Street
Manitowoc, Wisconsin 54220
(414) 684-1332

Marshfield Clinic
Adolescent Section and Clinic
1000 North Oak
Marshfield, Wisconsin 54449
(715) 387-5413 or 387-5251

Milwaukee Children's Hospital Adolescent Clinic
1700 West Wisconsin Avenue
Milwaukee, Wisconsin 53202
(414) 344-7100

Planned Parenthood Association of Wisconsin
1135 West State Street
Milwaukee, Wisconsin 53233
(414) 271-8181

Planned Parenthood of Sheboygan
635 West Center Street
Sheboygan, Wisconsin 53081
(414) 458-9401

Planned Parenthood of Washington County
320 South Fifth Avenue
West Bend, Wisconsin 53095
(414) 338-1303

CANADA

Adolescent Clinic
c/o C.O.P.C.
Kingston General Hospital
Kingston, Ontario, Canada

Ste.-Justine Hospital
3175 Cote Ste.-Catherine
Montreal, Quebec, Canada
(514) 731-4931

Adolescent Unit
Allan Memorial Institute
1025 Pine Avenue, West
Montreal 112, Quebec, Canada

Adolescent Unit
Montreal Children's Hospital
2300 Tupper Street
Montreal, Quebec, Canada

Adolescent Clinic
Moose Factory Hospital
Moose Factory, Ontario, Canada

Ambulatory Service
Adolescent Clinic
Hospital for Sick Children
Toronto, Ontario, Canada M5G 1X8
(416) 597-1500

I.O.D.E. Children's Centre
4001 Leslie Street
Willowdale, Ontario, Canada M2K 1E1
(416) 492-3836

Crisis Counseling

There are more than 300 agencies nationwide that are affiliated with the Family Service Association of America. These offer individual and family counseling at low cost as well as a variety of other family services.

For the agency nearest you, check your telephone directory under the following listings:

Family Service Association
Council for Community Services
County Department of Health
Counseling Clinic
Mental Health Clinic
United Fund

Or contact the New York office:

Family Service Association of America
44 East Twenty-third Street
New York, New York 10010
(212) 674-6100

HOTLINES

There are several hundred crisis hotlines across the nation. These can offer on-the-spot crisis counseling by phone and/or may refer you to sources of further help in your community. Most hotlines report that a large portion of their calls come from young people. Most offer sensitive, nonjudgmental help.

We are listing a few *national*, toll-free hotlines first and then local hotlines, which are listed in alphabetical order by state and city.

The starred (*) entries indicate hotlines that are for teens exclusively, especially for those in runaway or very stressful home situations. These offer telephone crisis counseling, in-person individual or family counseling and, in most cases, temporary shelter if needed.

If your crisis stems from a special need—either disease related or sexuality related (for example, pregnancy, homosexuality, venereal disease)—you may find additional help in the Special Needs section of this Appendix, where special resources are listed.

NATIONAL, TOLL-FREE HOTLINES

National Operation Venus Hotline
(A VD counseling and referral service)
In Philadelphia, call: (800) 462-4966
Out of state, call: (800) 523-1885

NATIONAL RUNAWAY SWITCHBOARD

(A special service to runaways and their parents and to teens in stressful situations. They can refer you to help in your community.)
In Illinois, call: (800) 972-6004
Out of state, call: (800) 621-4000

ALABAMA

Crisis Center, Birmingham: (205) 323-7777
*XIIIth Place Crisis Line, Birmingham:
   (205) 252-4537

ALASKA

Suicide Prevention and Crisis Center, Anchorage:
   (907) 276-1600
*Youth Services Center Crisis Line, Anchorage:
   (907) 279-9544

ARIZONA

Crisis Intervention Hotline, Flagstaff:
   (602) 774-2727
Crisis Intervention Program, Phoenix:
   (602) 258-8011
Suicide Prevention Hotline, Phoenix:
   (602) 275-3667
*Open-Inn Crisis Line, Tucson: (602) 790-2200
Suicide Prevention and Crisis Center, Tucson:
   (602) 327-6501

ARKANSAS

*Crisis Center, Little Rock: (501) 664-8834

CALIFORNIA

*Crisis Line, Alameda: (415) 522-8383
 Crisis Hot Line, Bakersfield: (805) 323-4357
*Helpline Youth Counseling, Bellflower:
   (213) 920-1706
*Berkeley Youth Alternatives, Berkeley:
   (415) 849-1402
*Youth Emergency Assistance, Chula Vista:
   (714) 422-9294
*Diogenes Crisis Line, Davis: (916) 756-5665 or
   446-4884
 Crisis Counseling Center, Encino: (213) 784-9406
 Suicide Prevention Emergency Line, Fremont:
   (415) 471-5500
*Odyssey Crisis Line, Fullerton: (714) 871-5646 or
   871-9365
 Suicide Prevention Center for Halfmoon Bay:
   (415) 726-5581
 Suicide Prevention Emergency Line, Hayward:
   (415) 351-3333
 Helpline, Los Angeles: (213) 620-0144
 Suicide Prevention Center, Los Angeles:
   (213) 381-5111

*Crisis Line, Newberry Park: (213) 529-2255
Cri-Help Drug Hotline, North Hollywood:
   (213) 985-8323
Crisis Counseling Hotline, Oakland: (415) 530-5433
Suicide Prevention Emergency Line, Oakland:
   (415) 849-2212
Los Alamitos Hot Line, Orange County:
   (213) 596-5548
West Orange County Hotline, Orange County:
   (714) 898-5150
Helpline, Orange County: (714) 894-4242
Suicide Prevention Center for Redwood City:
   (415) 367-8000
*Youth Service Center, Riverside: (714) 683-5193
Crisis Clinic, Sacramento: (916) 453-3696
Crisis Intervention Hotline, Sacramento:
   (916) 488-2100
Suicide Prevention Center, Sacramento:
   (916) 441-1135
*Crisis Line, San Anselmo: (415) 453-5200
*Crisis Line, Santa Barbara: (805) 963-8775
Hotline Crisis Telephone Counseling, Santa
   Barbara: (805) 963-8808
Crisis and Suicide Prevention Service, San
   Bernardino: (714) 886-4889
*The Bridge Crisis Line, San Diego: (714) 291-5222
*Project Oz Crisis Line, San Diego: (714) 272-3003
Crisis Line, San Francisco: (415) 673-6799
*Huckleberry House Crisis Line, San Francisco:
   (415) 731-3921
Suicide Prevention, Inc., San Francisco:
   (415) 221-1423
Suicide and Crisis Service, San Jose: (415) 287-2424
Suicide Prevention Center for San Mateo:
   (415) 877-5600
Sonoma County Sex Information Hotline, Sonoma:
   (707) 527-8585
*Youth Services Crisis Line, South Lake Tahoe:
   (916) 541-8500
Crisis Clinic and Drop-In Center, Yuba City:
   (916) 673-8255

COLORADO

*Crisis Center, Aurora: (303) 751-3010
Suicide Referral Service, Colorado Springs:
   (303) 471-4357
*Crisis Counseling for Young Adults, Denver:
   (303) 222-3344
*Prodigal House Crisis Line, Denver: (303) 831-8600
*Southwest Runaway Help, Denver: (303) 934-6510
Suicide and Crisis Control, Denver: (303) 756-8485
   or 789-3073 If no answer: (303) 757-0988

CONNECTICUT

*Stand, Inc. Crisis Line, Derby: (203) 735-6203
*Net Crisis Line, Glastonbury: (203) 633-8333
*The Rufuge Crisis Line, Willimantic: (203) 423-7731

DISTRICT OF COLUMBIA

Hotline: (301) 261-1616
Saja Crisis Line: (202) 462-5210
(See also Maryland and Virginia listings)

FLORIDA

*Youth Alternatives Crisis Line, Daytona Beach:
   (904) 252-6550
*Boys Time Out, Fort Lauderdale:
   (305) 764-6985
Crisis Intervention Center, Fort Lauderdale: (305)
   523-8553
*Girls Time Out, Fort Lauderdale: (305) 764-1091
Crisis Center and Suicide Prevention Hotline,
   Jacksonville: (904) 384-2234
*Jacksonville Youth Center, Jacksonville:
   (904) 354-0400
*Bay House Crisis Line, Miami: (305) 373-6161
Crisis Center for Women, Miami: (305) 270-1512
Crisis Service and Suicide Prevention Hotline,
   Miami: (305) 324-7520
*Miami Bridge Hotline, Miami: (305) 371-6211
Crisis Intervention Service, Orlando: (305) 628-1227
*YMCA Youth Home Crisis Line, Tallahassee:
   (904) 877-7974
Suicide and Crisis Center, Tampa: (813) 253-3311
*YMCA Youth Hostel, Tampa: (813) 251-8437

GEORGIA

*The Bridge Crisis Line, Atlanta: (404) 881-8344
Crisis Center, Atlanta: (404) 892-1358
*Salvation Army Girls Lodge, Atlanta:
   (404) 881-6953
Suicide Counseling, Atlanta: (404) 572-2626
*Truck Stop Boys Lodge, Atlanta: (404) 875-0184

HAWAII

*Hale Kipa Crisis Line, Honolulu: (808) 955-3591
Suicide Crisis Center, Honolulu: (808) 521-4555

IDAHO

Hot Line, Boise: (208) 345-7888
*Youth Service Bureau Hotline, Boise:
   (208) 345-3000

ILLINOIS

*Youth in Crisis Hotline, Berwyn: (312) 484-7400
 Crisis Line-Suicide Prevention Hotline,
   Champaign: (217) 359-4141
 Crisis Intervention Center, Chicago: (312) 794-3609
*New Life Hotline, Chicago: (312) 271-6165
*Aunt Martha's Youth Service Center, Park Forest:
   (312) 747-2701 or 747-2702

INDIANA

*Youth Service Bureau Crisis Line, Evansville:
   (812) 425-4355
*Shepherd's Inn Crisis Line, Fort Wayne:
   (219) 423-2461
*Switchboard Runaway Center, Fort Wayne:
   (219) 456-4561
*Stopover Crisis Line, Indianapolis: (317) 635-9301
 Suicide and Crisis Intervention, Indianapolis:
   (317) 632-7575

IOWA

*Shelter House Crisis Line, Ames: (515) 233-2330
 Crisis Line, Cedar Rapids: (319) 362-2174
 Crisis Line, Des Moines: (515) 266-8673
 Iowa Runaway Service Hotline, Des Moines:
   (515) 243-4906

KANSAS

Suicide Prevention Center, Kansas City:
   (913) 831-1773
Can Help-Suicide Prevention, Topeka:
   (913) 235-3434
Suicide Prevention Service, Wichita: (316) 686-7465
*Youth Alternatives, Inc. Hotline, Wichita:
   (306) 262-5273

KENTUCKY

Crisis and Suicide Prevention Hotline, Louisville:
   (502) 589-4313
*YMCA Shelter House, Louisville: (502) 635-5234

LOUISIANA

Crisis Line and Suicide Prevention, New Orleans:
   (504) 523-2673
*The Greenhouse Crisis Line, New Orleans:
   (504) 944-2477
 Hot Line, Shreveport: (318) 226-6060

MARYLAND

Hot Line, Annapolis: (301) 263-0330
Hot Line, Baltimore: (301) 269 6323
*Grassroots Crisis Line, Columbia: (301) 730-3090
*Second Mile House Crisis Line, Hyattsville:
   (301) 927-1386
*The Link Crisis Line, Rockville: (301) 762-0300

MASSACHUSETTS

*Project Rap Crisis Line, Beverly: (617) 922-0000 or
   927-4506
*The Bridge Crisis Line, Boston: (617) 227-7114
 Hot Line, Boston: (617) 267-9150
*Project Place Crisis Line, Boston: (617) 536-4181
*Crisis Center, Inc., Worcester: (617) 791-6562

MICHIGAN

 Crisis Counseling and Suicide Prevention, Ann
   Arbor: (313) 761-9834
*Ozone House Crisis Line, Ann Arbor:
   (313) 769-6540
*Cory Place Crisis Line, Bay City: (517) 895-8532
 Crisis Center-Six Area Coalition, Detroit:
   (313) 383-9000
*Crisis Line, Detroit: (313) 821-8800 or 821-8470
 Suicide Prevention/Drug Information, Detroit:
   (313) 875-5466
 Crisis Center-Suicide Prevention, Flint:
   (313) 235-5677
 Hotline Center, Flint: (313) 742-1230
*The Bridge Crisis Line, Grand Rapids:
   (616) 451-3001

Crisis Intervention and Suicide Switchboard,
Grand Rapids: (616) 774-3535
Crisis Intervention Center, Lansing: (517) 337-1717
*The Sanctuary Crisis Line, Pleasant Ridge:
(313) 547-2260
*Interlink Crisis Line, Saginaw: (517) 753-3431
*Link Crisis Intervention Center, St. Joseph:
(616) 983-6351

MINNESOTA

*Crisis Shelter, Duluth: (218) 724-5182
*The Bridge Crisis Line, Minneapolis:
(612) 333-5401
Crisis Intervention Center, Minneapolis:
(612) 347-3161
Suicide Prevention Center, Minneapolis:
(612) 347-2222

MISSISSIPPI

Crisis Center Hotline, Jackson: (601) 355-3070

MISSOURI

Suicide Prevention Center, Kansas City:
(816) 471-3000
*Youth in Need Crisis Line, St. Charles:
(314) 724-7171
Suicide-Crisis Intervention Hotline, St. Louis:
(314) 868-6300
*Youth Emergency Service, University City:
(314) 727-6294

MONTANA

Crisis Center-New Hope, Billings: (406) 248-3621
Crisis and Suicide Prevention Center, Great Falls:
(406) 453-6511
Crisis Center Hotline, Missoula: (406) 543-8277

NEBRASKA

*Crisis Line, Lincoln: (402) 475-6261
*Whitman Center Crisis Line, Omaha:
(402) 553-3337

NEVADA

Crisis Call Center, Carson City–Reno:
(702) 323-6111
*Focus Crisis Line, Las Vegas: (702) 382-4762
Suicide Prevention Center, Las Vegas:
(702) 736-4357

NEW JERSEY

Suicide Prevention Hotline, Atlantic City:
(609) 561-1234
Crisis Intervention HelpLine, Newark:
(201) 623-2323
*Operation Junction Crisis Line, North Wildwood:
(609) 729-1663
*Youth Haven Crisis Line, Paterson: (201) 345-8454

NEW MEXICO

Crisis and Suicide Prevention Center,
Albuquerque: (505) 265-7557
Crisis Counseling, Albuquerque: (505) 265-6787
Crisis Intervention Center, Santa Fe:
(505) 982-2771

NEW YORK

Crisis Center, Albany: (518) 434-1202
*REFER Crisis Line, Albany: (518) 434-1202
Community Youth Program Crisis Line, Bronx:
(212) 294-5252 or 731-8066
*Compass House Crisis Line, Buffalo:
(716) 886-0935
Crisis Services, Buffalo: (716) 838-5980
Outreach Crisis Line, Middletown: (914) 342-5633
*Contact Crisis Line, New York City:
(212) 533-3570
*Covenant House Crisis Line, New York City:
(212) 741-7580
Crisis Intervention Center, New York City:
(212) 662-8630
Suicide Prevention Hotline, New York City:
(212) 462-3322
Suicide Prevention League, New York City:
(212) 736-6191
*Seabury Barn Crisis Line, Stony Brook:
(516) 751-1411

Suicide Prevention Center, Syracuse:
(315) 474-1333
Suicide Prevention Service, White Plains:
(914) 946-0121

NORTH CAROLINA

*The Relatives Crisis Line, Charlotte: (704) 377-0602
Crisis Control Center, Greensboro: (919) 275-2852

NORTH DAKOTA

Suicide and Crisis Prevention Center, Bismarck:
(701) 663-6575 If no answer, call: (701) 255-4124.
Hot Line, Fargo: (701) 235-7335
Suicide Prevention Center, Fargo: (701) 232-4357
Crisis Intervention Service, Grand Forks:
(701) 775-0525

OHIO

Suicide Prevention Center, Akron: (216) 434-9144
Crisis Intervention-Suicide Prevention Center,
Canton: (216) 452-6000
Crisis Center-Rape Crisis Hotline, Cincinnati:
(513) 381-4430
*The Lighthouse Crisis Line, Cincinnati:
(513) 621-1522
Suicide Prevention Center, Cincinnati:
(513) 621-2273
Crisis Center, Cleveland: (216) 631-5800
Crisis Clinic, Cleveland: (216) 921-6631
Suicide Prevention Center, Cleveland:
(216) 229-4545
*Huckleberry House Crisis Line, Columbus:
(614) 294-5553
Suicide Prevention Center, Columbus:
(614) 221-5445
*Daybreak Crisis Line, Dayton: (513) 461-1000
*Stay Center Crisis Line, Hamilton: (513) 893-2730
*Walden Crisis Line, Lancaster: (614) 654-4500
*Together Crisis Line, Oxford: (513) 523-4146
*Daybreak Crisis Line, Youngstown: (216) 746-8410

OKLAHOMA

Crisis Center, Oklahoma City: (405) 325-6963
Hotline Crisis Service, Tulsa: (918) 583-4357

OREGON

*Sunflower House Crisis Line, Corvallis:
(503) 753-1241
Hotline, Eugene: (503) 484-9402 or 484-9408
*Looking Glass Crisis Line, Eugene: (503) 689-3111
Suicide and Personal Crisis Service, Portland:
(503) 227-0403

PENNSYLVANIA

*COMAC Youth Service Crisis Line, Abington:
(215) 885-6655
Crisis Intervention, Allentown: (215) 434-8268
*Valley Youth House Crisis Line, Bethlehem:
(215) 691-1200
Suicide Prevention Center, Philadelphia:
(215) 686-4420
*Voyage House Crisis Line, Philadelphia:
(215) 735-8406
*Amicus Crisis Line, Pittsburgh: (412) 621-3653

RHODE ISLAND

Hot Line, Providence: (401) 222-7525
*Sympatico Crisis Line, Wakefield: (401) 783-0650 or
783-0772

SOUTH CAROLINA

Crisis Counseling Center, Charleston:
(803) 577-0520
Hotline, Columbia: (803) 777-4256
Crisis Intervention and Suicide Prevention,
Greenville: (803) 271-0220

TENNESSEE

Suicide Prevention and Crisis Help, Knoxville:
(615) 637-9711
*Runaway House Crisis Line, Memphis:
(901) 276-1745
Suicide and Crisis Intervention Service, Memphis:
(901) 726-5531
Crisis Call Center, Nashville: (615) 244-7444

TEXAS

Crisis Intervention, Operation Drug Alert, and
  Suicide Prevention, Amarillo: (806) 376-4251
  If no answer, call: (806) 376-4442
Hot Line to Help, Austin: (512) 472-2411
Suicide Rescue, Inc., Beaumont: (713) 833-2311
Crisis Intervention and Suicide Prevention, Corpus
  Christi: (512) 883-6244
Suicide Prevention Center, Dallas: (214) 521-5531
Crisis Line, El Paso: (915) 779-1800
Crisis Intervention-Suicide Prevention Hotline,
  Fort Worth: (817) 336-3355
*Galveston YWCA Crisis Line, Galveston:
  (713) 763-8861
Hotline, Galveston: (713) 765-9416
Crisis Help Line, Houston: (713) 488-7222
Crisis Hotline of Houston: (713) 288-1505
*The Family Connection Crisis Line, Houston:
  (713) 523-6825

UTAH

Crisis Line, Provo: (801) 375-5111
Crisis Center, Salt Lake City: (801) 355-2846

VIRGINIA

*Alternative House Crisis Line, McLean:
  (703) 356-6360
Crisis Center, Norfolk: (804) 399-6393
Hotline, Richmond: (804) 358-9191

*Oasis House Crisis Line, Richmond: (804) 359-1647
*Roanoke Valley Trouble Center Crisis Line,
  Roanoke: (703) 563-0311

VERMONT

*Spectrum Crisis Line, Burlington: (801) 864-7423

WASHINGTON

Crisis Clinic, Seattle: (206) 325-5550
Crisis Information and Referral, Seattle:
  (206) 323-2100
Eastside Crisis Clinic, Seattle: (206) 641-3111
Crisis Services and Suicide Prevention, Spokane:
  (509) 838-4428

WEST VIRGINIA

Hotline, Charleston: (304) 348-4811
Suicide Prevention, Charleston: (304) 346-0826

WISCONSIN

Briarpatch Crisis Line, Madison: (608) 251-1126 or
  257-1436
Crisis Intervention Service, Madison:
  (608) 251-2345
*Pathfinders Crisis Line, Milwaukee: (414) 271-1560
Suicide Prevention for Waukesha County,
  Milwaukee: (414) 547-3388
*Youth Emergency Hot Line, Racine: (414) 637-9557

Special Needs Resources

ALCOHOL AND ALCOHOLISM

The National Clearinghouse for Alcohol Information
Box 2345
Rockville, Maryland 20852

Alcoholics Anonymous
Box 459
Grand Central Annex

New York, New York 10017
(Or consult your local telephone white pages for the
nearest chapter.)

Al-Anon Family Group Headquarters
115 East Twenty-third Street
New York, New York 10010
(Or consult your local telephone white pages for the
nearest chapter.)

ALLERGIES

Allergy Foundation of America
801 Second Avenue
New York, New York 10017
(212) 684-7875

National Institute of Allergy and Infectious Disease
Information Office
Bethesda, Maryland 20014

ASTHMA

The National Asthma Center
1999 Julian
Denver, Colorado
(303) 458-1999

BIRTH DEFECTS

Prevention and research:
The National Foundation-March of Dimes
P.O. Box 2000
White Plains, New York 10602
(Or consult your local telephone directory for the chapter nearest you.)

CANCER INFORMATION

24-hour, toll-free information hotline:
National Cancer Institute
(800) 638-6694

American Cancer Society
219 East Forty-second Street
New York, New York 10017
(Or consult your local telephone directory for nearest office.)

CHRONIC AND/OR CATASTROPHIC DISEASES

The City of Hope National Medical Center offers help at no charge (with physician referral) to those with cancer; heart, blood, and respiratory diseases; lupus, diabetes, and other metabolic problems; and disorders of the endocrine system. For more information, write to:

Office of Admissions
City of Hope National Medical Center
1500 East Duarte Road
Duarte, California 91010

DEPRESSION/MENTAL ILLNESS INFORMATION

National Association for Mental Health
1800 North Kent Street
Arlington, Virginia 22209
(703) 528-6408

DIABETES

American Diabetes Association
600 Fifth Avenue
New York, New York 10020

Juvenile Diabetes Foundation
2200 Benjamin Franklin Parkway
Philadelphia, Pennsylvania
(215) LO 7-4307

Pioneering center in diabetes research:
The Joslin Diabetes Foundation
15 Joslin Road
Boston, Massachusetts 02215

DIET

A group diet-exercise-behavior modification plan:
Weight Watchers®
(For the nearest class, check the white pages of your phone book.)

A group behavior modification plan:
Overeaters Anonymous
P.O. Box 6428
Torrance, California 90504
(Send a self-addressed, stamped envelope for address and phone number of the class nearest you.)

DRUG ABUSE INFORMATION AND HELP

Addicts Anonymous
Box 2000
Lexington, Kentucky 40507

National Association for the Prevention of Narcotics Abuse
305 East Seventy-ninth Street
New York, New York 10021

When a family member has a drug problem:
Families Anonymous, Inc.
P.O. Box 344
Torrance, California
(Send for the $1.00 kit telling how to contact your nearest group.)

Narcotics Education
6830 Laurel Avenue
Washington, D.C. 20012

EPILEPSY

American Epilepsy Society
Department of Neurology
University of Minnesota
Mayo Memorial Building
Box 341
Minneapolis, Minnesota 55455

For information and referral to local chapter, write to:
Epilepsy Foundation of America
1828 L Street N.W.
Washington, D.C. 20036

GAY SERVICES

There are many gay hotlines and counseling centers across the nation. The following are only a selection. For more information, check local telephone listings under "Gay," "Homosexual," or "Lesbian."

For information about gays or related self-help groups:
The Gay Switchboard
(215) 978-5700

Integrity (Gay Episcopal Forum)
National Information
701 Orange Street, No. 6
Ft. Valley, Georgia 31030

Gay Community Services Center
1213 North Highland
Hollywood, California 90028
(213) 464-7485

San Francisco Metropolitan Community Church
Rev. Charles W. Larson, M. Div., Pastor

1076 Guerrero
San Francisco, California 94110
(415) 285-0392

Tampa Metropolitan Community Church
Rev. Elder John H. Hose, Pastor
2904 Concordia Avenue
Tampa, Florida 33609
(813) 839-5939

Metropolitan Community Church of Greater St. Louis
5108 Waterman Avenue
P.O. Box 3147
St. Louis, Missouri 63130
(314) 381-7284

Homosexual Community Counseling Center
30 East Sixtieth Street
New York, New York 10021
(212) 688-0628

National Gay Student Center
2115 S Street N.W.
Washington, D.C. 20008
(202) 265-9890

HYPERTENSION (High Blood Pressure)

National High Blood Pressure Education Program
National Heart and Lung Institute
Washington, D.C. 20015

MEDICAL SERVICES

Besides adolescent clinics and Free Clinics that may exist in your area, you can get medical help and services at your local Department of Public Health. Consult your local phone directory under state, county, or city "Health Department" listings.

Your Department of Public Health offers a variety of services, including pregnancy testing, birth control, diabetic screening, immunization clinics, well-baby clinics, and VD clinics. Fees vary according to ability to pay.

MIGRAINE

For information about doctors or clinics in your area, write to either of the following:

The National Migraine Foundation
2422 West Foster Avenue
Chicago, Illinois 60625

American Association for the Study of Headache
5252 North Western Avenue
Chicago, Illinois 60625

PARENTHOOD

Breast-feeding class information:
La Leche League International
9616 Minneapolis Avenue
Franklin Park, Illinois 60131
(312) 455-7730

Help and information for prevention of child abuse:
Parents Anonymous
2810 Artesia Boulevard
Redondo Beach, California 90278
(Write to above address for group nearest you.)

National Committee for Prevention of Child Abuse
Box 2866
Chicago, Illinois 60690

Support groups for young and/or single parents:
National Association Concerned with School-Age
   Parents
7315 Wisconsin Avenue
Suite 211-W
Washington, D.C. 20014
(Write to above address for group nearest you.)

Children's Home Society Rap Groups for Mothers
In California, check your local white pages. There are
24 CHS rap groups throughout the state.

PARENTHOOD/NONPARENTHOOD

For would-be nonparents:
Write for free literature on whether or not to become
a parent, have one child or none, and explore nonparenthood as a viable life option:
National Organization for Non-Parents
3 North Liberty Street
Baltimore, Maryland 21201

PREGNANCY

For abortion referral:
Check the white pages of your telephone directory for
local listings of

The Clergy Counseling Service
Planned Parenthood
National Organization of Women
Department of Health

For alternatives to abortion:
Check the white pages of your telephone directory for
local listings of
Birthright
Florence Crittenton Association
Children's Home Society (in California)

For prenatal care, counseling, or childbirth class information:
Look in phone book white pages under city, county,
or state "Department of Public Health."

For information about genetic counseling centers
throughout the United States, write to the following
address:
The National Genetics Foundation
250 West Fifty-seventh Street
New York, New York 10019
(212) 265-3166

For information about closest Lamaze training class:
International Childbirth Education Association
Box 5852
Milwaukee, Wisconsin 53220
(414) 476-0130

SICKLE-CELL ANEMIA

The National Genetics Foundation
9 West Fifty-seventh Street
New York, New York 10019

SEXUAL ABUSE

If you are raped, check your local listings under
"Rape Crisis Center" or "Rape Crisis Hotline."

If you are a victim of sexual (or other physical) abuse
from a friend or family member, check your local
white pages (or ask the Operator for help) for your
local Children's Protective Services.

WOMEN'S HEALTH CONCERNS

HealthRight, Inc., is a women's health education and
consumer advocacy organization. This group re-
searches and publishes pamphlets on women's health

concerns as well as a quarterly newsletter. They also run a Patient Advocacy program and conduct "Know Your Body" courses.

For a list of available pamphlets or more information, write to:

HealthRight, Inc.
Women's Health Forum
175 Fifth Avenue
New York, New York 10010
(212) 674-3660

Books

The following is a list of books that we recommend for further information on a variety of topics. You may find these at your local bookstore or in the library.

DIET

Act Thin, Stay Thin by Dr. Richard B. Stuart (W.W. Norton & Company, Inc.). In this excellent, recently published psychological weight-loss guide, Dr. Richard Stuart, famous for his research about eating behavior and as the psychological director of Weight Watchers International, offers help in dealing with feelings that cause you to overeat. This book shows how you can change your behavior with a variety of sensible techniques, lose weight, and keep it off!

A Diet for Living by Dr. Jean Mayer (David McKay Co.). One of the nation's foremost authorities on nutrition talks in an interesting, readable fashion about food facts and fiction, vitamins, weight control, buying and preparing foods.

Dr. Schiff's Miracle Weight Loss Guide by Martin M. Schiff, M.D. (Parket Publishing Company, Inc.). Although we object strongly to the title (there are no miracles in weight loss—only hard work and motivation!), the book's weight-loss work program has a great deal of merit, as Dr. Schiff helps the reader to examine feelings behind eating behavior and to find alternate plans of action.

EXERCISE

The Complete Runner by the Editors of RUNNERS WORLD Magazine (Avon). This book covers the psychology and physiology of running with special material for the young runner. There is also additional information on avoiding injuries, choosing proper footwear, running techniques and nutrition tips. It's a potpourri of useful facts for beginning and experienced runners.

The Runner's Handbook: A Complete Fitness Guide For Men and Women On the Run by Bob Glover and Jack Shepherd (Penguin). This fascinating new book was written by a professional running coach (Glover) and an award-winning writer (Shepherd) and is particularly valuable for beginning runners. It contains many useful suggestions—from having fun with running to how to do essential stretching exercises to avoid injuries. Details on injuries, diseases, nutrition and special running advice for women are included as well as a guide to running spaces in more than 25 American cities. It's a valuable guide for young people on the run!

MEDICAL

From Woman to Woman: A Gynecologist Answers Questions About You and Your Body by Lucienne Lanson, M.D. (in hardback and paperback from Knopf, Inc.). Any questions that a woman could have about her body, menstrual cycles, birth control, pregnancy, and common gynecological disorders are answered in this fascinating book that manages to be warm, informative and, at times, even entertaining!

How to Be Your Own Doctor . . . Sometimes by Keith W. Sehnert, M.D., with Howard Eisenberg (Grosset & Dunlap). This book is not meant to replace your physician, but to make you more conscious of your health and a more conscientious medical consumer. It has an excellent first aid and common illness guide, complete information on how to choose and work with a doctor, and a back-of-the-book family health record.

Our Bodies, Ourselves by the Boston Women's Health Book Collective (Simon & Schuster). Although this excellent softbound book is by and for women, it may be helpful to everyone—men included—with its extensive coverage of sexuality and general health concerns, like nutrition and common health problems.

MENTAL HEALTH (AND ADOLESCENT SURVIVAL!)

Compassion and Self-Hate: An Alternative to Despair by Theodore Isaac Rubin, M.D., with Eleanor Rubin (David McKay Co.). In this excellent book, Dr. Rubin (author of many previous books including the famous *Lisa and David*) examines what he sees as the root of much unhappiness: self-hate. This book offers valuable suggestions for learning to recognize self-hate in your own life and how to conquer this with compassion.

How to Be Your Own Best Friend
How to Take Charge of Your Life
Both of these books are by Mildred Newman and Dr. Bernard Berkowitz and both are available in paperback from Ballantine. The titles of these popular, warmly written, practical, and inspiring self-help guides are self-explanatory. These books may be especially helpful for young people who are trying to build confidence, self-acceptance, and independence.

How to Survive the Loss of a Love (58 Things to Do When There Is Nothing to Be Done) by Melba Colgrove, Ph.D., Harold H. Bloomfield, M.D., and Peter McWilliams (Lion Press, Simon & Schuster). This unusually warm and comforting self-help book was written by a psychiatrist (Bloomfield), a psychologist (Colgrove) and a poet (McWilliams). It has a lovely blend of poetry and practical advice on accepting a loss, grieving and, most important, growing to forgive.

The Book of Hope: How Women Can Overcome Depression by Helen De Rosis, M.D., and Victoria Y. Pellegrino (in hardback from Macmillan Publishing Co.; in paperback from Bantam). Although this excellent self-help guide for dealing with depression, loneliness, anxiety, shyness, boredom, and inertia was written for women, it has insights that may be beneficial for men, too, and for young people in particular.

The Womansbook by Victoria Billings (in paperback from Fawcett-Crest). This commonsense guide to the changing role of women may be particularly helpful for young women (and men, too!), with discussions on feelings and independence, equality, self-image, love relationships, friendships, and sexuality.

Why Am I So Miserable if These Are the Best Years of My Life? by Andrea Boroff Eagan (in hardback from Lippincott; in paperback from Pyramid Books). This is another book that was written for young women, but it contains a great deal of helpful information that would be beneficial for a male, too. This excellent book covers the whole spectrum of adolescence—from friendships and the psychology of changes to sexuality and self-determination. The last chapter—"Going on from Here"—is a terrific, up-to-the-minute guide to sorting out life options.

YOU! The Teenage Survival Book by Dr. Sol Gordon with Roger Conant (Quadrangle/New York Times Book Co.). A self-help work (and fun) book, *YOU* is a uniquely personal book, covering all aspects of adolescent survival—from sexuality to school, from emotional growth to love relationships and family life. It also has special material on developing your creativity.

PARENTHOOD/NONPARENTHOOD

A Baby? Maybe . . . A Guide to Making the Most Fateful Decision of Your Life by Dr. Elizabeth M. Whelan (softbound, from the Bobbs-Merrill Company). This well-written, nonjudgmental book offers help in making the parenthood/nonparenthood decision. It doesn't take sides, but discusses the pros and cons of each choice with intelligence and insight.

The Parent Test: How to Measure and Develop Your Talent for Parenthood by Ellen Peck and Dr. William Granzig (G.P. Putnam's Sons). Should you or shouldn't you have a baby? Before you decide, measure your aptitude for parenthood via the tests and suggestions in this new book.

PARENTING AND PREGNANCY

Preparing for Parenthood: Understanding Your Feelings About Pregnancy, Childbirth and Your Body by Dr. Lee Salk (David McKay Co.). This excellent book by the noted child psychologist talks about all aspects of parenting—from mixed feelings about being a parent, breast-feeding versus bottle-feeding, postpartum blues, meeting your child's emotional needs, *and* the importance of building a life of your own away from your baby!

Parents' Yellow Pages: A Directory by the Princeton Center for Infancy, Frank Caplan, general editor (Anchor Books). This is a comprehensive guide to sources of help for emergencies and nonemergencies, problems and happy possibilities.

Your Baby, Your Body: Fitness During Pregnancy by

Carol Stahmann Dilfer (in cloth and paperback from Crown Publishers, Inc.). This new, how-to guide to fitness during pregnancy not only includes a fitness program, but also tells how your body changes during pregnancy, how to relieve aches and pains, how to avoid getting fat—and much more!

SEXUALITY

The Birth Control Book by Howard Shapiro, M.D. (St. Martin's Press). This is a complete, in-depth and sensitive guide to birth control (with material on male contraceptives and abortion as well as the usual female methods). Dr. Shapiro, a gynecologist, is medical adviser to chapters of the National Organization for Women and Planned Parenthood.

Facts About Sex for Today's Youth by Dr. Sol Gordon (The John Day Co.). A practical, concise, lavishly illustrated book, *Facts* manages to cover all aspects of sexuality in only 50 pages.

Gay: What You Should Know About Homosexuality by Morton Hunt (Farrar, Straus & Giroux). Written for teen-agers and young adults, this excellent book attempts to dispel some common fears and misunderstandings about homosexuality. It is candid, yet not sensational, and offers reassuring insights into sexual feelings, needs, and preferences—for homosexual *and* heterosexual readers.

Learning About Sex: The Contemporary Guide for Young Adults by Gary F. Kelly (Barron's Educational Series, Inc.). An honest, nonsexist guide to all aspects of sexuality—from physical development to growth beyond traditional sex roles—this book offers a lot of nonjudgmental, up-to-date information.

Let's Make Sex a Household Word: A Guide for Parents and Children by Dr. Sol Gordon (The John Day Co.). Although this fascinating book seems to be slanted most toward parents, it offers a lot of excellent material for teen-agers as well and may help many parents and teen-agers begin to communicate about sex. Dr. Gordon has some excellent communication tips. We were also very impressed with two of the chapters contributed by sex educator Elizabeth Canfield: "Rights and Responsibilities for the Sexual Adolescent" and "A Skeptics Glossary."

Films

The following informative, nonjudgmental films explore various aspects of adolescent survival, feelings, and/or sexuality. You can see the films. They are, generally, available for purchase or rental to schools, churches, youth groups, etc. Unless noted, all are 16mm films.

Little Red Schoolhouse
119 South Kilkea Drive
Los Angeles, California 90048

Sex, Feelings and Values is a series of six, open-end films for high school, college, or adult audiences. Among the topics discussed by young people in this series are: sex miseducation, moral attitudes toward sexual behavior, how parental influences affect this behavior, sex fears, homosexual fears, and sex games.
Purchase Price: $900   Rental (3-day): $100

The Date is a gentle look at human relationships. The open-end film explores what boys and girls want from each other. It is aimed at a junior and senior high school audience.
Purchase Price: $300   Rental (3-day): $35

Perennial Education, Inc.
477 Roger Williams
P.O. Box 855 Ravinia
Highland Park, Illinois 60635

A Baby Is Born (Film #1015) is a film of an actual hospital delivery. It is designed to inform future parents about normal childbirth and the joy, fear, pain, and new responsibilities felt by these young first-time parents.
Purchase Price: $300   Rental: $30

A Far Cry from Yesterday (Film #1022) is designed to educate teens about making responsible choices regarding their sexuality. The film follows a young unmarried couple as they deal with an unplanned pregnancy, decide to keep the baby, and find their life disrupted by the baby. The film explores the near-tragic consequences of their decision to keep their baby.
Purchase Price: $275   Rental: $28

Are You Ready for Sex? (Film #1065): High School students show differing points of view in this film on

responsible sexual decision-making. Through discussions and dramatizations, sexual responsibility, communication, peer pressure, personal values, sexual intercourse, and birth control measures are examined.
Purchase Price: $300   Rental: $30

Birth of a Family (Film #1051): This film shows preparation for childbirth with scenes from childbirth classes *and* labor and childbirth.
Purchase Price: $300   Rental: $30

Four Young Women (Film #1044) is a documentary about four women who decide to have abortions for very different reasons. No easy answers or solutions are offered. The film looks closely at the personal values and emotional factors involved in the decisions. Medical aspects of abortion and the importance of effective contraception are also discussed.
Purchase Price: $285   Rental: $28.50

Hope Is Not a Method (Film #1005) offers straightforward information about birth control with up to date information on all methods.
Purchase Price: $250   Rental: $25

Human Growth III (Film #265): This film shows adolescent sexual development as part of a normal physical, emotional, and social process. Biological facts—and feelings—are discussed by young people from fifth grade to young married couples.
Purchase Price: $280   Rental: $28

It Couldn't Happen to Me (Film #1023): Premarital sex, birth control, and pregnancy are the topics discussed in this film. Interviews with pregnant teenagers, a girl who gave her baby up for adoption, a girl who had an abortion, and three physicians explore reasons for nonuse of contraceptives.
Purchase Price: $300   Rental: $30

Lavender (Film #256): This is an honest and sensitive film dealing with the lives, thoughts, and feelings of two young Lesbians named Carol and Diane.
Purchase Price: $170   Rental: $17

Teen Sexuality: What's Right for You? (Film #1056): A group of high school students candidly discuss many aspects of human sexuality including masturbation, homosexuality, boy-girl relationships, friendship, love, and mutual respect. In the film, many of their questions are answered by three doctors.
Purchase Price: $300   Rental: $30

Venereal Disease: Why Do We Still Have It? (Film #1067): Designed for junior high school students, this film talks about VD from a medical standpoint while introducing issues of personal values, behavior, and responsibility.
Purchase Price: $300   Rental: $30

What's Good to Eat? (Film #691) discusses the importance of good nutrition, a balanced variety of foods in our diets. It shows how the body uses nutrients and how the four food groups provide a balanced diet.
Purchase Price: $225   Rental: $22.50

When Love Needs Care (Film #1036) is a documentary that portrays the actual experiences of two teenagers being examined and treated for venereal disease. The boy and girl are nervous but honest. The doctors are supportive while talking frankly about the importance of detecting VD early and of contacting sex partners who may be infected.
Purchase Price: $175   Rental: $17.50

Whole Body Manual (Film #1074): Fitness, exercise, and good nutrition are the key points of this film that shows through striking, innovative photography how efficient and agile a healthy body can be and what simple choices are necessary to maintain it.
Purchase Price: $280   Rental: $28

Young, Single and Pregnant (Film #1043): This documentary focuses on four young women who decided on four different solutions to unplanned pregnancies: adoption, abortion, marriage, and single parenthood. The film stresses the individuality of each woman's decision.
Purchase Price: $265   Rental: $26.50

Your Pelvic and Breast Examination (Film #1050) is a sensitive film that helps to dispel the fears and the mystery that too often surround routine examinations, showing how simple and painless these procedures can be. Here we see a breast self-examination, a pelvic exam, Pap test, and gonorrhea culture. The film discusses the importance of regular breast self-examination and annual visits to a physician.
Purchase Price: $175   Rental: $17.50

Walt Disney Educational Media Company
500 South Buena Vista Street
Burbank, California 91521

Good Sense and Good Food (Set 63-8064S; filmstrip) is humorous and teen-oriented, looking at nutrition, vitamin research, and the effects of protein and vitamin deficiencies in humans.
Purchase Price: $81

Growing Up (Set 63-804S; filmstrip): This series describes the male and female reproductive systems, the changes of puberty, menstruation, and the feelings and pressures involved in growing up—including sibling rivalry, peer pressure, struggle for approval, and much more.
Purchase Price: $81

Children's Home Society
Public Affairs Department
5429 McConnell Avenue
Los Angeles, California 90066

Growing Up Together: Four Teen Mothers and Their Babies is an award-winning film that shows the hardships and joys of single parenthood via an in-depth look into the lives of four teen mothers: Annie, 16; Criss, 16; Anne, 18; and Lynn, 19. Candid interviews with these young mothers and their families and scenes from typical days in the lives of these young mothers highlight the film.

Growing Up Together has been shown on public television and in many classrooms and group meetings as well. For more information on the film's availability, write to the above address.

"Self-Incorporated"
Agency for Instructional Television
Box A
Bloomington, Indiana 47401

Self-Incorporated is a classroom television/film series designed to help the young teen to cope with the emotional and social problems of growing up. The series consists of fifteen 15-minute programs on emotional health and life-coping skills.

Among these programs are

Trying Times takes a look at peer pressure versus wanting to be part of the group as Meg feels pressure to smoke and drink because her cousin Julie and the rest of the crowd do.

No Trespassing examines every individual's need for privacy and the feelings that arise when such privacy is denied. Alex, who lives with his parents and three siblings in a crowded apartment, sets up a private place for himself in an abandoned building—only to be joined by some friends!

Getting Closer explores the fears of being rejected by others, especially by those of the opposite sex, as we watch shy Greg try to ask Laura to dance.

Down and Back looks at failure and ways to cope in a constructive way as it tells the story of Terri, who worked and wished very hard, but did not make the cheerleading squad.

Pressure Makes Perfect: Through the experiences of Nan, a young musician, this film examines the effects that pressure to achieve can have on a young person's life and the need for learning how to cope constructively with such pressures.

Different Folks is a contemporary look at changing sex roles. Matt, whose mother is a veterinarian and whose father, a free-lance illustrator, does most of the housework, feels pain and confusion when his friends tease him about his father's so-called femininity.

Changes is designed to help teens understand the feelings related to physical changes and social situations that also stem from such changes.

For more information about these and the other "Self-Incorporated" programs, write to the Agency for Instructional Television at the above address.